The Quantum Leader

Applications for the New World of Work

SECOND EDITION

Kathy Malloch, PhD, MBA, RN, FAAN

President
Kathy Malloch Consulting Services, Inc.
Glendale, Arizona

Clinical Professor, Master of Healthcare Innovation,
College of Nursing and Healthcare Innovation
Arizona State University
Phoenix, Arizona

Member, Arizona State Board of Nursing

Consultant, api software, Inc.
Hartford, Wisconsin

Tim Porter-O'Grady, DM, EdD, APRN, FAAN

Senior Partner
Tim Porter-O'Grady Associates, Inc.
Atlanta, Georgia

Associate Professor and Leadership Scholar,
College of Nursing and Healthcare Innovation,
Arizona State University
Phoenix, Arizona

JONES AND BARTLETT PUBLISHERS

Sudbury, Massachusetts

BOSTON   TORONTO   LONDON   SINGAPORE

World Headquarters
Jones and Bartlett Publishers
40 Tall Pine Drive
Sudbury, MA 01776
978-443-5000
info@jbpub.com
www.jbpub.com

Jones and Bartlett Publishers
Canada
6339 Ormindale Way
Mississauga, Ontario L5V 1J2
Canada

Jones and Bartlett Publishers
International
Barb House, Barb Mews
London W6 7PA
United Kingdom

Jones and Bartlett's books and products are available through most bookstores and online booksellers. To contact Jones and Bartlett Publishers directly, call 800-832-0034, fax 978-443-8000, or visit our website, www.jbpub.com.

Substantial discounts on bulk quantities of Jones and Bartlett's publications are available to corporations, professional associations, and other qualified organizations. For details and specific discount information, contact the special sales department at Jones and Bartlett via the above contact information or send an email to specialsales@jbpub.com.

The authors, editor, and publisher have made every effort to provide accurate information. However, they are not responsible for errors, omissions, or for any outcomes related to the use of the contents of this book and take no responsibility for the use of the products and procedures described. Treatments and side effects described in this book may not be applicable to all people; likewise, some people may require a dose or experience a side effect that is not described herein. Drugs and medical devices are discussed that may have limited availability controlled by the Food and Drug Administration (FDA) for use only in a research study or clinical trial. Research, clinical practice, and government regulations often change the accepted standard in this field. When consideration is being given to use of any drug in the clinical setting, the healthcare provider or reader is responsible for determining FDA status of the drug, reading the package insert, and reviewing prescribing information for the most up-to-date recommendations on dose, precautions, and contraindications, and determining the appropriate usage for the product. This is especially important in the case of drugs that are new or seldom used.

Production Credits

Publisher: Kevin Sullivan
Aquisitions Editor: Emily Ekle
Aquisitions Editor: Amy Sibley
Associate Editor: Patricia Donnelly
Editorial Assistant: Rachel Shuster
Associate Production Editor:
  Amanda Clerkin

Marketing Manager: Rebecca Wasley
Manufacturing and Inventory
  Control Supervisor: Amy Bacus
Composition: Spoke & Wheel
Cover Design: Kristin E. Ohlin
Cover Image Credit: © Ali Mazraie Shadi/
  ShutterStock, Inc.

Printing and Binding: Courier Corporation
Cover Printing: Courier Corporation

Library of Congress Cataloging-in-Publication Data

Malloch, Kathy.
 The quantum leader : applications for the new world of work / Kathy Malloch, Tim Porter-O'Grady. — 2nd ed.
    p. ; cm.
 Includes bibliographical references and index.
 ISBN 978-0-7637-6540-8 (pbk.)
 1. Leadership. 2. Nursing services—Administration. 3. Psychology, Industrial. I. Porter-O'Grady, Timothy. II. Title.
 [DNLM: 1. Leadership. 2. Nursing, Supervisory. 3. Psychology, Industrial. WY 105 M255q 2009]
 HD57.7.M348 2009
 658.4'092—dc22

                        2008029805
6048

Printed in the United States of America
12 11 10   10 9 8 7 6 5 4 3 2

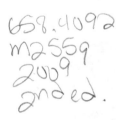

Contents

Chapter 4   Confronting Crisis: The Leadership of Constant Change   65

Chapter 5   The Vulnerable Leader   95

Chapter 6   Innovation Leadership: A New Way of Being   111

Preface

Since the work of leadership is ever changing and yet still the same in many ways, this second edition of *The Quantum Leader* is written for both current and aspiring leaders as a means to gain an appreciation of the complexities faced today. New strategies, new behaviors, and of course, new vulnerabilities are required to practice in the evolving world of technology, while healthcare leaders are challenged to consistently sustain system infrastructures that support the essential caring and therapeutic behaviors of the healer.

In writing this book, the interconnectedness of myriad leadership concepts and behaviors was both challenging and revealing. Writing about behaviors that were undeniably connected and intertwined challenged us as we attempted to clarify concepts without creating artificial boundaries between them. Necessarily, a vulnerable leader must be courageous as well as a peacemaker who is continually challenged to minimize toxic behaviors. Coaching in the new age requires full engagement in order to achieve therapeutic and value-based services.

The Quantum Leader is written for both experienced and aspiring healthcare leaders but has applications to leadership in any discipline that is accountable for the work of facilitation of others, coaching for achievement, elimination of toxic behaviors, and leading into the future. We invite leaders in all organizations to share in our work and as always to share ideas and suggestions to improve the work of the quantum leader.

Kathy Malloch
Tim Porter-O'Grady

Acknowledgments

Writing the second edition of *The Quantum Leader* has again reaffirmed that taking a risk to write about non-traditional leadership topics is a needed service for healthcare leaders. I have continued to expand my thinking about leadership and to appreciate the importance of competent and authentic leaders in the rapidly emerging information age. My journey in health care has been blessed with a most supportive family and very special friendships of the best and brightest professionals. Much recognition goes to Bryan E. Malloch, DO, my best friend, my confidant, and my husband. He has never wavered in his support and recognition of my endeavors—even those classified as wild hairs! Having Tim Porter-O'Grady as a mentor, colleague, and friend is a gift that I cherish every day, and I am continually learning from his wisdom, love of excellence, and willingness to listen to new ideas. Finally, I would like to acknowledge my mom, Jean Fox, who remains a constant source of strength. She is a role model of patience, balance, and honesty in a way that is uniquely special and inspirational. Thank you, mom, for always being there.

Kathy Malloch

My thanks and appreciation to Mark Ponder who continues to exemplify the best in caring and nursing, demonstrating the reality that gender has nothing to do with sensitive and excellent nursing care. And to Kathy Malloch my professional partner, my thanks for her friendship, talent, intellect, and commitment to what is best for those we serve. My thanks to my mother Margaret Black who still, after 12 children, 33 grandchildren, and 17 great-grandchildren and a lifetime of giving, has the energy to encourage the best in her firstborn. To all my professional colleagues, I thank you for your courage, caring, and encouragement to me and all nurses in meeting the challenges of caring for others, regardless of how the world changes before them.

Tim Porter-O'Grady

Making Sense of Transformation: Quantum Realities in a New Age

CHAPTER OBJECTIVES:

Upon completion of this chapter, the reader will:

1. Make sense of complexity concepts as applied to health organizations.
2. Translate complexity notions into leadership processes.
3. Apply concepts of quantum and complexity thinking into decision making, practice roles, and organizational realities.

INTRODUCTION

The cycle of change seems to have quickened and intensified. The problem with current change is twofold. First, the pace of change has quickened so much that it is difficult to keep up, and second, the changes themselves are filled with so many other changes and increasing levels of complexity that they are difficult to understand. People are finding change challenging and difficult to cope with.

The leader's role is directed toward understanding the complexity of change and translating it in a manner that can be understood by those upon whom it impacts. First, however, the leader must find her or his own meaning embedded in the change, to translate it from a personal perspective with both passion and coherence. Given its current complexities, a different understanding regarding change and its function in the world is unfolding. In today's world, driven by increasing technology, globalization, fiber optic connectedness, and the machinations of complexity science, the leader has much to contend with in translating realities into the common work experience of those he or she leads.

Chaos and complexity as a systems dynamic address elements of the universe as they affect all living systems. As we leave the industrial age, with all that implies, we leave an age that was defined more by the mechanistic elements of function and relationship than by its relational elements. In the sociotechnical age, the understanding of reality operates on a much broader and significantly different premise. Much of the structures, format, and activities of the industrial frame were defined

> **Gem**
>
> Change never begins nor does it end—it is the fundamental reality of the universe. People don't start to change or stop changing. Change simply is!

> **Newtonian-Age Characteristics**
>
> - Reductionistic
> - Vertical
> - Mechanical
> - Hierarchical
> - Compartmental
> - Whole as the sum of its parts

by Newtonian realities. Isaac Newton saw the universe as a great machine. Deeper and richer research since then has indicated that the universe, instead of being a great machine, is an even greater set of intersections and relationships (a great thought). Instead of understanding the universe and its systems and subsystems as a great machine viewed independently, compartmentally, and discretely, the universe can now be understood as something wider ranging and more intensely related than previous Newtonian-based science and research indicated.

Quantum or complexity science is a group of theoretical constructs that look at the universe and its elements as complex adaptive systems. Quantum science seeks the relationship between and among all things and attempts to define the nature of that

Quantum-Age Characteristics	
• Multilateral	• Intersecting
• Multidirectional	• Interacting
• Relational	• Integrating

relationship and its action and impact on all life experiences. Because of the intensity of relationships intersecting between multiple disciplines, questions of complexity are not simple, nor are they easy to answer. Although still in its infancy, complexity science is beginning to provide a broader base of understanding for the actions and intersections of life everywhere in the universe. From the broadest frames of reference to the narrowest and most minute elements, complexity and quantum science looks for themes and the intersections between them.

Perhaps one of the best ways of understanding complexity science is recognizing in it a polarity with apparently existing opposites, each playing a definitive and critical role. In the more traditional linear worldview, there are specific assumptions used to represent the overuse of one pole, thereby skewing what would otherwise be a balance in worldview assumptions. Out of complexity science comes emerging worldview descriptors in a wide variety of arenas and disciplines such as holism, observer in the observation, complex adaptive systems, nonlinear relationships, polarity thinking, quantum physics, variation, morphogenesis, self-organization, pattern analysis, etc.

Quantum science looks at change: how it works, what it means, from where it moves, and to where it is going. Quantum science is actively interested in adaptation, integration, interaction, probability and prediction, and the continuous dynamics of movement.

UNDERSTANDING COMPLEXITY

Newtonian Conflict

Frank was busy trying to sort out the organizational chart for the hospital. He felt that if he could get people configured on the chart in the right manner, efficiency would result. Alignment of related jobs and responsibilities with the right department was key. Yet, he was finding it difficult to create such alignments because different relationships needed to emerge at different times and with changing players. Such structuring worked well with large chunks of the organization, but it was problematic when he got to more functional levels of the system. Relationships were fluid and ever changing, depending on the circumstances, and alignments needed to be more fluid. The organizational chart with its hard lines and boxes didn't seem to address that everyday reality.

The leader must know how to incorporate into her or his understanding of leadership this application of multifocal complexity. Furthermore, a leader must apply these notions of quantum reality and complexity to the leadership role and workplace interactions. Within quantum reality, it is increasingly understood that, although the individual is very important, the relationship between and among individuals and their collective relationship to the system is even more critical. The ability to integrate group activities, to cross group boundaries, and to see all systems as a fundamental set of relationships is a critical skill set for the contemporary manager. This leader must reflect an understanding of the independent and interdependent activities that are necessary to create effectiveness and sustainability in systems.

In complexity applications, the leader knows the importance of interpreting and applying network topology in systems and relationships looking at the arrangement or mapping of the links, nodes, and elements of these networked relationships in a way that emphasizes the physical and logical connections between nodes in a complexity. This network topology is one application of complexity having significant implications with regard to types of relationships, the intersections of interactions of these relationships, and the necessary leadership supports that facilitate them. In these models the leader is able to distinguish between network topologies such as point-to-point, buss, star, rain, mesh, tree, hybrid, etc. Furthermore, the leader is able to recognize which leadership capacities are appropriate and viable when applied to specific network or relational topographies.

Rather than exhibit unilateral control, this leader recognizes that control must be distributed across the network/system. This distribution is entirely dependent upon the work, accountability, the authority necessary to undertake the work, and expectations for performance. The leader also recognizes that there must be a goodness of fit between context, content, and outcome. Great change is achieved through small and successful increments of change that, when aggregated, lend themselves well to the success of greater and broader change. This kind of change is nonlinear and does not represent many past strategies that have been used to undertake change. The quantum leader knows that the relationship between the expenditure of energy and the input of work will not always relate to the breadth and depth of the output. In short, the vagaries associated with work may have little to do with how much work one does, but rather have more to do with the intensity of fit between the activity, the intent, and the outcome. Clearly, the leader must have a new understanding of this complex and dynamic relationship between workers and work.

The nonlinearity of complex adaptive systems tends to favor continuous and dynamic innovation and creativity over stability, a strict format, and unchanging structure. The notion of *attractors* is important in quantum systems. In the Newtonian model, the notion of attractor relates to instantaneous rest patterns or regions, such as the rest moment of a pendulum on a clock. Attractors tend to draw specific energy to them. They are also where the system's action or pattern is energized and bounded. This concept is important because rather than looking at barriers to action, process, or change, the leader begins to look at the inherent energy of the system and asks how to act in concert with it.

Overcoming the machine metaphor in leadership is tricky work. The notion of *machine* is so intensely tied to all our leadership experiences and models that it will be difficult to shift from them. The leader may often find that dependence on the machine model of organization, relationship, or interaction is an impediment to undertaking a more effective leadership role in a quantum format. Combining micro and macro concepts will be equally important.

Emerging science related to the human genome is a classic example of the growing importance of microbiological studies in the future management of disease. On the other hand, human macroevolutionary dynamics have had a tremendous impact on the multiplication and adaptation of the human species. Both of these forms of transformation, micro and macro, have equal importance in understanding health care, and exercising the role of a health service provider requires the ability to embrace both.

For the leader, there are important skills that are necessary for applying complexity principles in the expression of the leadership role. In an excellent work outlining the application of complexity theory to health care, called *EdgeWare* (Zimmerman, Lindberg, and Plsek, 1998), the authors enumerate nine basic principles that influence the leader's role in health care. Each one of these principles forms a firm foundation upon which to both conceive and unfold the quantum role of leader. Using these nine principles as a frame, we have explored them with our own unique quantum perspective, and we discuss them next.

Kaleidoscope

An easy way to "see" complexity is through the lens of a kaleidoscope. The interfacing and interweaving elements of the constantly changing intersection of parts that continuously "dance" together as they mold new shapes and configurations best represent the components and wholeness of complexity. What is important in viewing the kaleidoscope is the requirement of movement and intersections. Both are necessary for the unending formation of new forms and the unlimited arrangement of possible configurations and relationships in the ever-changing shapes. What a powerful tool for seeing quantum visions.

Creativity Over Stability

In the quantum world, stability is a synonym for death. Stability means no movement, which is synonymous with a dead system. Think of how many people and organizations "lust" for the peace and safety of stability in a universe that does everything it can to upset the stable and create the conditions for movement and change.

Stability Signposts

- Policy
- Procedure
- Ritual
- Routines
- Organization charts
- Titles and positions

Quantum Leader Characteristics

- Fluid
- Flexible
- Mobile
- Reflects synthesis
- Works from the whole
- Coordinates the intersection

Principle 1

The leader looks at every activity in the organization through the eyes of quantum systems.

The leader has a great deal of work to do to overcome the existing structures and models of organization in her or his work setting. The machine metaphor has been inculcated in both the design and restructuring of clinical work. In quantum thinking, the leader is fully aware that the compartmentalization and vertical orientation of the organization is not adequate for the work being done there.

Clinical work requires strong levels and processes of integration and horizontal relationships. Because of the needs of patients and the clinical activities of the organization, it is critical for interaction and communication to be facilitated across the system. Most health systems, however, are designed to be more vertically integrated than horizontally linked. Although many clinical activities are linked, many of the organizational structures within which they unfold are not connected in the same way. In effective healthcare systems, linkages, integration, and interface of clinical and support activities operate continuously and dynamically throughout the organization. The leader, therefore, is continually struggling to accommodate this reality, and sometimes leaders must focus on overcoming the organizational impediments to accomplishing the leader's work and the work of those who provide care.

Many existing Newtonian systems reflect a high need for control. However, clinical providers need great latitude for individual and collective integration, information, and relationships in the exercise of their clinical work. The leader recognizes this and makes sure that all clinical systems and structures are able to support a more dynamic and interactive frame of reference.

The clinical work of health care is a complex mosaic of intersections and collective activities that requires heavy emphasis on relationship building, communication networks, and well-coordinated interfaces between professionals and structures in the workplace. This is the central focus of the leader's organizing work. Yet the leader also works to see the hidden intersections and connections in all relationships and where they exist in all organizational and human activity. The leader's focus is predominantly on the intersections and relationships between individuals and functions, support structures and work, organization and clinical activity, and practice and practitioners. This multifocal approach to understanding and applying the leadership role is critical to both effectively seeing the role and applying the necessary skills for facilitating the interactions and confluences to assure that the work is effective and achieves its desired results.

In this set of circumstances, the leader begins to conceptualize a change in her or his view of the organization and of the work. The more the leader sees individual activities from the perspective of the whole, noting the common elements embedded in all activity, the more likely the leader will have an accurate perspective of actions and responses necessary to obtain sustainable outcomes. In this way, the leader begins to think about process as a part of structure, structure as

---

Quantum Control

So much of management is historically about control. In the quantum world, control is not an issue; change is. Everything is in constant movement, shifting and becoming. The wise leader recognizes that the role of leadership is in managing the relationship of people to the constant movement of the dynamic of change. It is in managing people's response to this constant movement that the leader can then ensure creativity, innovation, and relevance remain the fundamental core of all work.

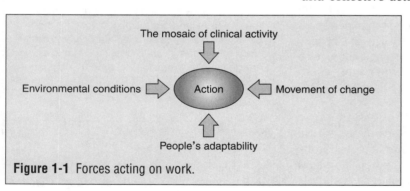

Figure 1-1 Forces acting on work.

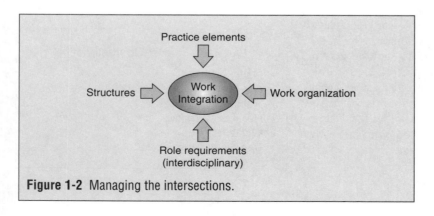

Figure 1-2 Managing the intersections.

embedded in all processes, and both structure and process as fundamental components of obtaining outcomes and creating the conditions for positive relationships and sustainable processes.

Principle 2

Create the broadest possible vision with any number of variables in which people are free to form and unfold new ways of working and creating.

All systems have a high level of unpredictability embedded in them. This reflects an understanding in complexity and quantum science that simple constructs lead to complex behaviors. The tendency of leadership is to be overly specific and detailed in setting of agendas, developing strategies, or pursuing directions for the organizations and for people's work. In contrast, in quantum reality, overspecifying work and activities interferes with the ability of the system to adapt quickly and easily to changing conditions and circumstances as well as to shifts in work and projects. Indeed, as projects and work unfold, the work itself changes. Doing the work acts as a catalyst for future changes that can only be anticipated as the work unfolds. In this case, experience itself changes the conditions and circumstances of the work. Systems are continually flexible, adaptable, and inherently innovative if allowed to unfold in unpredictable and uncertain ways. The leader must be aware of this confluence of interactions and forces as a profound and essential part of unfolding goals and objectives as well as project outcomes.

The leader must be aware that innovation and creation at work respond specifically to environmental and contextual forces. These forces influence much of the contents of programs and projects. The leader must become a good signpost reader, aware of the environmental and conditional circumstances operating and influencing the conditions and activities of work. Any change in the payment structure for healthcare services automatically creates a change in the emphasis, content, and character of those services. A change in social policy regarding confidentiality, for example, has a direct impact on the design, implementation, and management of clinical and business information systems. A new technological discovery in the practice or clinical service creates a new technique and methodology for clinical intervention, changing the mechanism for intervention, the way in which patients are cared for, the way in which processes are paid for, and the supporting infrastructure related to delivering the new service.

What is also helpful for the manager is to recognize the virtuality of complexity and its embeddedness in every level and component of human dynamics and life activity. Processes and interactions are dynamic, not completely dependent on any one function or structural element in the organization. In fact, much of this action goes on out of view, almost at the level of the unconscious, forcing the leader to be aware of the dynamics operating in a higher level than that which is immediately visible. The leader must look at means, threads, or even pictures moving across the backdrop of activity that are clear indicators of process and progress. These indicators may even be activities themselves. In this set of circumstances, the leader is looking for the connections, the points of convergence between efforts and activities, and is attempting to identify the "noise" that indicates they are not working well together or that the confluence of forces are not merging in a way that will create the conditions for integration, operation, practice, and functional success.

It is also wise for the leader to recognize that a good vision, set of objectives, or focus can lead to a broad base of related effective and essential activities. For example, taking

> **Gem**
>
> Leaders recognize that their relationship is with the whole system, not with the department with which they are frequently aligned. Leaders manage their services by bringing their unique service perspective to the whole system and linking and integrating it with other perspectives in order to address the needs of the whole.

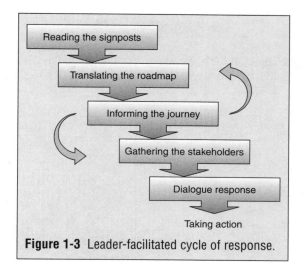

Figure 1-3 Leader-facilitated cycle of response.

> **Dynamic Processes**
>
> Leaders and staff often conclude that there is an end to particular effort or work process. The leader must take on a new mantle of thinking about beginnings and endings. In quantum change, all process is dynamic and continuous; it neither begins nor ends. The leader is continuously engaged in interacting with the constant ebb and flow of all process. The good leaders simply ascertain at what place in the flow specific processes unfold and how those activities lead to the goals being sought.

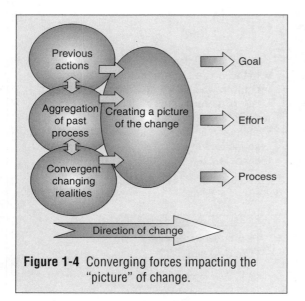

Figure 1-4 Converging forces impacting the "picture" of change.

on a new diagnostic technology can have considerable impact across the system. If the diagnostic technology provides an opportunity to diagnose the potential for disease early on, it may eliminate or limit the use of currently employed technology that addresses the same disease when discovered in its later stages. The new technology changes or limits the need for and application of technology that may historically have been a source of great service and revenue for the organization. The implication is that the choice of new technology has a broader impact on the effectiveness and focus of the system than simply the individual diagnostic activity of the technology itself. This example is a small indicator of the effect that specific choices might have on other activities in the organization. The leader is always aware of this and is continuously looking at the broader-based implications related to any unilateral, simple, or focus set of choices.

In creating a vision, it is important for the leader to recognize that a simple, broader-based vision may itself transform all the functions and activities in an organization. If, for example, a clinical organization's vision changes from providing good high-quality bed-based services to providing equally high-quality outpatient and ambulatory care services, implications will be considerable regarding the organizational infrastructure, support systems and their priorities, capital planning activities, and financial and revenue considerations. In fact, each and every one of these functional elements will be transformed in ways that are significant for both the viability and the future success of the organization. A simple change in a broadly delineated vision creates complex changes across the system. This holds true with almost any undertaking related to setting visions or goals at any level of the organization.

What is critical for the manager and leader at any level of the organization is his or her reflection of the global impact of simple changes in goals, direction, or priorities at any place in the system. These changes, regardless of where they occur, can have broader-based implications for any and all other parts of the system. It is important for the leader to realize that, regardless at what level of leadership he or she operates, he or she has considerable impact on the organization as a whole when making decisions, regardless of the level of the system at which these decisions are made. In quantum complexity, decisions made at any place in the system can have tremendous implications and impact on decisions and activities unfolding at any other place in the system. While this should not be a frightening consideration, it should be a sobering realization

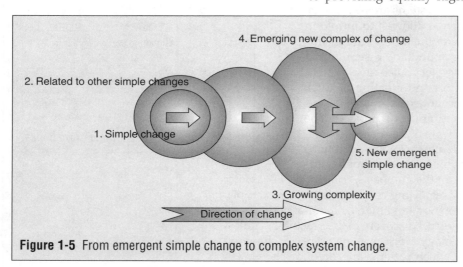

Figure 1-5 From emergent simple change to complex system change.

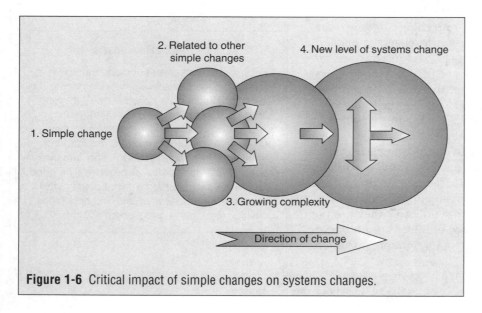

Figure 1-6 Critical impact of simple changes on systems changes.

with regard to the implications and impact of decisions that occur at a unit level or any organizational level within the human work system.

Principle 3

Create a balance between structural and mechanical formality and relational and intersectional dynamics, recognizing the contribution of each to the other and of both to the whole.

There clearly is always the need for structural formation in undertaking and functioning in human organizations. However, what is important to recognize is that structural formats are tools that give form and discipline to the far more variable and dynamic processes associated with human action. The leader must recognize that balance needs to be obtained between structural elements in the organization and the dynamic elements of human action.

The relationship between structure and human dynamics is not constant or rigid. Additionally, one is not an outflow of the other. What occurs in any given point in time is a continuous "dance" between structure and human action to changes in its cadence, outflow, interaction, and music as the relationship unfolds. The leader maintains a high level of awareness regarding the nature and content of the interaction between structure and human dynamics at any given point.

What often occurs in the dance between structure and action are changes in circumstances, conditions, and external forces in the environment that create a set of new conditions. These conditions now change the circumstances or the context influencing the dance between structure, process, and the relationships of work. The leader in this set of circumstances looks carefully at the mix of these influences and forces and what it says about appropriate action or response at any given moment. The environmental and contextual indicators related to the immediate situation provide more information than a simple assessment of the current situation or activities. Here the leader asks what she is indicating with regard to where the organization is within her context and what signposts are revealed with regard to appropriate response and specific direction. Through reading these contextual factors well, the leader can see better and make a better and more appropriate response with regard to direction, priorities, and action choices.

While the leader must maintain appropriate attention to building good supporting infrastructure, he or she must also be aware of the relationship and confluence of forces that are always indicators of any change moment. Those forces provide information regarding the dynamics of the journey, the elements of change, and the ascending priorities at any given moment that indicate a need for different strategies, a change in direction, or the establishment of new priorities or processes. Structure is modified by the dynamic of the dance of change. The leader recognizes the need to modify, alter, adjust, or even transform structures in order to make the organization more adaptable and more effective in its response to the demands of a given moment or specified change events.

Historically, the greatest problem for organizations has not been their power or influences or economic significance but instead has been their inability to quickly and nimbly adapt to the subtle and sometimes small changes that can transform their circumstances, their conditions,

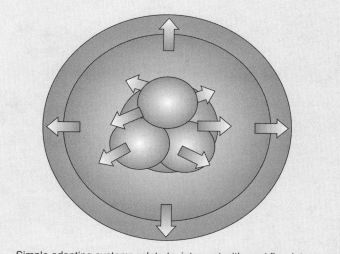

Simple adapting systems relate to, intersect with, and flow into other simple systems and, when aggregated, create broader, more complex systems in a continuous and dynamic "dance" between them.

Figure 1-7 The outflow and interaction between simple and complex elements of a system.

Quantum Guide

The wise leader is always driven by a relationship focus. This leader constantly seeks to better see and configure the interaction between people, processes, and structures. It is this critical interface between these elements upon which the constant forces of change are acting.

Responding to and adjusting relationships, decisions, and actions within the context of people, processes, and structures disciplines the activity of the leader and keeps leadership action focused on the dynamics that lead to sustainable systems change.

Gem

Absolute stability in quantum awareness is a synonym for death. The persons and organizations that fail to continuously adapt and grow are doomed to die. For the leader, it is important to translate this message to all people in the organization: "adapt or die." In this set of circumstances, all work is change and change is the work. This message is the centerpiece of good leadership and the requisite in all leadership performance.

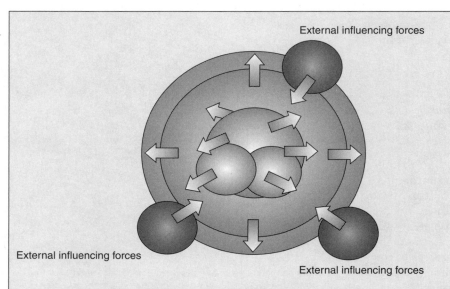

External influencing forces

External influencing forces

External influencing forces

This mosaic of forces and influences, internal and external, are constantly interacting with and upon each other. Each intersection and interaction creates a confluence of effort converging at defined moments to create a new set of conditions and circumstances that, when aggregated, leads to a new reality.

Figure 1-8 Internal and external forces in the activity of exchange interacting to create a new reality.

Quantum Scenario

Jim was in a quandary. Important changes needed to be made in his department, and staff was holding on desperately to past rituals and routines. Jim needed to create a set of circumstances that would make it no longer safe for them to remain with their past practices. He was concerned with whether he should create a critical event by undertaking an immediate change or help them slowly transition toward a change in behavior.

Jim decided in favor of an immediate and dramatic change, creating sufficient chaos to make past practices no longer tenable and forcing the staff to confront the demand for work change. Jim knew that this approach would create immediate reaction and significant "noise." However, he recognized that chaos and noise are essential constituents of all meaningful change, and that, as a leader, it was not his role to avoid the pain of immediate change but, instead, to help staff with their adaptation and the development of new tools and processes that would help them adjust to new ways of working.

and ultimately their ability to thrive. The good leader makes sure changes in human dynamics are not sacrificed on the altar of form and structure. To the contrary, structure and format should be disciplined by creativity, innovation, and the organization's ability to quickly adapt and adjust to changes. The leader is vital in facilitating this critical dance and assuring that it unfolds in meaningful ways for people as well as the organization.

Principle 4

The leader must maintain tension between the chaotic and the orderly in managing information, human dynamics, differences, linkages, and environmental and contextual circumstances.

The core of good leadership is always related to achieving balance between sometimes competing and at other times confluent forces. None of the elements identified here have precedence or priority over the others. Weighting of forces such as information management versus organizational structural control is not the point of good leadership. Each component of human activity is required in order to effectively coordinate, maintain, and integrate the systems' response to the demand for movement and change. The leader should be able to determine the appropriate balance of activities and action at any given time in relationship to the demands on the organization for action or for change.

Biological researchers reveal that absolute patterns of regularity are critical indicators of decline and even death. A certain amount of chaos is required for all life processes to operate effectively. The biological and the universal complex adaptive systems require a certain amount of chaos in their processes to sustain the presence of life. The struggle here is between the degree of chaos necessary to sustain life and the point of chaos beyond which the chaos itself contributes to the decline of life and action. Finding this balance is one of the critical roles of the leader.

Analysis provides a frame of reference for looking at what is. However, analysis alone is not sufficient to be able to address all the issues or forces influencing a particular direction or action. It is a mechanical process for looking at structure, form, circumstances, and conditions and drawing judgments with regard to what responses are appropriate. Analysis plays a role only in determining what the focused action should be. In quantum systems, change lies at the core of all life and function. This care of change creates a demand for a much broader and deeper balance of activities that may include analysis but is not limited to it.

A balance of tools and processes is necessary to understand the broad mosaic of influences and circumstances that is critical to the role of the leader. The leader recognizes information, not as a thing but as a dynamic, which itself indicates the elements of flow and change. Information is like a river flowing through the human experience and through the organizational structure. Every person in the structure requires information in order to adequately and accurately unfold his or her own work. All individuals must be able to get into the river and gather from it the information and tools necessary to adequately unfold their role in conjunction with the roles and processes of others along the river's edge.

This notion of a flowing, dynamic river of information is critical to understanding the application of information in making decisions, undertaking action, producing outcomes, and evaluating effective performance. Recognized as a part of this flow is the understanding that different points along the river of information require different kinds of resources that are available in a changing format. They alter emphasis and even content depending on the need for information and the point at which that data is gathered. It is the complex interplay along the river's flow that brings value to the use of information. Clearly, different people require different information at different points along the information flow. However, once gathered, all the information creates a composite or aggregate of information that in one way or another will speak to the health, the integrity, and the viability of the organization as a whole. The leader acts as integrator, facilitator, and coordinator of the information flow, linked information, and its application as a tool for evaluating the effectiveness and the efficacy of the organization's journey.

While we have used information as one example of the management of flow and of handling change in interacting with chaos, what is important to remember is that the organization, if it is successful, is continuously living on the edge of chaos. Effective, viable, healthy, and alive organizations are those that walk that tightrope between stability and chaos with a tendency to favor the essential chaos embedded in their own necessary changes.

Organizations must be committed to their own change. In order to make those changes, there must be in organizations and human systems a connection to the chaos, a willingness to engage its realities, and a process that incorporates the vagaries and uncertainties that chaos brings into the dynamics of planning, strategizing, and acting for the future of the organization. The leader represents this ease with chaos in her or his own role. This person recognizes the essential value of the change dynamic and the chaos that change brings with it and represents well an engagement with and embracing of the realities and elements of chaos. The leader recognizes the levels of functions and structure that are present in the organization. This leader also

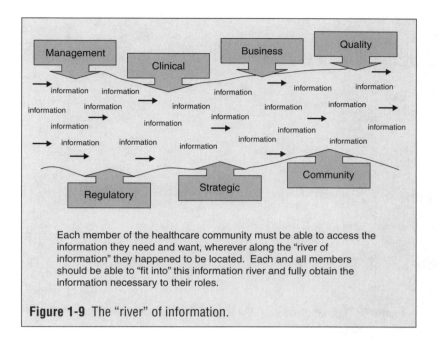

Each member of the healthcare community must be able to access the information they need and want, wherever along the "river of information" they happened to be located. Each and all members should be able to "fit into" this information river and fully obtain the information necessary to their roles.

Figure 1-9 The "river" of information.

The Tension Tightrope

Change can never occur in the presence of high levels of satisfaction. It is incongruous to expect that people will change those things from which they are enjoying great satisfaction. The leader, then, must manage people at the tension between satisfaction and dissatisfaction. The wise leader recognizes the level of balance in motivating the staff to change between their level of satisfaction and dissatisfaction in the attempt to have staff respond to the need for change. Finding this place of critical tension is challenging, yet it is necessary if staff is to engage their own journey of change.

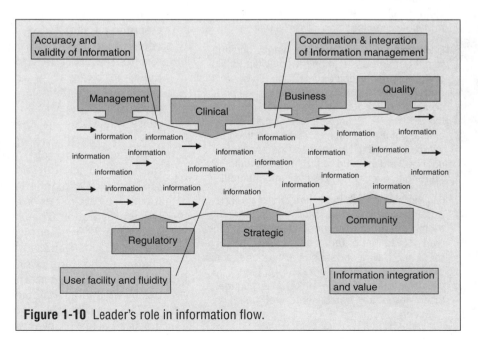

Figure 1-10 Leader's role in information flow.

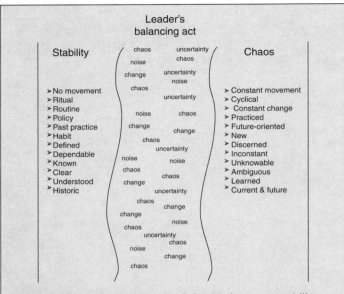

Figure 1-11 Leader walking the tightrope between stability and chaos.

The Chaotic Paradox

Nancy was struggling with two groups of people in her organization; one group was eager to undertake the new changes in practice, and the other was equally as strongly committed to current practices. Nancy knew that changes had to occur; she just wasn't clear exactly what changes were appropriate and what practices should remain the same.

Confronted with this paradox, Nancy decided to get both groups into one room. Using a flip chart, she undertook an intensive dialogue between both groups around the issues and concerns related to the needed change. Using the flip chart to document all thoughts and critical points. Nancy was able to identify the values needed to be retained, the challenges of change, and insights regarding what changes needed to occur and how they might unfold.

By combining both the purveyors of change and those who valued stability and engaging them both around the need for change, Nancy was able to use paradox as a tool for discernment and built a consensus around a specific direction for change. Furthermore, Nancy was able to engage the stakeholders in the discernment and establishment of their own direction for change.

recognizes that the more the organization is available for the challenges and dynamics of change that foreshadow its future and define its journey, the more successful it will likely become.

Principle 5

The uncertainty of transformation in change brings with it the necessary engagement of both tension and paradox.

The leader recognizes the need to maintain a specific level of tension in the organization. However, this tension is not related to distress or high levels of painful relationships. The tension embedded in quantum leadership is one that is intentionally maintained between creativity and complexity on the one hand, and peoples' need for stability and regularity on the other. The leader recognizes the fundamental need for stability in the organization and incorporates it into the structural elements and components of unfolding work, as well as the relationships necessary to support both the work and the worker. However, the leader does not sacrifice the fundamental tension between order and chaos just to guarantee worker comfort.

A part of sustaining successful activities and the future of the organization is recognizing the tension between current systems functions and operations and the environment, which is continuously creating the conditions that change current realities. The leader, as the major signpost reader, anticipates the fundamental and essential changes embedded in all movement in human systems. That individual has the responsibility for communicating the movement of change, the impact of that movement on current functions, and the need to prepare for the very next thing. In this, the leader manages the timing, processing, and case for change in a way that balances the stability and integrity of people in the organization with the growing demand for change in the way of doing business.

In dealing with the continuous dynamics of change, the leader learns to master paradox as a way of moving change. The leader recognizes the essential paradox between the fundamental need for stability and the equally fundamental drive for adaptation and change. In managing these realities, the leader uses paradox as a tool for making change. For example, the leader might suggest to a group most reluctant to change how they might maintain their stability and order by radically altering their work processes as a way of ensuring that stability. Clearly, this makes little sense, but it does challenge people to use existing notions and concepts as a vehicle for addressing specific required adaptations and changes.

In living comfortably with paradox, the leader must be willing to raise paradoxical questions as a part of unfolding her or his role in guiding people to undertake essential change. Furthermore, the leader must inculcate in her or his own personal behavior the willingness to live with paradox. The leader asks herself or himself questions about leading and how that might be undertaken without providing control and order as a framework for leadership. How does the leader direct change without initiating that direction herself or himself? How does the leader integrate acceptance of essential change and change activities by modeling acceptance within the context of the leader's role?

The leader creates the conditions and circumstances in which paradox is a part of problem solving and change making. For example, the leader might gather complex groups together with highly divergent opinions in an effort to create sufficient diversity to make any one solution or points of view untenable. The paradox is used as a frame of reference for helping people identify and address essential change. Using the need for stability can form a foundation upon which paradoxical, radical, and significant change can be undertaken in the workers' efforts to maintain their stability and good order. Such processes call the leader to not only embrace the need for paradox but also use paradox as a tool for challenge and change.

Principle 6

Ambiguity and uncertainty are fundamental conditions for effective change: you don't have to be sure to be successful.

Evolution, heredity, and adaptation are all rife with examples of how uncertainty is essential for the ability to thrive. Indeed, without the necessary diversity and uncertainty of species and the highly variegated environmental conditions of the earth, there would not have been sufficient differentiation to support life as we know it. Uncertainty is an essential constituent of all adaptation.

Organizations have difficulty with uncertainty. The mechanical foundations of organizational structure and activity exist to remove as much uncertainty as possible from the conditions and circumstances of organizational behavior. By so doing, these organizations contribute to their own lack of adaptation and ability to thrive. One of the fundamental roles of the leader is to assure the organization does not become so enamored of its stability, form, and function that it fails to be aware of the fundamental need to shift and adapt all processes, reflecting the contextual changes that are driving it to thrive in a new or emerging reality.

The leader is constantly aware of the environmental forces and external influences that are creating the conditions for change within organizations. Indeed, the leader's role is to translate the fundamental forces of change into the language of the organization so that its people are continually aware of the action of these forces and their lives. These conditions create the uncertainty that is so much a part of life's experience. It is not that uncertainty is untenable or inappropriate; it is more that uncertainty is frequently ignored, as organizations concentrate more on their function and the stability they so desperately seek.

The leader always lives at the point of uncertainty. In fact, the leader is often a boundary walker, looking down at the issues, concerns, and actions of the organization from its "balcony." From this perspective, the leader begins to gain a better insight of the broad diversity of forces that act in concert to create the conditions for successful change. Nevertheless, the leader knows that no one choice or action unilaterally drives effectiveness or success.

In staying on the periphery of the organization, the leader avoids the temptation to become absolute, certain, and specifically clear about the single most correct action. In fact, good leaders tend to favor experimentation and innovative processes. This ties a number of different approaches to one solution and is a mechanism for finding the best

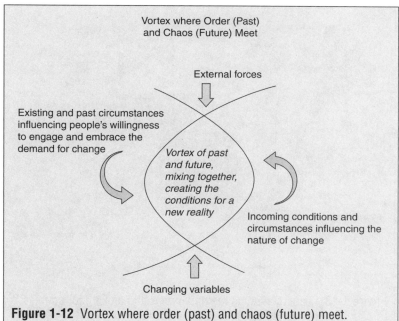

Figure 1-12 Vortex where order (past) and chaos (future) meet.

Within the figure:
Vortex where Order (Past) and Chaos (Future) Meet
External forces
Existing and past circumstances influencing people's willingness to engage and embrace the demand for change
Vortex of past and future, mixing together, creating the conditions for a new reality
Incoming conditions and circumstances influencing the nature of change
Changing variables

Gem

Certainty can never be obtained to a sufficient enough degree to eliminate ambiguity. Uncertainty will always be a condition influencing human judgment and decision making. The leader will never have sufficient information or data upon which to know with absolute certitude what choices are right. Information can indicate factors influencing decision making and, when aggregated, can indicate the appropriate direction for choice. However, judgment must still be rendered, risk faced, uncertainty confronted, and action taken. That is the work of leadership.

Quantum Guide

Leaders make time in their schedule to periodically go to the "balcony." Distancing themselves from their own role and workplace, leaders go far enough away to broadly scan the environment, conditions, and circumstances that affect the lives of people and their organization. This is an essential role of the leader if the leader is not to be drawn into a narrow frame of reference for experiencing change and shifts in roles and performance. The leader is then better able to return to the staff and translate accurately to them the conditions and characteristics of the broader journey. This brings a deeper understanding to their own work experience and acknowledges their particular contributions to the organization's success as a citizen journeying in a larger world.

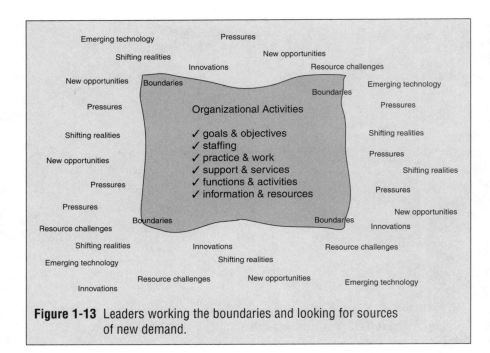

Figure 1-13 Leaders working the boundaries and looking for sources of new demand.

fit between selected processes and an effective outcome. This availability to a variety of approaches and solutions provides a better frame of reference for focusing on those mechanisms that span the possibility of being more successful than simply strategizing, deciding, and directing a solution based on consensus or unilateral decision making.

The good leader clearly defines the frame of reference, constructs, or conditions that relate to a solution. But what this leader does not do is find a specific single response or action that will be necessary to a situation's resolution. Instead, the leader gathers individuals around various solutions with the intent of finding in each of them those elements or processes that might lend themselves to addressing an issue or concern in a more meaningful way. Through this availability, process, experimentation, or innovation, the leader increases the possibilities of good choice and extends that availability to a variety of elements that may impart a sustainable solution or a whole new set of processes to better advantage the organization and its work.

Principle 7

The informal organizational networks are critical to an organization's success, as are the formal networks.

Leaders intuitively know that the informal communication and action network of organizations and systems are highly effective tools of communication and information generation. However, this is often not formalized into the ongoing operational reality of the organization. In short, these informal networks are looked at as anomalous, rather than as normative operating processes of human dynamic systems. In formal networks, gossip, story sharing, personal life experiences, and so forth are all a part of the essential constituents of the communication system. Often these informal networks or informal groups of individuals have a greater significance to the effectiveness of the work of the system than do the formal structures and communication networks.

It is perhaps in these informal or shadow networks that much of the creativity and innovation of the organization is located. Indeed, Art Kleiner's new research on core group theory (2004) indicates that many of these powerful individuals and groups are not located within the formal organizational and leadership structure. Yet these individuals and groups have a huge significance with regard to the organization's effectiveness and creativity. Located throughout the system, these core individuals and groups often form informal networks where ideas, notions, innovations, and significant changes are discussed. Any number of stories have been told with regard to how creative and innovative processes have unfolded, not from the ordinary and usual format and structures of the organization, but rather from the serendipitous actions and activities of individuals and groups having gathered informally for purposes other than those defined by work. The leader accommodates

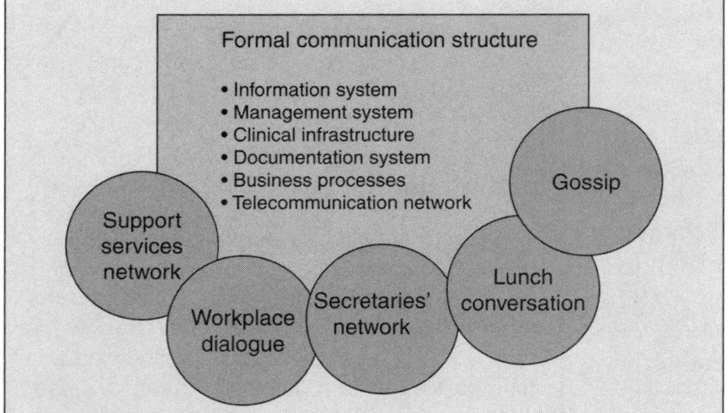

Figure 1-14 Formal and informal communication networks.

this reality and recognizes that through informal networks, much creativity and innovation upon which the future of the organization depends gets discussed in a safe context.

Leaders not only value these informal networks, they use them. The good leader tries to access and maintain relationships with some of the better-known components of the informal networks, such as secretaries, unit clerks, housekeeping, and security services, as well as the wide variety of lunchtime gatherings, where the real issues and concerns of the organization are addressed with a great deal of specificity and clarity and in ways not usually permitted within the normal organizational constructs. This leader recognizes these gatherings as fundamental tools of innovation, creativity, and truth telling that help the organization in its own growth and adaptation as well as its orientation to current reality.

The leader recognizes these informal networks hold opportunities to truly problem solve and obtain ideas and notions that might not otherwise be obtained in the formal system. Because of the complexity and compartmentalization of much of the structures of health care, leaders would be advised to join, indeed, create informal networks that operate outside the formal structure. This will provide access to the highest levels of creativity and diversity, and leaders can then better apply ideas generated there to the work and dynamics of the organization.

Principle 8

The most important part of systems is their intersections: larger systems should be the aggregation of successful smaller systems.

In quantum reality, all systems are aggregations of smaller systems. Smaller systems clump together in a dynamic of interaction and intersections to create larger systems when such clumping provides value

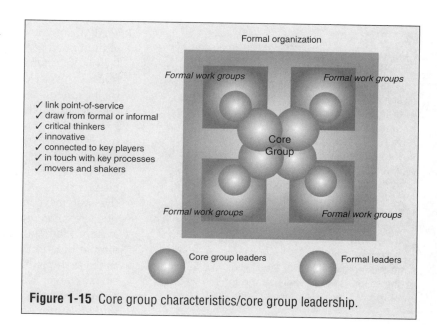

Figure 1-15 Core group characteristics/core group leadership.

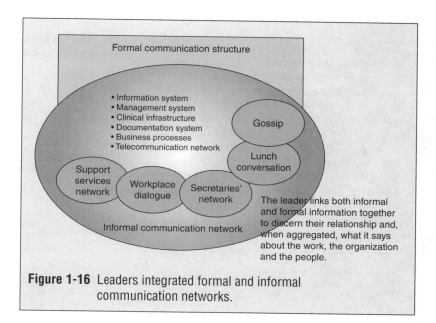

Figure 1-16 Leaders integrated formal and informal communication networks.

and meaning for the smaller systems. This reflects a principle that, regardless of the size of the system, "systemness" is always present, from the smallest measures of intensity to the largest measures of complexity. Indeed, if one wants to understand a large, complex system, it is better to look for the simplicity that lies at its center.

If one looks at the Internet, it becomes clear exactly how systems operate. As an individual uses the Internet, he or she creates personal intersections, interfaces, networks, and an information complex based on what he or she seeks to do or to accomplish. An individual system that meets the specific needs of that individual is created. However, to interact with the Internet, individuals access a part of a broader, more complex system within which their unique body of information becomes a part of a larger chain and complex of information and access points (Internet networks or communities). This makes it possible for others to draw from the Internet what they need from it. Continuing this dynamic throughout the whole human community, one can begin to see the narrow simplicity and broad-based complexity of interactions and intersections that make the Internet the complex yet simple system that it truly is.

All of complexity is a result of cross-referencing, crossover, and integration of a broad complex of sometimes unrelated sets of elements or factors, that, when aggregated, create increasingly complex organizations. Whether computers, the human body, or even the universe, all their elements make up both simple and complex systems. The notion of advancing between the simple elements and the aggregated impact they have on all elements is a metaphor for understanding complex adaptive systems. For the leader, the only way to truly understand complex systems is to be able to effectively make simple systems work well in themselves and then interface well with other simple systems that are also working well. Through this complex integration of simple, effective systems, complex systems are built and sustained. A failure of any one system is ultimately a failure in the entire complexity of the larger system. Here the leader recognizes that assuring the effectiveness of the simple functional system and addressing its successful interface with other systems builds the complex array of intersections necessary to sustain larger systems and to assure that simple systems and the larger array of complex systems work in concert to be mutually self-sustaining and life affirming.

Principle 9

All creatures both compete and cooperate for resources and for the opportunity to live.

Competition is embedded in the very fabric of life experience in this principle, exhibited at all levels of life from the cellular to the most complex organisms. Competition is a normative and universal experience. Cooperation and mutuality are equally essential to the ability to thrive. Whole communities of creatures at all levels of evolution work in concert to assure their mutual survival.

However, competition is also vital to life. In this paradox, competition is as important to adaptation and sustainability as are mutualism and symbiosis. At all levels of liability in life experience, examples of cooperation between and among species, organisms, and environments is as much an example of the activities and structures of life as is competition.

In nature, competition between animals is the most visible representation of the competition built into life. When species prey or feed upon each other in order to sustain life, they are clearly representing competition. Yet at the same time, cooperation between species is also often necessary to mutually support life. For example, African wrens live on the backs of water buffaloes, eating ticks that would otherwise irritate and infect the skin of these animals. In the ocean, smaller fish often accompany unrelated larger fish in order to feed off the creatures that would

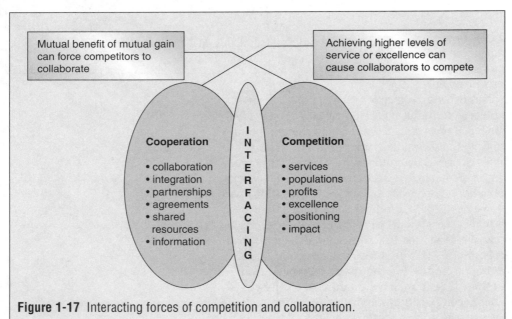

Figure 1-17 Interacting forces of competition and collaboration.

otherwise infect or endanger the life of larger fish. At all levels of existence, examples of both cooperation and competition are evident in every degree of complexity.

The leader looks for opportunities to visualize complexity and seeks to find the points of competition and cooperation that must exist in equal degrees in order for work to be successful or for the workplace to thrive. In fact, competition may contain within it the seeds of cooperation between competitors when mutual advantage is at stake. The leader may be aware of the need to produce incentives for cooperation even with those with whom he or she may most directly compete. The leader must also incorporate the possibility of forming alliances around specific issues with competitors without sacrificing the other arenas within which the leader would continue to be competitive with another organization.

Neither competition nor cooperation predominates in quantum systems. Whether one prefers to cooperate during competition is an indication of a higher-level issue affecting potential resonance in the system. This does not mean that competitiveness is eliminated as a condition or circumstance of one's life experience; instead, it means that where cooperation is possible and can advance the integrity of systems and systemness, it should be the preferred strategy. Here again, however, competitiveness and cooperation are not constant variables. The degree of competitiveness and cooperation may change, depending on the set of circumstances, issues, or frame of reference within which relationships are established. Since these are in themselves a dynamic, they may adjust or shift, ultimately changing the ratio of cooperation to competition. The leader exemplifies an awareness of these changing circumstances and can accommodate them, adjusting the degree of competitiveness and cooperation depending on conditions and circumstances reflected in the relationship between them.

CONCLUSION

Complexity management is simply another tool available to the leader to both understand and apply systems processes in order to effectively guide and lead people and organizations on the journey. Although chaos and complexity models are in their infancy, there is much already available to further our understanding of the application of complexity models in leadership decision making and the design of organizations. Every good leader will develop a growing understanding of the application of complexity and chaos in

Competing for Quality

Marie and Fred are managers at St. Anywhere's Hospital. They have both been leaders in the hospital for a number of years and have worked diligently to assure the hospital success even in tough times when resources were short. However, although they both cooperated and collaborated extensively in advancing the interests and success of the hospital, they maintained an ongoing competition with regard to measures of clinical quality and service excellence. Marie and Fred constantly competed with each other to see who could achieve the best service and quality scores in the organization. Invariably their departments exchanged measures of excellence as they continue to compete with each other for higher levels of quality.

Marie and Fred present an example of both collaboration and competition expressed in a way that serves as a means to support the system. In this case both collaborated to sustain the success of the hospital, but each also competed over performance measures. Their accomplishments benefited each department, yet at the same time advanced the interests of the system. Theirs is an example of a continuous and dynamic interplay of the forces of both competition and collaboration.

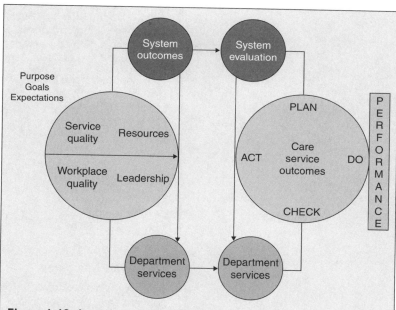

Figure 1-18 A continuous dynamic for strategy and goal achievement.

Gem

Complexity science calls us to understand the unpredictable, chaotic, and uncertain influences and circumstances that guide the action of all life in the universe. While the leader looks for order and symmetry in the workplace, just beneath the surface lies the chaos and complexity that are the foundations upon which the next order and symmetry will unfold. It is this continuous dance between order and chaos, simplicity and complexity, and leadership and systems that guides the unfolding of the future role of the leader.

the exercise of leadership. This new critical concept will have increasing influence over the design and structure of work in the quantum age. Understanding the impact of complexity on decision making, organizational design, relationships, and work and applying it in the exercise of leadership will be essential to the success of the leader in the 21st-century workplace.

SCENARIO-BASED FUTURES PLANNING

As the future becomes increasingly important but remains basically unclear, it becomes vital to be involved in processes that help organizations and people discern their preferred future. However, rather than predicting the future, it is important to look at the signs (vectors) that, when converged, indicate the pathway or journey to the future, rather than the future itself. Leaders must use a number of creative processes and mechanisms for both gathering stakeholders around their own futures journey and defining the actions and activities that will be necessary to create a preferred future.

Scenario-based approaches define possible conditions and circumstances and the factors that may emerge if those conditions or circumstances unfold. The specific organization or people affected by a given scenario explore the potential responses and actions. Usually three kinds of scenarios are identified: (1) the scenario that emerges if nothing changes, (2) the scenario that exists in the worst possible case, and (3) the scenario that will emerge if all positive factors converge to create an ideal set of conditions or circumstances. Building scenarios is like constructing stories reflecting specific and defined elements and components that, when aggregated, give a picture of life within the derived scenario.

Scenario leaders use the following processes in the group's exploration of possible futures:

Brainstorming
Conceptual block busting
Vectoring
Data interpretation
Technology assessment
Financial projecting
Community planning
Demographic shifts
Pattern management
Future search technologies
Consensus decision making

Scenario Exploration

Gather a small group of formal and informal leaders around a single issue, such as patient care, new technology, length of stay, quality or cost control, and so on. Using the single issue as the driver, use the above techniques to attack the issue under the umbrella of a different scenario format: whether conditions remain the same, worst-case options, and best-case options. Identify how your world would operate with regard to the specific issue under each one of these scenarios. Remember that current elements, data, circumstances, and conditions provide the backdrop for the scenario as it unfolds. When scenarios are completed, they can be adjusted with regard to action planning, which will direct the organization to create a preferred future based on the preponderance of the evidence with regard to which scenario appears most appropriate and demands the most specific response.

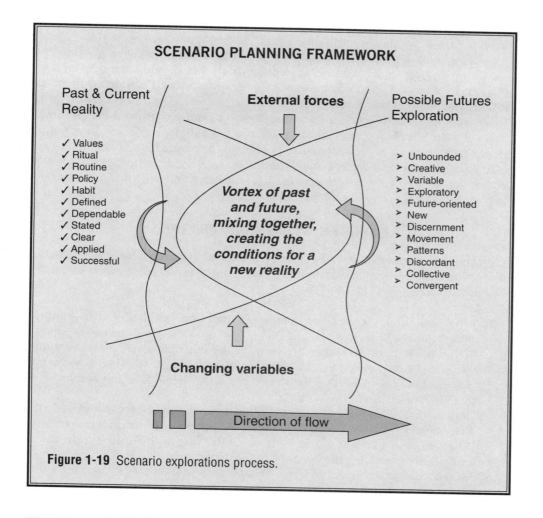

Figure 1-19 Scenario explorations process.

COMPLEXITY CASE STUDY

Sandra has been the clinical manager in critical care for 10 years. She has noticed that there has been an increasing level of changes in technology and clinical practice in the past 5 years. This new technology has created a different way of treating patients and has called clinical providers to adjust the way in which they deliver care for those patients. Because of the new technology, patients who are more seriously ill are now receiving higher levels of complex and intense care. At the same time, the demand to reduce the length of stay has accelerated as costs have increased and the revenue margin has tightened.

Staff have been reasonably responsive to the demand for change. However, there is a large number of staff members who are finding it difficult to let go of past practices and patterns of clinical behavior. At the same time, there is a large number of staff members who are eager to embrace the challenges of new practices and to incorporate them more quickly on the service. Sandra notes that this diversity of behavior is present in the medical staff as well. She's finding it hard to determine whether she needs to take a decisive lead and direct the staff to address these new changes or if she should take the additional time required to engage them in dialogue and group process so that together they might determine the best methods of action. Time is of the essence, yet all must be involved.

A group of the critical care staff have been meeting informally over lunch to talk about some of the issues in the service and to discuss matters of concern with regard to changing practice and new patient care demands. They have come up with many creative suggestions and are eager to begin implementing them as soon as possible.

Sandra appreciates their contribution but is beginning to feel as though she's losing control and now is no longer the source of providing direction in her department.

Administration, using a future-search approach, has developed a new strategic plan and set of goals and objectives for the health system. Each department has fully participated in the development of the strategic process and now must begin to incorporate the strategic goals into the operation and activity of the department. Every department must give evidence of advancing the strategic goals of the organization, a part of which is departmental competition for advancing quality and service excellence. Sandra must begin to build this initiative in her department. She is feeling challenged and is unsure how to manage all of this work and still implement new sets of priorities and actions in her department.

Complexity Case Study Questions

Using quantum examples from the principles outlined in this chapter, review Sandra's leadership case study and respond to the following questions that reflect leadership in a quantum age.

1. What are three elements of complexity that can be identified in Sandra's circumstances?
2. Is there conflict or resonance between the organization's method of creating a vision and direction and Sandra's obligations to do the same in her department?
3. How certain does Sandra need to become about her issues and responses to them before she undertakes action?
4. Does Sandra have issues around controlling information, the content of work, the distribution of power, and the management of personal and institutional anxiety?
5. What are the paradoxes Sandra is now confronting in the course of providing clinical care and doing the business of the department?
6. Sandra must act on multiple levels. What are those multiple circumstances and levels of action that must occur in order for the unit to continue to grow and to thrive?
7. What is the emerging power of the informal system? Has the core group changed the dynamics of leadership and the movement of change?
8. What is the relationship between the larger organization (larger, complex system) and the department (smaller complex system), and how is the tension and resonance between them now managed differently?
9. What are the elements of competition and collaboration that are reflected in the departmental goals and staff activities?

Application

Take the same questions and apply them to your own department's concerns or issues. Begin your discussion of your own department's issues by focusing on a particular problem or concern currently confronting the service or the department. In the context of group dialogue use the questions above to explore the issues and concerns. Try to establish a different frame of reference for answering them and a new set of processes for responding to them. Remember, there are no limitations or parameters, so exploration, innovation, and creativity are the tools that should be applied to this group process.

REFERENCES

Kleiner, A. (2004). *Who really matters: The core group theory of power, privilege, and success.* New York: Currency.

Zimmerman, B., Lindberg, C., & Plsek, P. (1998). *Edgeware: Insights from complexity science for health care leaders.* Irving, TX: VHA Publishing.

SUGGESTED READINGS

Battram, A. (1998). *Navigating complexity.* London and Sterling, VA: The Industrial Society.

Goldsmith, M. (2003). *The many facets of leadership.* Upper Saddle River, NJ: Financial Times/Prentice Hall.

Griffin, G. S. (1996). *Complexity theory in construction management.* Unpublished doctoral dissertation, Colorado State University.

Hazy, J., Goldstein, J., & Lichtenstein, B. (2007). *Complex systems leadership theory: New perspectives from complexity science on social and organizational effectiveness.* New York: Vintage Press.

Janssen, M. (2002). *Complexity and ecosystem management: The theory and practice of multi-agent systems.* Cheltenham, UK: Edward Elgar.

Lewin, R., & Regine, B. (2000). *The soul at work: Listen, respond, let go: Embracing complexity science for business success.* New York: Simon & Schuster.

Lewin, R., & Regine, B. (2001). *Weaving complexity and business: Engaging the soul at work.* New York: Texere.

Lissack, M. (2002). *The interaction of complexity and management.* Westport, CT: Quorum Books.

Mainzer, K. (2004). *Thinking in complexity: The computational dynamics of matter, mind and mankind* (4th rev. and enl. ed.). New York: Springer.

McElroy, M. W. (2003). *The new knowledge management: Complexity, learning, and sustainable innovation.* Boston: KMCI Press.

Miller, J., & Scott, P. (2007). *Complex adaptive systems: An introduction to computational models of social life.* Princeton, NJ: Princeton University Press.

Olson, E.E., & Eoyang, G.H. (2001). *Facilitating organization change: Lessons from complexity science.* San Francisco: Jossey-Bass/Pfeiffer.

Ragsdell, G., West, D., & Wilby, J. (2002). *Systems theory and practice in the knowledge age.* New York: Kluwer Academic/Plenum Publishers.

Samad, T., & Weyrauch, J. (2000). *Automation, control, and complexity: An integrated approach.* New York: Wiley.

Shan, Y., & Ang, Y. (2008). *Applications of complex adaptive systems.* Hershey, PA: IGI Publishing.

CHAPTER 2

Leading in a New Age

CHAPTER OBJECTIVES:

Upon completion of this chapter, the reader will:

1. Understand the new requisites of leadership.
2. Identify the critical elements of competent clinical leadership.
3. Name the characteristics of new-age leaders and the changes in the expression of the role.
4. Enumerate the changes in the 21st-century workplace influencing both the work and worker and forming the context for new-age leadership.

INTRODUCTION: A DIFFERENT AGE

Periodically in the course of human history there have been dramatic social, cultural, and economic shifts that, when they occur, alter the human experience in radical ways. From the medieval age into the age of enlightenment, the Victorian age, the industrial age, and, now, the sociotechnical or digital age, human experience has been radically altered. At the time of the shift between two ages, we will call it a paradigmatic moment (a series of peaceful interludes punctuated by intellectually violent revolutions leading to the replacement of one conceptual worldview by another) (Kuhn, 1996), elements of chaos, uncertainty, loss, transformation, and the constant dynamic of continuous movement occur in a dynamic of interaction that creates the necessary conditions for successful transition into a new reality—a new age.

Everything is different as we enter the new age. As we leave the industrial age, everything about work and leadership is changing. The leader must be aware that older skills and talents gained from experiences in previous learning are newly subject to question. Work now represents a whole different set of values, interactions, and intersections and requires the ability to integrate, coordinate, and facilitate these dramatic changes in work.

The problem of all this change is that much of what leaders have learned in the past for addressing change is no longer adequate for

> ### Gem
>
> It's a new world for organizations. No longer can the old institutional models of work and workplace govern how and what people do. It is now time to rethink the very foundations of work.

> ### New-Age Characteristics
>
> - Mobile
> - Portable
> - Fast
> - Fluid
> - Flexible
> - Systems driven
> - Digital
> - Relational

today's emerging demands for leadership. As a result, leaders are often frustrated with a lack of skills to address the changing character of work, and employees are uncomfortable with the quality and content of the work of those who lead them. As a workplace changes, so does the need for leadership. However, in order to lead well, the leader must gain new insights and skills, change the talents and abilities acquired over a lifetime of experience, and adapt and adopt new behaviors and patterns of leadership to better reflect the context for work in today's environment.

Along with significant technological innovations, changes in communication, and the globalization of work, leaders also must adjust to instant communication, unbounded relationships, the globalization of economics, a shifting political landscape, high-tech clinical processes, new mechanisms of knowledge management, and a host of other challenging and daunting changes in the way in which human beings relate and interact together. All this has a dramatic impact on the ability of the leader to provide meaning, value, and a clear direction within the context of the 21st century.

Simply dealing with the context of leadership and the drama of new emerging work realities can frequently be overwhelming for leaders. Indeed, it is overwhelming for organizations. The pace of change and the demands of that pace are so challenging that it appears almost beyond human competence to be able to address these changes in a meaningful way. As a result, leaders and those they lead must now live more comfortably in the ambiguity and the challenges of continuous change, which is often called "permanent whitewater."

This notion of continuous and endless change as a dynamic for work is an important concept upon which the leader must build. Construction of new leadership must occur within the context of emerging new frames of reference for work. The leader must recognize that change is itself the work. Understanding the notion of change as a permanent human condition, rather than as a set of circumstances that can be managed and manipulated, is an important first step. They must conceive change as a permanent, contextual and conditional circumstance of all work. Recent research on complexity indicates that change is the normative condition of the universe. Human beings do not create or make change; instead, they give change its form—the way in which change can unfold in realistic stages, applying meaning to the human experience. Change is a lived experience, forever "dancing" across the consciousness on the landscape of human experience.

The leader must engage change with the expectation that it is a permanent condition. Leaders must exemplify in their own role a constant and continuous engagement of change as a fundamental part of their leadership experience. Within their own behaviors and adaptation, leaders exemplify a living accommodation to the constancy of change. Representing this reality as a personal leadership example and model of engaging change is a critical part of the leader's role in helping others to both understand and adapt to the permanent condition of change.

All people desire some level of stability in their lives. The challenge for the leader exists at the point of tension between personal stability and the ever-evolving dynamic of change. A critical role that change plays in individuals' lives must be facilitated by the leader in a way that assures continuous growth for individuals while, at the same time, maintaining the comfort and calm often found in the ritual and routine of human experience. This is a special challenge. Leaders must be able to demonstrate in their personal lives and leadership the engagement with and embracing of change. They must be able, at the same time, to maintain sufficient calm, peacefulness, and adaptability so staff can

---

A Meaning for Work

The role of the leader is to provide a context for meaning. Workers need to get back in touch with the *why* of their work: the reason they do what they do. Work always changes, as it should. What should remain constant, however, is the value of the work and the meaning each individual brings to it. This meaning gives them their reason for doing work and their desire to keep growing and expanding their skill and their effort.

Change Is Forever

Change never changes! Leaders must understand that change is the work and will be the single constant in all human activity. Embracing this reality is the essential cornerstone to effective leadership. It informs the work of the leader and calls on leaders to incorporate the reality of constant change into all work relationships and action. Staff must know that they cannot stop change, nor slow it, or even alter it. They can only respond to it, giving it the form it will take, and addressing the impact it will express.

Chaos and Calm

Chaos does not always mean *noise*. Calm in the face of chaos exhibits a basic understanding of the work of chaos in changing our frame of reference, our direction, or our activity. Chaos serves a purpose and acts to challenge our insights and sensibilities, calling us to a new way of seeing and being.

Industrial Age Infrastructure

- Mechanical
- Functional
- Structured
- Reductionistic
- Vertical
- Compartmental

incorporate those qualities in their own roles as they confront life-changing events. In this way, leaders become conduits for change, instruments that staff can witness and themselves incorporate as an appropriate model of engagement and accommodation to change.

LEADING IN A FOREVER FLUID WORLD

Much of the institutional infrastructure of the industrial age represented a more mechanical application of work. As newer models of work emerge, driven by increasingly broad-based technological innovations, entire new constructs and frameworks for work also emerge. Leaders must now conceive of work as a highly fluid and mobile exercise, challenging old notions of fixed and compartmentalized structures and frames. Even the industrial notion of *job* presents a perspective of work that is individualistic, unilateral, nonaligned, and functionally focused. Job descriptions, the tools that have most articulated the content of work, are no longer adequate for defining work. Today, work changes so quickly in its content that identifying it becomes deceptive. Job descriptions no longer address expectations and performance clearly and specifically enough to have any meaning. In fact, the content of work is changing so quickly that codifying it becomes an exercise in futility. Now, instead of job functions, individuals must identify their work within the context of specific roles. Workers must look at their role in light of its intersections, relationships, and work demands. It is these interactions that provide better insight and understanding with regard to the content of work roles and the exercise of work. In short, people must recognize that work's role is better defined by its relationship to others and to outcomes than by any definition of permanent content.

The stable institutions of the 20th-century workplace no longer represent either the framework or the circumstances of work for the 21st-century workplace. The old bricks and mortar institutionally fixed settings and structures for work are not the prevailing reality for the form and context of 21st-century work. Fluidity, mobility, the ability to do work at any time, any place across the globe exemplify the contemporary vision of work. Cellular phones, laptop computers, wireless networks, and global accessibility all reflect changing conditions that challenge our notion of work. Historically, work required a specific time and place and was much more structured and formal and bounded with more clearly delineated parameters. Now work can be performed anywhere on the globe. Workers connect across the globe using contemporary technology, changing the very nature of interaction and communication as well as work performance. As a result, the locus of control for work, decision making, and relationships is now shifting from fixed work sites to highly mobile work processes.

This shift in the locus of control reflects a change in the nature of work, the nature of work relationships, and new intersections between worker and workplace. Leaders must recognize that the worker is becoming increasingly competent in controlling and managing the variables associated with his or her own work. The locus of control for content of work and the relationships necessary to sustain it are moving inexorably from manager to worker. This creates conditions and circumstances that allow the worker to be more self-directed, the work to be more decentralized, and the workplace to be more fluid.

Several new elements emerge as a result of this change that permanently alter the social conditions of work. There's a greater desire and need for workers to have more highly technical skills. There is also a need for the more educated worker, a desire for more technically prepared workers, and a better interface between the unique technical

---

New-Age Infrastructure

- Wholistic
- Relational
- Synthesis
- Multifocal
- Multidirectional
- Integrated

No Role for Job Descriptions

In a time of great change, the role for job descriptions diminishes considerably. Changes in function, activity, purposes, and goals of work shift so quickly that describing them in job categories no longer suffices. Descriptions and definers of work now require a clearer identification of the purposes and the outcome of work rather than the functions and processes of any work category. More importantly, the confluence of work efforts and the integration of individual roles within a team context is a more important delineation of the characteristics of work than job descriptions can ever provide.

Workers Control the Means of Work

- Local decisions predominate.
- Decisions are made where they are implemented.
- The work is knowledge work.
- Quality depends on who does the work.
- Efficiency requires competent decisions.
- Clinical decisions require ownership by clinicians.

skills of each worker. In this set of circumstances, the leader must align all of these skill sets in a way that advances the outcomes of work. The social challenge embedded in this is the reduction in demand and need for nonskilled or uneducated workers, forever changing the landscape of work. As with everything in a complex world, the interactions and intersections of the work demands creates social and political circumstances that require a change in the infrastructure that supports human activity.

NEW LEADERSHIP, NEW EXPECTATIONS

It is clear that traditional, industrial-age skill sets operating in the framework of institutional models of work are no longer sustainable. These work models cannot operate successfully in a highly mobile work environment. The globalization of work alters notions and processes such as job descriptions, performance expectations, job compliance, management-driven decision making, and hierarchical structures. The vertical constructs for decision making and the command-and-control structures are no longer the means by which managers can assure the work is appropriately done and outcomes are achieved. This more mechanical notion of the relationship between worker and work as well as worker and workplace can no longer be sustained. The relationship in the new workplace is far more dynamic, interactive, and increasingly interdependent. It is in this developing frame of reference within which the role of the leader must now unfold.

Leaders need to recognize that their role is predominantly transformational and reconceptual as they confront the vagaries of the new age. It is in this reconceptual and transformational change, especially in its initial stages, that the leader must be able to demonstrate an understanding of the content of change, translate it, and redefine it along with enumerating the impact that change will have on the worker and the workplace. In this first stage, leaders must exemplify a level of frankness and honesty that at times may appear painful and challenging to those who must hear about the radical nature of work changes. Leaders must persuade followers to embrace the imperative of change in their own work and the need for immediate behavioral and role adjustments. Leaders must exemplify that competency is always shifting depending on demand. In order to remain continuously competent, workers must be continually engaged in addressing the content and influences of their own work. As technology creates new means of working and demands on the work itself, workers must shift their emphasis. This is especially critical when one considers the degree of technological shifts and their impact on therapeutic care and treatment of patients and rendering healthcare services.

Much of the education of the practitioner is now dependent on immediately meeting patients' needs over shorter lengths of stay. As a result, caregivers have less time to render the same kinds of service that they once provided over much longer periods of time. Caregivers must now raise work-related issues about what activities are critical to care, what activities must be left behind, and what new activities are emerging, created by the demand for applying new technology. This new work changes the nature of the relationship between patient and provider. It requires leaders to address the meaning of the change, the content of the activities of work, and the time frames needed for accomplishing the clinical work in a way that is effective, efficient, and meets the needs of the patient. It is the leader's role to make sure that the elements and fundamental circumstances of a change in emphasis and priority are part of the deliberation and decision making of the clinical staff. The leader must help the staff confront those things that are no longer usual and ordinary, including the clinical activities to which they have been accustomed. Often the staff must give

---

Shared Decisions

- Decentralized
- Team-based
- Horizontal
- Inclusive
- Engaging
- Accountable
- Point-of-service based

Command and Control

- Centralized
- Unilateral
- Vertical
- Directed
- Superordinate
- Hierarchical

Leadership Honesty

- Direct
- Frank
- Disclosing
- Open
- Vulnerable
- Exploratory
- Discourse friendly

Leadership Dishonesty

- Secretive
- Polarizing
- Noninclusive
- Exclusive
- Controlling
- Selective
- Incomplete

over old ways of doing business in order to adapt to new applications and technologies and do so quickly and efficiently.

Adaptation is critical to the staff's ability to succeed. In order to help staff adapt, the leader, constantly living in the potential, anticipates the changes that will affect work and translates those changes in language the staff can understand. Furthermore, the leader helps the staff in applying new concepts and notions of work, by making it safe to risk, experiment, challenge, and evaluate new methods of clinical performance. The leader in this set of circumstances exemplifies in the role an individual commitment to adaptation and change by making risk and experimentation safe and appropriate strategies for organizational and individual adaptation.

Because the leader anticipates the next cycle of change, he or she keeps an eye on the broader frame of reference for all work activities. Leaders look for meaning in change to guide its translation into the lives of workers in a way that can be understood and applied. For example, much health care today requires providers to rethink service delivery and how to make it more portable, fluid, and easy for the patient to access and use. Increasingly, patients are healing in places other than healthcare institutions and now require a level of information and access to clinical support that was once available to them from their caregivers when that support was provided directly by caregivers in hospitals. Leaders now must translate this set of circumstances and guide their followers to make decisions about how skills once offered in the institution can now be provided to patients in other settings. This role of translation of change is a vital part of the role of the leader, as new concepts and notions of service must be defined and incorporated within the context of the emerging contemporary role of the caregiver.

In inaugurating a new paradigm for work, the leader must emphasize a different set of principles. Delineating a new set of rules for staff, the leader needs to create a different framework and way of thinking for staff that helps everyone understand the emerging new demands for work.

1. *The leader must be able to address the inner resources and wisdom of both leader and follower.* The leader can't know everything about change or the impact of change on work. Good leaders access collective wisdom and utilize it in helping teams adapt and adjust to whole new ways of doing business. Leaders must engage all participants in the system to develop a level of interpersonal competency and contribution that helps the work and learning team find common ground, share mutual and unique competencies, meet the challenge of change together, and develop new patterns of work and relationships. This requires high participant approaches to the application of leadership. In this case, the leader is essentially a gatherer, making sure the right stakeholders are at the decision-making table with regard to work and its exercise.

The leader recognizes that no work is essentially independent. All work activities have a level of interdependence that recognizes the impact of anyone's role on all other roles. This essential interdependence requires in the leader a broad competence in applying systems thinking in decision making at all levels. Furthermore, the leader must be able to articulate in the followers' roles his or her own understanding of the impact of individual action on others. Leaders must translate their understanding of collective wisdom and the intersection of all efforts in the roles of each provider. What must result in the workplace is the respect and understanding of the value and importance of the unique contribution

---

Gem

There is a new relationship between the patient and the caregiver requiring a new level of honesty about what is or is not going to happen. Caregivers must now realize that they have to reteach the patient what to expect in a different model for service delivery. Remember, much might have changed since the patient's last experience, except for the patient's own expectations. These expectations now must be changed to match the current reality for service if patient satisfaction is to ever be achieved.

Adaptation

Fluidity and flexibility are now a requisite of all work. Holding onto past practices and nonrelevant traditions that do not better serve the patient is a failure strategy. The leader must require a new way of both seeing and doing the work and provide a safe context for clinical change. Stoking the expectation for changes in practice is a minimum requirement for good leadership.

User-Controlled Health Care

The system in which most providers were "born" was designed to be provider-driven and controlled. With the introduction of the Internet and mass customization, the user is being empowered to control more aspects of choice and action, forever changing the rules governing service and decision making. Users are taking control. The obligation of the provider now is to make sure the user becomes competent in exercising control and to do whatever is necessary to make the user competent.

Building Interdependence

The leader's primary role is to build a real and sustaining sense of team. The interdependence now necessary to good service is such that care cannot be successful without team-based commitment to designing a delivering service. The following core elements of interdependence must be inculcated into all work:

- Collaboration
- Integration
- Consensus based
- Dialogue driven
- Clearly delineated roles
- Common goals (negotiated)
- Mutuality of function

Creating the Service Mosaic

- Remember that all roles are linked.
- Define the intersections.
- Clarify the boundaries.
- Define the mutual expectations.
- Identify commonly agreed-upon goals.
- Be open to continuous learning and adaptation.
- Establish a frame for resolving conflict.

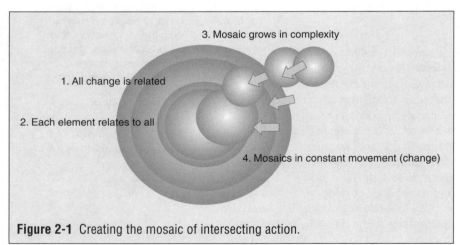

1. All change is related
2. Each element relates to all
3. Mosaic grows in complexity
4. Mosaics in constant movement (change)

Figure 2-1 Creating the mosaic of intersecting action.

of each worker and the collective integration of those contributions in making a substantive difference in the care of patients.

Leaders represent a deep understanding that all work reflects a mosaic of interfaces that when pulled together act as a whole in moving to achieving sustainable outcomes. Reflecting this understanding in the application of the leader's role creates an appreciation in the follower with regard to the value of the worker's own efforts. Rather than seeing unilateral action as desirable, this systems reality creates in the worker an understanding that individual action must fit with the collective enterprise. The resulting mosaic of individual actions must substantially link and integrate in a way that ultimately has a meaningful impact on the patients served. This wisdom calls all workers to a different level of understanding with regard to the meaning and relationship of individual work versus the work of the team. This realization affects decision making, collaboration, and clinical action at every level of application. It is the leader's role to make sure this reality is constantly before the staff, continually reminding them of this synthesis of activity as a means of integrating and investing staff in the work of the whole.

2. *It is the leader's role to acknowledge the interconnectedness of everyone and everything.* Everything that all people do has some relationship to everything everyone else does.

There is always and everywhere a continuing dynamic and synthesis of activities that ultimately relate to all other activities. This results in a perpetual interface of motion and process acting in concert with the movements and flow of life. One of the cognitive competencies of leadership now is the application of systems thinking to problems and issues, and indeed, to the work itself.

Self-management and servant leadership are now essential characteristics influencing the role of the leader. Collective effort doesn't diminish the impact of individual effort; it simply indicates the value of that effort when aggregated with the whole. Leaders are challenged to create much stronger team-based and relationship-driven work systems. The contemporary leader must focus not only on individual performance, but also on the interconnectedness and intersections of performance and the collective products of good work performance.

Individuals can no longer be encouraged to solve problems in isolation. Leaders must actively search for opportunities to build the proper connections, collective creativity, positive human relationships, and the use of intuitive processes for problem solving. The leader uses tools of participation, relationship, and interpersonal interaction. The skilled leader must have well-honed interpersonal and interactional competencies. Not only must this leader be able to express these competencies, but he or she must also be able to translate them well for followers so that they express these competencies in the exercise of their own roles.

The role of the leader must also reflect change in the dynamics of application of the role. Leaders must see themselves as servants to those who do the work, as well as to the organization. This notion of servant leadership creates a different model of the application of the leader role. It calls leaders to see themselves in the context of the service role rather than from the traditional hierarchical position of the manager. Positional considerations for the role are no longer as valuable as relational considerations. In this new context, the application of the leader's role represents a facilitation and access to resources, systems, supports, and information in any way that advances the viability of the work of the staff. While this is not a new concept, it is no longer optional. The expression of the role calls for deeper notions of partnership, collateral relationship, horizontal decision making, and collective problem solving. Here again the leader must exemplify these skills, first in the role of the leader, and through its application create exemplars for the staff so that the same behaviors can be found in staff roles, too.

3. *Hierarchies must be deconstructed.* People can no longer only focus on specialized and defined tasks. While efficiency is certainly obtained through specialization and work focus, effectiveness is sustained by recognizing the integration of all activities around a common goal. What hierarchies do support is the differentiation and compartmentalization of work in decision making. What often happens is that flexibility, fluidity, innovation, risk taking, and challenge are designed out of responsive creative action. The hierarchical configuration of systems and work processes creates a significant management structure and legitimizes that structure to undertake decision making and evaluation of work and performance.

Often an organization's departments that could be identified as servant structures, such as finance, human resources, and information systems, become decision points guiding and directing organizational decision making in ways that are ultimately inappropriate and nonproductive. Rather than playing a servant's role, they provide a primary decision-making role, hijacking legitimate and effective decision making. In the transformative organizational context, those services that most represent the core business of the organization play the predominant decision-making and application role. However, what is required in this set of circumstances is that those departments (such as finance, human resources, and information services) must make sure that these primary decisions are informed by specialized information available in support departments.

Of course, this calls for a whole new way of looking at relationships and roles. These intersections between support and service call for reframing interaction and decision making. A huge reformatting of the structural integration of support and service systems will be required as well to properly configure health-care organizations in a way that focuses on service, quality, and value. Indeed, value will only be fully achieved through a massive overhauling of the structure and organization of health care in a way that reorients the operational priorities to better support core services and the obtaining and advancing of clinical and service value. No organization that sacrifices its core business has ever survived. How many times have hospitals done that in the past 2 decades alone? Perhaps, on a more detailed review, the current nursing shortage is the result of "turfing" nurses out of hospitals during the days of reengineering, when they were replaced with more functional and less skilled workers. Certainly this is a heavy price to pay, as the complex demands of care today require more resources with a higher level of skill and competence and fewer nurses are available.

The Servant Leader

- Lateral role with the staff
- Seeks to support staff decisions
- Provides information for staff decisions
- Open to staff direction
- Uses group process
- Facilitates challenging decisions
- Advocates for staff leadership

Servant Leader Skills

- Vulnerability
- Openness
- Adaptivity
- Inclusiveness
- Directness and honesty
- Group dynamic skills
- Great role modeling

Deconstructing Hierarchies

- Bring decisions to the staff
- Disclose necessary information
- Develop group skills in staff
- Develop shared decision-making processes
- Build staff ownership of issues and solutions
- Have staff confront normal conflict
- Create staff social cohesiveness (celebrating)

Gem

A leader should never allow staff to transfer decisions and accountability for action to the leader. Staff ownership of all issues is critical to accountability, which cannot be sustained if the leader acts for the staff. The leader must never own decisions and actions that belong to the staff and must make sure staff never transfers them out of their own locus of control.

Leadership at that time would have required great courage on the part of nurse executives and managers in the face of overwhelming demand from their administrators to cut staff in order to comply with the prevailing cult of reengineering.

It is precisely this disoriented hierarchy that places the clinical decision-making process beneath the financial and operational decision structure, even though these clinical services are the core of the work of the healthcare system.

NEW CORE COMPETENCIES FOR THE HEALTHCARE LEADER

The leader must be able to evidence the engagements of significant change in his or her own role. While not blinded by past success or limited by it, the new leader must reconceptualize the worldview of the staff and renew a focus on their core values, beliefs, practices, and notions. Indeed, the leader must do that for herself or himself. Healthcare leaders must change not only the way they think but also the way they act and how they engage others in decision making and in clinical action.

Therefore, specific competencies that are critical to the unfolding role of the leader include conceptual, participation, interpersonal, and leadership competencies. Each has critical elements that are important to their expression and has a significant impact on the role of staff. The leader must be able to demonstrate facility in the expression of these skills if staff are to be able to perform well within the context of a new work reality.

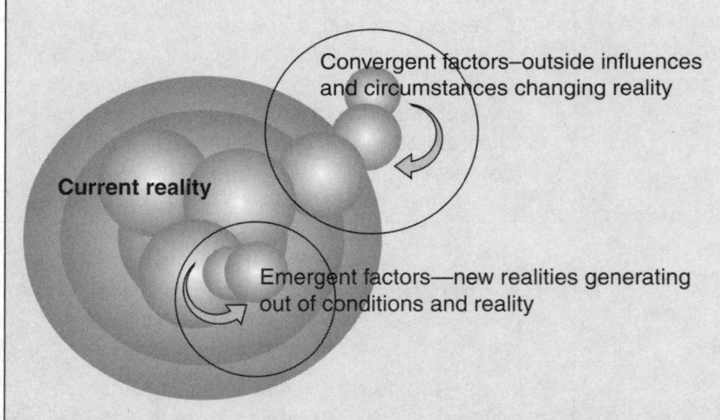

The expression of management knowledge gives evidence of the mind maps or conceptual schemes that leaders reflect. Leaders create context for others' work. Therefore, the leader must be able to translate concept into reality for staff in a language that they can understand. The leader must create a sort of mind map that becomes for the staff both process and outcome. The use of these leadership mind maps assists in leadership action planning and helping staff through new experiences. Using these mind maps, leaders can help staff rethink and reconceptualize their activities and their work within the context of the new format for that work. Through the stages of development, such as direction setting, decision making, communicating processes, structural design, interpersonal and interdisciplinary interaction, and consensus building, the leader guides the staff to a different and higher level of practice. The leader recognizes that no change is going to occur unless the staff is able to articulate and incorporate it within their own understanding. The leader must not only develop strong conceptual competency but strong translation skills as well.

While mind maps provide a strategic framework for directing action, they can also be limiting. The leader must be constantly aware of the accuracy and timeliness of her or his own conceptions and mental models. Outdated or inaccurate concepts or notions of clinical work or the context of work can prevent concerted and meaningful action. Furthermore, they can limit the leader's ability to identify social and organizational cues, which can lead staff in the wrong direction rather than provide support for them. The leader must remember that critical cues reflect the leader's own ability to see them. Therefore, the leader must constantly check and recheck the mental map

---

Leadership Courage

Courage is a fundamental skill necessary to all leadership. It is the one thing that can only be demonstrated through the behavior of the leader. There are signs that the staff need to see in the leader to indicate he or she acts courageously, such as:

- Does not hold back negative news
- Speaks up in controversies
- Does not fear sharing views
- Is direct with others
- Can express countervailing views
- Does not shy away from noise
- Engages change directly

Gem

Remember, it is more effective to act your way into a new way of thinking than to think your way into a new way of acting.

Figure 2-2 Use of new mental models and mind maps for creating new realities.

that is used for decision making to make sure that it is congruent with the shifts and changes in the context within which work unfolds.

The most important conceptual skill for the leader today is the development of true systems thinking. The systems thinker doesn't simply look at healthcare delivery as an organized group of services, compartmentalized and configured to meet patient needs. Instead, the leader sees care delivery as an integrated set of service configurations and interfaces that operate together along a continuum of health and illness to advance the interests of the patient. The leadership role is grounded in accountability and managing core interactions rather than simply operating at the level of control. In this case, problems are not seen in isolation from each other but are a necessary part of a larger universe of interactions and intersections that must be addressed. Problems and medication administration or patient care can be looked at, not simply as the fault of an individual but within the context of a system of delivery. This system of delivery is affected by workload, knowledge, resources, workflow, and a set of standards and practices that guide the delivery of medication. The leader sees all these elements in concert and addresses them within the context of one great relationship rather than in iterative and functional segments. The healthcare leader recognizes that the whole is greater than the sum of its parts, the power of language and expression reflects the conceptual foundations the leader maintains, and the leader's own ability to translate concept into reality depends fundamentally on his or her relationship with others.

The 21st-century leader struggles with all the confusion and chaos that affects the ability to translate concept into action. In the past, leaders have been taught to equate control with order. We know, however, through quantum thinking, that stability is a metaphor for death. Innovative and creative environments require equally innovative solutions, which cannot be obtained without confronting the vagaries and noise of instability, chaos, and uncertainty. This level of being overwhelmed is a constant condition in the process of change and is often reflected in followers' reactions. The leader must model an ability to deal with chaos by partnering with it, engaging its energy, and sorting through the information it is attempting to generate with regard to how things are changing. The leader attempts to reap the deep meaning from the chaos and to rescue from the flux and movement of chaos the inherent order, appropriateness, and concerted action that must be taken to continue the movement forward.

Certainty is not required for action. This does not mean that the leader has permission to act without thinking or without verifying the collective wisdom in any given pursuit. However, uncertainty calls the leader to sort through the confluence of forces (the vectoring) to determine what direction is indicated by the convergence of the vectors. In order to do this the leader must exhibit several ways of thinking:

1. *Openness to surprises as opportunities for new ideas.* The leader must always be aware of the temptation to use existing or old mental models to look at new sets of circumstances. The leader's own mental model must also shift as the context tells a different story about experiences, reality, and the shift in emphasis or action.
2. *Situation testing in the validation of new information.* The leader is always testing assumptions, insights, and knowledge against a changing context. This contextual shift creates a demand to recognize that what one knows is not always constant. Information,

---

Systems Thinking Requisites

- Seeing the whole, not just one piece
- Recognizing flow in all events
- Building larger systems from small ones
- Integrating everything
- Looking for fit
- Creating a common vision
- Building relatedness

Systems Thinking Applications

- Interdisciplinary
- Interdepartmental
- Facilitates whole thinking
- Inclusive engagement
- Looks for linkages
- Seeks common ground
- Frequently looks outside the box

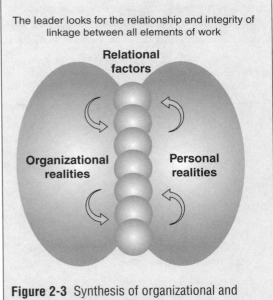

The leader looks for the relationship and integrity of linkage between all elements of work

Relational factors

Organizational realities

Personal realities

Figure 2-3 Synthesis of organizational and personal realities.

Quantum Leadership Process

- Testing assumptions
- Reading signposts
- Stretching the limits
- Pushing perceptions
- Creating new mental models
- Reaching for the potential
- Behaving with boldness

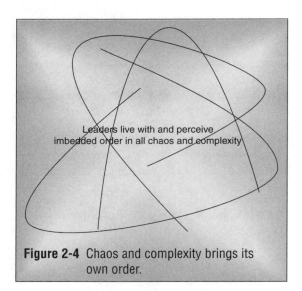

Figure 2-4 Chaos and complexity brings its own order.

Gem

Risk is embedded in every action. No change can occur at any level of the organization without a willingness to engage risk and maximize the benefit that lies secretly and deeply within.

---

data, and insights must be obtained as they arise and are applied to the emerging situation so that there is a connection between context and action that is highly congruent and leads to good flow and appropriate action.

3. *Making accurate assumptions about new levels of uncertainty and inherent risk.* There are no risk-free actions. The leader must recognize that risk is embedded in every human activity and cannot be fully eliminated. Thus, the issue for the leader is a matter of degrees of risk rather than the elimination of risk altogether. Looking at levels and intensities of risk against required action gives the leader a sense of what will be required in terms of staff energy, commitment, understanding, and concerted personal action. This risk testing is a constant part of the leader's decision skills.

4. *Evidence is in the action.* While the leader must consider all stages of decision making and consideration, ultimately, action is required. Most problems of leadership lie between the decision and action phases. Risk is embedded in all action taken. If no action is taken, then risk can be minimized or avoided, at least over the short term. However, there is a long-term price to be paid if action is delayed beyond the time of its demand. The leader looks at applying action at the right time. Timing is a critical strategy in facilitating and advancing vital change. Knowing when to act and how to act are as critical as the action itself.

PATTERN RECOGNITION

Relying on outdated mental models and mind maps results in an inadequate orientation to the realities of the time. Entrenched thinking and outdated models are the result of not having kept up with changes in contextual issues and in patterns of work. Recognizing patterns is an important conceptual talent because it provides the leader an opportunity to understand what action is effective and when to take it. It helps keep the leader from undertaking polarized action or applying incomplete information to decisions. The leader who can recognize patterns in any given situation and synthesize the information those patterns demonstrate will make more accurate decisions. In this process the leader looks at the why of issues and sorts through the multiple arrays of information, determining what values and seminal elements can be drawn from it. The leader uses the aggregation of data and other complexes of information to create a mosaic, out of which can be drawn indicators of direction or supports for particular decision making.

SYNTHESIS

As leaders become more expert in systems thinking, they acquire the ability to synthesize many pieces of information into an integrated whole. Through analysis and integration, bits of information, pieces of data, elements of insight, and components of process can all be pulled together

- Seeing themes
- Setting direction
- Assessing the movement
- Relationship in motion

Figure 2-5 Patterns indicate direction.

to help guide the imagination and thinking of the leader. Leaders take the various elements of information and draw relevance from them to guide their decision making and action. This synthesis of processes uses multiple sources as a way of drawing conclusions and taking action. The transforming leader applies systems thinking proficiently, moving past compartmentalization, incrementalism, and vertical models of thinking and planning to better delineate a goodness of fit between demand and action. Integration of thought and action are critical talents for the leader. Moving seamlessly through thought and application, the leader links as much data to current demand as possible so that action is always informed by the most vibrant and applicable supporting data possible.

Leadership Continuous Learning
1. Confronting the ritual and routine
2. Stimulating creative skills
3. Aggregating information resources
4. Applying all learning
5. Experimenting actions
6. Innovation thinking and application
7. No boundaries, lots of brainstorming
8. No permanent solutions or behavior
9. Using ambiguity to stretch assumptions
10. Evaluating outcomes and values

LEADERSHIP AND CONTINUOUS LEARNING

How often have managers confronted what appears to be "brain-dead people?" These are people who have become so addicted to ritual and routine they have no creative and responsive behaviors left to respond to the demand for change. Here again the leader represents in the context of his or her own behavior a commitment to continuous adaptation and growth. In short, the leader indicates a personal availability to continuous learning.

Effective leaders continuously remain open to new ideas and approaches. In fact, they so live their availability to new ideas and approaches that it becomes their way of life. They represent to those they lead a living commitment to openness and learning. However, even leaders can experience information overload. With so much data unfolding at every moment of the workday, it can be hard to keep up with what the data is presenting. Often, the data itself becomes demanding, requiring time away from the usual activities of work just to be able to assimilate it and to organize it to make it useful. It is important to sort through desired information and useful information. The leader recognizes that there will be greater amounts of information available than individuals can use. It becomes the responsibility of the leader, therefore, to sort through the many sources of data and to discipline information flow so she or he can focus on those pieces of information that are important to particular moments or processes of decision making. This way, the leader prevents data backlogs and information overload. In the management of information, the leader uses time effectively by prioritizing the information that is critical to the work being done. Instead of simply reading journals, the leader pulls from the journal those articles that mean something in the context of the role or the demand of the time.

Openness to Learning
• Availability to the new
• Looking past today
• Moving past ritual
• Questioning everything
• Insatiable curiosity
• Having more questions than answers

Data smog is an important issue for leaders. Not all data has value. Often data is generated to meet the needs of those sending it, rather than those receiving it. The recipient of data must make some decisions with regard to its value, meaning, and appropriateness to work demands. Leaders recognize information as a support service, not an end in itself. Careful management of what kind of information, what form the information takes, and what information has impact are basic requirements for making information usable. Leaders will find that most of the information generated has limited value. In fact, most of the information received will not contain anything of value at any given moment. Information, in fact, changes its value depending on the issues. It is the role of the leader to make sure that there is a goodness of fit between information used and the decisions made.

Leaders also need to sort in ways that help discern information that is real and that which is simply informative. It is wise to look at information from a questioning perspective, recognizing that information itself can be a source of problems. Information can be incomplete, inaccurate, or even biased. Leaders themselves can read

Managing Data Smog
• Sorting through the nonrelevant
• Scrapping the unnecessary
• Finding core information
• Relating data elements
• Using all the tools well
• Not accepting the pieces until you've seen it all

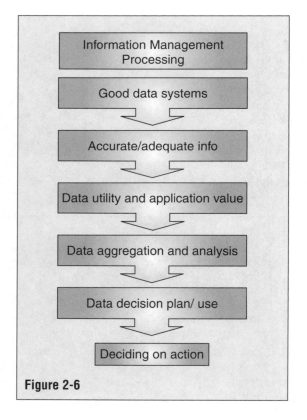

Figure 2-6

information through biased eyes and therefore skew it in ways that reflect a particular perspective. There are critical differences between information management, developing knowledge, and obtaining a real understanding from appropriate utilization of data. Poor data and poor data management can get directly in the way of effectiveness and good decision making, especially if it crowds out good reflection, vertical thinking, appropriate dialogue, and openness to new learning.

Information tends to be seductive. Often, the more information one gets, the more seduced one is. What results can be an inability to recall or to recognize sources of information and to remember what information served as a basis for making specific decisions. There are several things a good leader does to compensate for the inappropriately dramatic impact of too much information:

1. *Discusses and compares information and data.* The good leader looks for opportunities to share information and insights, to obtain others' views, and to debate the veracity and impact of specific information on particular elements of work. This dialogue can offset dependence on e-mail, cell phones, message machines, and other mediums not requiring direct interaction.
2. *Makes time for personal reflection.* Understanding information calls for individuals to spend time with it to delineate its meaning. This level of meaning calls for a higher degree of reflection and discernment when one puts the information in the context of where and how it will be used.
3. *Looks to others to explain data that is difficult to understand or can only be comprehended through a different frame of reference.* Whenever there is information that is unclear, complex, or beyond easy understanding, the leader goes to those who can clarify and develop understanding in order to assure that the information always remains useful.
4. *Always asks how useful information is.* Getting information is not as important as having the right information and making use of it. As mentioned previously, sifting through information in order to find the riches that it provides requires that priorities be set with regard to meaningful information, avoiding seeking information that is not useful in the work or cannot be used for good decision making.
5. *Never allows herself or himself to be bombarded or held hostage to all the bits of information.* There is a level of insecurity that comes with not knowing everything. One of the obligations of social interaction is often being considered with it or in the loop regarding what's going on. The temptation to be drawn into this frame of reference is significant, especially considering the need for membership, inclusion, and social intercourse. Leaders, however, are constantly aware of the difference between that which is fashionable and that which is wise. The wise leader knows what needs to be known, relates that level of knowledge to the work and action that must be undertaken and the decisions that must be made. By keeping focused on this reality, the leader fails to be sucked into superficial knowing and fashionable response.

Fear is also a major impediment to openness and availability and to learning leadership. Fear usually generates from a few major sources. It is usually a response to an anticipated threat, discomfort, pain, or death. Fear can be so mobilizing that it can cripple appropriate decision making and action. Leaders recognize that fear is a constant companion in the human experience; it cannot be completely eliminated from our consciousness. However, fear can be either a motivator or an immobilizer.

Leaders should think about how they use their time and how their use of time reflects their confidence in how they deal with their own fear of taking action. Good leaders ask consistently: How do I do my job? What values about work and self were taught during my childhood? How was I dealt with in school? How did my peers perceive me and interact with me? Is my concept of self consistent with the demands on my role and my time? Am I skillful at prioritizing? Do I feel in control of my life and my time? How do I use my time to make sure that it is most effective? Self-reflection and the ability to think about values, meaning, and purpose have an impact on the legitimate expression of the leader's role. Dealing with the personal anxieties of creating consonance between one's self-image and the expression of the leader's role is a critical process in advancing leadership effectiveness and obtaining leadership excellence. The leader who is not good at self-reflection is generally not good at leading others to make changes in their lives.

The strong leader makes self-reflection an active exercise and regularly schedules that as part of his or her leadership learning development. In this process the leader safely yet positively seeks information and support regarding skills, styles, and expression of the role. Good leaders accept the consequences of their own role and behavior, exhibiting a willingness to engage those consequences and to undertake action to compensate for whatever deficits or challenges must be addressed. Good leaders are familiar with the no-excuses approach to learning. Nothing on the leader's agenda makes it difficult or increases the anxiety of confronting learning opportunities in a way that will produce meaningful personal and collective change.

PARTICIPATION COMPETENCE

In health care, professionals must be fully involved in the decisions that affect their practice and those they serve. Participation competencies require the fostering of good communication skills and the development of purposeful behaviors that promote professional commitment and action. Professional and personal goals must emerge so the level of congruence between the action of the professional and the goals of the organization can occur. High involvement is a requisite, not an option. People rarely become involved in those things that do not provide meaning for them. Restructuring organizations, changing the workplace, redefining work, or altering standards of work all have a direct impact on professionals attempting to do the work. Undertaking any of these actions without the concerted investment of those whom they impact is not a wise strategy for leaders.

High regard for engagement and inclusion is reflected in the role of the leader who emphasizes shared decision making and deliberate involvement of others in decisions. Embracing decisions independently is no longer an option in interdisciplinary and multifocal delivery systems. Large bodies of research exist that demonstrate that engaging and including professionals in making decisions improves the quality information processes, the application of good thinking, and the effectiveness of decisions and their implementation. The ability of the leader to view power within the context of the shared relationship is a vital notion to effective decision making in today's complex work systems. Work or involvement isn't an option for decision making; it is a mechanism for effective decision making that requires good skills and excellent process. The struggle is in moving out of parental behaviors and the leadership model that is based on hierarchical structures and parental frames of reference.

Information Leaders' Problems

- Being bombarded
- Faced with internal bias
- Subject to nonobjective review
- Faced with unlinked pieces
- Subject to piecemeal presentation
- Receive selective information
- Have incomplete data

Gem

Fear is like blinders over the eyes and the mind, binding you to past insights, practices, and experiences. Fear cripples the imagination and binds the spirit such that availability to the creative and the new is lost in the darkness of immobility.

Self-Reflection

The strong leader recognizes that an important part of information management is reflection. This self-assessment should include personal biases, desires, and preferences. Looking past personal perspectives and reviewing the data within the context out of which it arises deepens the objectivity and clarity with which the leader can observe and assess the data. Critical components that should be carefully accommodated in this reflective self-assessment are:

- Personal biases
- Current mental models
- Individual needs
- Past practices
- Self-fulfilling expectations
- Wish listing
- Prescriptive deliberation

Finding Meaning

We seek to find meaning in all we do.

- Look past the work and find the reason for doing it.
- Seek the values embedded in action.
- Reflect on the purposes related to doing the work.
- Share insights with trusted others to give values a voice.
- Challenge your beliefs regularly to validate them.
- As leader, find others to explore new realities and insights.
- Review values continuously.

The Leader as Role

Leaders are simply playing a role they do not need to live every moment of their lives. However, every moment they are in the role they cannot pretend that they are not. Those they lead have a right to expect that they are leaders and will lead effectively.

Since it is a role, the leader may find time away when leadership is not expected in a place and time that is appropriate and away from work.

Interpersonal Competence

- Leadership is all about relationships.
- Leadership requires emotional balance.
- Conflict is present in all relationships.
- Communication skills are not leadership optional.
- The leader never owns others' issues nor resolves other people's problems.
- Accountability means the leader sees that defined outcomes are attained.
- Leaders have no friends among those they lead; it is not a component of the role.
- The leader keeps no secrets, in fact, favors disclosure.

Leaders have to examine their own beliefs as well as their attachment to certain behaviors and practices that may preclude equality and collaborative relationships in the workplace. Leaders must recognize that they are differentiated by role, not by position. Considering this, the leader recognizes that engagement in decisions that affect practice, work, or patient care must include those who are accountable for those activities. If high-quality outcomes are to be assured, those who do the work to achieve them must be fully invested in the decisions that affect them. Empowerment, accountability, and ownership are no longer additions to the excellent exercise of affective work. Leaders who are unable to incorporate such practices and behaviors into their own role simply cannot be successful in sustaining worker confidence and investment in advancing clinical care.

INTERPERSONAL COMPETENCE

Empowerment and participation cannot exist in practice if interpersonal facility is missing in the leader. In order to function well in the facilitating, coordinating, and integrating roles, a leader must be a masterful communicator. Interpersonal communication includes a wide array of relational and communication skills that result in constant investment and engagement and inclusion of individuals in decisions and actions that affect their work and their future.

Methods of communication and the framing of words and language are the major skills in communication and information management. Leaders are meaning makers and, thus, spend their lives translating strategies, decisions, and actions in the language of those who must live with the impact of the decisions of others. Reframing concepts and notions or reorienting language to express strategies and direction becomes a talent that the leader must develop to a high degree. This process of inclusion and relationship building is essential to the very ability of the organization to thrive. Negotiating, listening, setting others in internal compasses, reframing incorrect notions, reengaging others' principles, and translating strategy and direction into the language of practitioners are all basic skill sets of good leadership.

Facilitation and coaching skills require that the leader be able to form relationships with individuals and groups in which counseling, teaching, and mentoring is aimed at improving performance and more deeply investing the worker in the meaning and value of the work itself. Coaching and facilitating requires that the leader evaluate process rather than employee; sort through confidence, competence, and understanding to see that they are present in action; and identify and clearly enumerate performance problems as a way of developing insights into obstacles for good performance and developing tools for overcoming them.

LEADERSHIP COMPETENCE

There is no one set of activities or competencies that can fall under the rubric of leadership competence alone. Leadership competence is the sum of all the activities related to the expression of leadership covered in this chapter. Besides communication interaction, directing, discerning, dialoguing, and coaching, the leader's ability to have a technical understanding of work and its application is clearly an important corollary to the expression of leadership. While it should not be the leader's expectation to be fully technically competent in all the elements of practice, or even of his or her discipline, it is important to be aware of the technical specifics that impact work. Staff have a tremendous appreciation for the exceptionally clinically skilled leader who not only expresses the role of the leader with great insight but can do it well within the context of the work expectations of clinical practice. This is a critical element of understanding what facilitates the positive impact of the leader's role.

Perhaps at the core of working with others are skills that relate to building and maintaining meaningful relationships and sustaining those relationships around the demands of work. Interdependence is a critical notion for successful leadership. Recognizing that all clinical activity is relationship dependent and fundamentally collaborative in nature, the leader ensures that such behaviors are consistently present. Leaders cannot avoid conflict (see Chapter 3). Relationship management and the intersections and interactions between individuals and disciplines are the critical centerpieces of all clinical activity. Leaders continually facilitate these intersections and broaden the frame of reference of those at the intersections. Bringing purpose, strategy, objectives, and a directional frame of reference to the work of staff helps connect staff to the broader journey of meeting the healthcare needs of the community. By doing this the leader maintains a meaning focus in the work of practitioners and makes that work congruent with the purposes of the health system.

Ultimately, from a systems perspective, the leader must continually integrate, facilitate, and coordinate between individuals and systems, seeking the highest level of convergence between making sure that the system supports the work of the individual and that the work of the individual fulfills the obligations of the system. All the support infrastructures, relationships, work processes, and clinical interactions must converge around the point of care in order to make sure that every effort interfaces in a way that meaningfully affects the delivery of patient care. It is there that good clinical leadership finds its fulfillment.

Facilitation Skills

1. Right people; right decisions
2. Good group-dynamic skills
3. Strong intuition regarding others' needs
4. Examines skill contribution of team
5. Mentoring and coordinating skills
6. Favors no personal relationship
7. Models behaviors expected in others
8. Defines expected behaviors in advance
9. Establishes group goals that are congruent with organization
10. Behaviors congruent with expectations

Quantum Leader Competence

- Technical proficiency in discipline
- Role understanding re: expectation
- Communication ability
- Discernment of direction
- Dialogue skill sets
- Coaching method and process
- Goal orientation
- Fiscal and goal congruence
- Systems facility and utility

Leading from the Quantum Intersect

- Integration of the disciplines
- Group problem solving
- Coordination of teams
- Integration of service
- Negotiating service boundaries
- Mediating normative stressors
- Generational integration
- Goals achievement/evaluation
- Facilitation of direction
- Integrating conflicting demands
- Continuous change management

REFERENCES

Kuhn, T. (1996). The structure of scientific revolutions. Chicago: University of Chicago Press.

SUGGESTED READINGS

Austin, D.M. (2002). *Human services management: Organizational leadership in social work practice.* New York: Columbia University Press.

Avolio, B.J., & Yammarino, F.J. (2002). *Transformational and charismatic leadership: The road ahead (Monographs in leadership and management).* Boston: JAI Press.

Bhal, K.T., & Ansari, M.A. (2000). *Managing dyadic interactions in organizational leadership.* Thousand Oaks, CA: Sage Publications.

Bryner, A., & Markova, D. (1996). *An unused intelligence: Physical thinking for 21st-century leadership.* Berkeley, CA: Conari Press.

Fairholm, G.W. (1993). *Organizational power politics: Tactics in organizational leadership.* Westport, CT: Praeger.

Henry, C.R. (1996). *A general reflects on leadership and management: Reorganizing, consolidating, downsizing.* Columbus, OH: Battelle Press.

Laub, J.A. (1999). *Assessing the servant organization: Development of the servant organizational leadership assessment (SOLA) instrument.*

Morrison, K. (2007). *Complexity leadership.* Charlotte, NC: Information Age Publishing.

Murensky, C.L. (2002). *The relationships between emotional intelligence, personality, critical thinking ability and organizational leadership performance at upper levels of management.*

Porter, L.W., Angle, H.L., & Allen, R.W. (2003). *Organizational influence processes.* Armonk, NY: M.E. Sharpe.

Romig, D.A. (2001). *Side by side leadership: Achieving outstanding results together.* Austin, TX: Bard Press.

Sagini, M.M. (2001). *Organizational behavior: The challenges of the new millennium.* Lanham, MD: University Press of America.

Stacey, R. (2007). *Complexity and the experience of leading organizations.* New York: Routledge.

Thompson, C.M. (2000). *The congruent life: Following the inward path to fulfilling work and inspired leadership.* San Francisco: Jossey-Bass.

Zaccaro, S.J., & Klimoski, R.J. (2001). *The nature of organizational leadership: Understanding the performance imperatives confronting today's leaders.* San Francisco: Jossey-Bass.Kuhn

APPENDIX

New Age Mythbusting

There are many who do not believe that the new age is here or that it is any different from any other time in history. In fact, there are those who would suggest that everything is simply a continuum of what has already occurred and that there are no real revolutionary elements that occur in the historical journey. Some even suggest that there is nothing new under the sun and that we have already experienced all there is to experience.

Of course, nothing could be further from the truth. The digital age has created a new level of reality, if not actually altered it forever. It is important for the leader to be able to perceive the drama of the changes confronting all of us and to engage its meaning and translate its application. But first, the leader must raise and confront the right questions about the myths and reticence before others will be willing to engage the transformation in their own lives.

Myth 1: There is no change!

Leader questions:

What is it that is not changing?

How is your work different from what it was 10 years, 1 year, or 3 months ago?

How would you describe the world differently from your parents when they were your age?

What is different about work today from it was 100, 60, 30, or 10 years ago?

Myth 2: Everything goes full circle and we end up doing it all over again, just like the last time!

Leader questions:

What exactly is it that we are doing that is the same as the last time?

Are the circumstances and conditions exactly the same as the last time, and will the response to them really be exactly the same?

How will we respond differently this time that will make the application of what we have already experienced unique to the time yet appropriate to the change?

Myth 3: I don't have to change!

Leader questions:

Can you remember what you looked like when you were 4 years old, 14, 24, 34, etc.? Do you look the same now?

Have you watched your children age, grow, change, and/or become adults? Are you exempt from that same process?

Work always changes; how do you change with it to continue to be relevant or valuable?

Myth 4: I dream of the good old days!

Leader questions:

Which one?

Are you willing to live without what wasn't available to you in the good old days?

Can you accept the bad as well as the good of the good old days?

Is it possible for you to visualize what things were really like in the good old days and place yourself in the midst of them? Describe everything those days represent.

Myth 5: Our quality of life is in decline!

Leader questions:

How is your quality of life less than what it was 50, 30, or 10 years ago?

Name the conveniences you have now that you didn't have 30, 20, or 10 years ago.

Name at least two medical treatments available today that weren't available 10 years ago.

What would you be willing to give up in your life that allows you to live better and more comfortably, if you went back 30, 40, or 50 years?

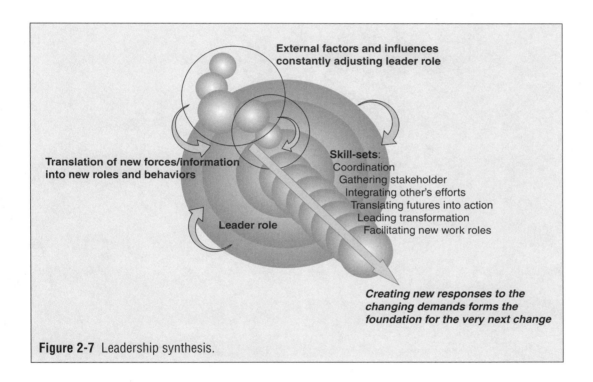

Figure 2-7 Leadership synthesis.

CHAPTER 3

Quantum Leadership: Effective Conflict

CHAPTER OBJECTIVES:

Upon completion of this chapter, the reader will:

1. Define the elements of conflict and the applications of each element to the work of leadership.
2. Outline the elements of response the leader must make to adequately address the components of conflict.
3. Develop the leadership role in normative conflict management by developing conflict processes as a tool for effectively managing differences.
4. Construct a program or approach to normative human conflict that is ongoing and operates as a fundamental part of conducting the business of providing health care.

INTRODUCTION

In making conflict normative, the leader creates a frame for conflict that turns it from an event to a process. The more conflict is looked at as a normal occurrence, one that reflects the usual vagaries of human interaction, the more likely it can be handled appropriately. This notion of normative conflict is a relatively recent understanding of the role conflict plays in organizational dynamics. Good leaders recognize that the tensions associated with normative human conflict simply represent the usual and ordinary differences that exist between people at all levels of the human community. Conflict itself is never a problem. However, *unresolved* conflict continues on a growth trajectory that becomes increasingly problematic to the extent that it is ignored or unaddressed. The wise leader, therefore, never ignores conflict; in fact, he or she searches for it in the human community and, always finding it, addresses it in an appropriate and timely fashion.

CREATING A CONFLICT-FRIENDLY CULTURE

The good leader recognizes that conflict cannot be avoided. In fact, this leader does everything not to avoid conflict. What the leader does is create an environment that provides a safe space for identifying and expressing conflicts. This leader recognizes

---

Gem

The best way to avoid conflict is to create a culture where conflict is accepted as a part of the way of interacting with each other.

Addressing Potential for Conflict

In this stage, leaders are required to:

- Develop their intuition and use conflict-resolving processes
- Keep an eye on what's going on
- Listen to staff clues of conflict
- Note the differences that are causing "noise"
- Remember always that the leader does not own the conflict
- Create an atmosphere of trust
- Remember that diversity is essential to all good dialogue
- Ensure that communication is open and honest

Intuitive Sense of Potential for Conflict

- Awareness of individual needs
- Sensing shifts in communication levels
- Notation of personality differences
- Noticing clique formation
- Seeing whispered conversations
- Hearing sarcastic comments
- Observing change in relationships
- Watching increased negativism
- Detecting decrease in satisfaction

---

that conflict management is the one fundamental obligation that he or she has in the leadership role. Knowing that conflict cannot be avoided, the leader makes it comfortable and safe to engage conflict at any stage. More importantly, this leader recognizes that opening the staff to the noise, ambiguity, and challenge of expressing differences creates a special milieu, which, in turn, can often be demanding for the leader to manage.

Good leaders are responsible for creating a positive context for work. Leaders are continually attempting to provide a framework for work that is positive, encouraging, and growth oriented. A good part of creating this context is building the kinds of relationships that evidence partnership, openness, and trust.

When conflict is considered a regular part of the manager's responsibilities, confronting it directly becomes a part of expressing the manager's role. The manager must begin to recognize that fear of confrontation is a significant impediment to resolving interpersonal and relationship-based conflicts.

The best time to address conflict is early in its expression. Seeing a conflict situation emerge is a forewarning that it is likely to blossom. The manager needs to know that conflict does not go away of its own volition. Since it is normal for almost all human interactions, conflict simply changes its form and emerges somewhere else or in some other kind of "wolf's clothing."

The longer conflict simmers, the more difficult it is to resolve. Conflict is not a static process that just sits there, failing to gather energy. On the contrary, it is not uncommon to watch unresolved conflict grow in intensity as it lies just below the surface collecting energy and building toward a cataclysmic eruption. Unresolved conflict always intensifies.

The good leader has an intuitive sense of the potential for conflict. This person knows that every interaction is rife with the seeds for conflict. Human differences drive its unfolding. If not recognized early, the conflict continues to gather potential and to grow in possibility until its expression becomes likely. The leader wants to do two things in the presence of the potential for conflict: address it early and address it appropriately.

SKILLS FOR ISOLATING CONFLICT

Leaders need to recognize that early engagement of conflict means recognizing it soon enough to address it without "noise" and/or overwhelming personal emotion. In the earliest moments of an interpersonal conflict, the beginning signs of the impending conflict are always present. An attitude of disrespect, an unkind word from one person to another, an offhand remark, or an inappropriate phrase can be early signs of the gathering storm of a conflict. The leader lets no remark or behavior that represents anger, misunderstanding, or personal apprehension go unaddressed. Each of these emotions is an indicator of an underlying set of concerns that begs to be addressed. Interrupting the course of a conflict in these early stages gets the real issues out in the open and raises the chance that addressing them will allay further opportunity for the conflict to accelerate.

In the earliest stages of conflict, the leader is constantly looking for people creating positions and taking sides. Indeed, in the earliest stages, the conflict-driven individual creates boundaries and limits to a view or position as a way of emphasizing the differences and becomes exclusionary or exclusive to perceptions or notions that represent the chosen position. Ownership and expression of the position and extreme defense of it create the initial conditions and circumstances upon which further conflict can build.

From constant awareness to listening carefully to the content of the conflict, the leader prepares to mediate the conflict in the right manner. It is important for the leader to be able to identify the key elements of the impending conflict situation. What most often appears in the conflict is usually the signpost that the real issues lie somewhere more deeply buried. The leader may need to dig further to find the critical source for the conflict. Often conflict language represents feelings, not circumstances. Feelings generally either get in the way of the truth or actually mask it.

The leader may need to go through the feelings in order to get to the underlying issues in order to really resolve conflict situations. There are trigger remarks that are indicative of intensity of feeling and perception that the leader will need to sort through. Often the leader will first hear the following feeling responses:

"She always does this to me."
"He is forever dumping on me."
"She never stops criticizing me."
"He makes me so angry."
"She makes me just want to scream."
"He swears at me all the time."

These comments are filled with reactive emotion. They represent feelings of anger and even helplessness. Sometimes they are accompanied by behaviors; sometimes they are merely expressive of feeling. Either way, they are powerful indicators of impending and irresolvable conflict.

Not all conflict can be addressed by the leader on the spot. Work requirements may mean that the conflict expression temporarily goes in the "parking lot" of response until it can be more reasonably addressed. Even so, if the leader hears the comments from the aggressor or from the offended individual, it is important that a response be identified regarding follow-up action. Short yet key responses to the individual(s) from the leader are advisable.

To the aggressor:

"I'm concerned about what I just heard; I'll need to talk with you about it after we finish this task (work, procedure, meeting, etc.)"

Or

"I hear what you're saying and I think we need to talk about it after we are done here."

Or

"I am very unclear about what you are saying and I think we need to talk about it right after we're done here."

The leader might respond to the offended person:

"I need to know more; let's talk when we're done here."

Or

"I'm concerned about how you're feeling right now. Let's talk when this task (meeting, procedure, work, etc.) is finished."

You'll note that the leader does not yet address the two (or more) individuals quite yet. There needs to be more clarity built around the conflict before any purposeful resolution occurs. Getting the facts and feelings straight from the outset will be a critical element in the resolution process. Perhaps the most important aspect of getting conflict straight is found in correctly gathering the right information. The good leader pays attention not only to what is said but also to what is felt. Getting to what is said is always best obtained by going through the individual's feelings first, so that those feelings have a route of expression, clear content, and the individual has an opportunity to be heard early in the process. Too often, leaders try to resolve the conflict early on, hoping that by doing so they

---

Isolating Conflict

The following indicate the potential for conflict:

- Anticipating differences
- Change in language
- Change in feelings
- New processes
- New employee
- Shifting priorities
- Critical event(s)
- Personality clashes
- New work demands
- Loss(es)

Creating a Trusting Context

Always keep an ear out for these emotional trigger words—they are telling the leader that conflict is emerging and feelings are growing more intense!

Gem

The leader is aware that conflict is always present regardless of the lack of evidence of its action. Anticipating the action of conflict is central to the role of good leadership. The leader never forgets the continuous and inevitable role of conflict in all human interaction.

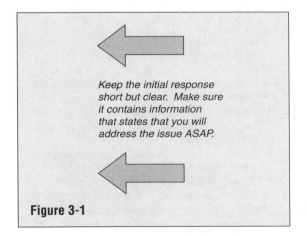

Keep the initial response short but clear. Make sure it contains information that states that you will address the issue ASAP.

Figure 3-1

Gem

Unresolved conflict always gathers energy and continues to grow in intensity. Always!

Gem

Do not resolve conflict too early in the process. If you fail to manage all the essential steps, the conflict will strike back later in a way, a time, and a place you never expected.

The Price of Distrust

- Untenable noise
- Lack of involvement
- Crisis in confidence
- Noncommunication
- Personal isolation
- Errors in practice
- No team consciousness
- No loyalty
- Limited accountability

Addressing Interpersonal Alienation

- Make sure expectations regarding communications are precise and clear.
- Include communication effectiveness as a part of the competency-based performance requirements.
- Make all staff accountable for communication and interaction problems between any staff members.
- Keep the team focused on its contributions and the individuals' value to the team.
- Do not let personal behaviors, agendas, and values impede staff members' ability to interact and communicate effectively.
- Address isolation and alienation behaviors immediately.

---

can short-circuit the conflict and keep it from escalating. As a result, leaders often fail to address strongly felt personal feelings that, if left unaddressed, ultimately affect the sustainability of conflict resolution.

CREATING A TRUSTING CONTEXT

Building a great conflict resolution process is the one thing that assures conflict is minimized. In health care, focusing on the patient requires a strong trusting relationship between and among all staff members. Staff members who work in an atmosphere of distrust do not collaborate or integrate with each other in providing care and reaching organizational goals. In the presence of rapid change, a level of distrust and uncertainty can quickly and easily emerge.

The willingness and ability the leader can gather to assure staff commitment, energy, and mutuality clearly affects the quality of staff members' work. There are specific behaviors that break trust between people and can create a milieu rife with conflict.

Unfair Procedures and Processes

Any time staff perceives that work rules are unfair or inappropriately applied, elements of mistrust emerge. In these circumstances, staff began to feel that their opportunity in providing input and making a contribution to the work is limited. This begins to interfere with their ability to communicate and interact confidently with each other. When the leader has her or his own agenda or undertakes individual action processes out of context with the rules of the organization, elements of mistrust emerge. Consistency, fairness, equal application of the rules, and open communication help maintain an environment of trust that encourages the staff to ask questions, approach the undiscussables, and explore difficult issues together.

Not Communicating Fully

When all staff members can openly communicate and share information interactively, they create a spirit of inquiry and open information sharing. In this way, all members have an opportunity to obtain and make use of all the information necessary to work well and to achieve meaningful outcomes. These behaviors actually facilitate trust and build a foundation for expanding trust between and among team members.

The leader must always be alert to the cues that indicate that openness in relationship and communication is not operating effectively between and among staff members. Some signs are:

1. Silent response to a statement or question
2. Nodding with no actual verbal acknowledgment
3. Labeling staff members as "non-team players"
4. Language games and jargon
5. Staff members disappearing in the presence of other staff members or the leader

These behavioral indicators tell the leader that trust is lacking between and among staff members and that further addressing of the environment of communication is required to adequately maintain effective communication and interaction.

Allowing Alienation Between Individuals

Relationships between and among staff members are important to their ability to work together effectively over the long term. Any problem or struggle in the relationship eventually breaks down the whole team's ability to communicate and work together. The leader wants to address any issues of discomfort, relationship problems, and ineffective communication as quickly as possible. As with all conflict, issues will grow into major problems fairly quickly. Emotional challenges that exist between individuals also reduce each person's opportunity to develop the trust they will need to effectively undertake their work.

Misguided Focus of Staff

Staff members have their own assumptions about what should be accomplished and how the work should be done. With professional staff, the notion of individual intent and professional self-direction often predominates. This may cause the individual staff to undertake action independently or individually in a way that is not appropriate or in the best interests of the organization and those it serves.

The leader must recognize this issue early in the staff behavior pattern. Unilateral and individual performance expectations or actions that are not in concert with standards or team expectations can create great interpersonal noise in the organization. The leader must be able to clearly recognize the individual professional staff members' need for self-direction and decision making, yet provide a context within which those decisions can be deemed appropriate and valid. Addressing these issues in advance of performance by using clear protocols, policies, and practices helps provide clear and effective parameters for individuals, which helps identify the boundaries of performance and individual behavior.

> **Creating a Trusting Context: Addressing Staff Misguided Focus**
>
> 1. Watch individual practice, making sure it is consistent with standards.
> 2. Listen to other staff members' complaints about an individual's performance.
> 3. Make sure protocols, policies, and practices are clear.
> 4. Identify limits and boundaries to practice or work.
> 5. Assure a model for mentoring and precepting is available to new staff.
> 6. Identify models and mentors for practice and relationship behavior.
> 7. Support staff who question and challenge practices and protocols and explore options to questionable practices and processes.

Eliminating Superior–Subordinating Behaviors

Health care is rife with historical hierarchical structures, roles, and relationships. These traditional practices have unfolded over a long period of time in health care and have created conditions and circumstances that result in master–servant relationships, behaviors, and patterns of interaction. Because control is such an integral element of hierarchical relationships, certain individuals reflect a higher level of need for control and controlling behaviors. Other staff members are more passive and are therefore more easily managed and controlled by others. In either case, the behaviors are inappropriate in any effective professional environment. Quantum leadership is about building relationships and intersections and establishing the patterns of communication and response that reflect the nature of these relationships.

It is important for the leader to ensure that these behaviors are not represented in her or his own leadership. The leader must be careful to remove maternalism/paternalism within the leader's own specific pattern of behavior. The leader must clearly articulate in personal behavior a pattern of partnership, collegiality, and professionalism. Through representing this pattern of behavior, this leader creates a milieu and a set of expectations with regard to the partnering behaviors asked of the staff. Eliminating old hierarchical behaviors is extremely challenging in an environment that has historically valued and embraced them. For the leader, it will always be a work in progress, exemplified by her or his own personal behavior and relationship with the staff.

> **Eliminating Superior–Subordinate Relationships**
>
> - Reduce or eliminate as much hierarchy as possible.
> - Emphasize partnership in communication and decision making.
> - Clarify expectations with regard to professional behavior.
> - Reduce and ultimately eliminate parentalism and leader behaviors.
> - Help staff develop increasing collateral interdependence in both decisions and professional actions.

Eliminating Word Games

Language is critical to the effectiveness of organizations. It is the means within which understanding is obtained, communication is advanced, and action is taken. Precision and clarity in the expression of language, especially in a professional environment, is essential to maintaining the value of the work. Often, however, in the work environment, language and words are not as deeply valued as they need to be. The careless use of language can lead to misunderstanding, errors, and missed opportunities for relationship building and team accomplishment.

Sometimes, purposeful distortions and misuse of the language can be undertaken by staff, and even leaders, ultimately distorting meaning. Using doublespeak as a means of deliberately clouding the message; jargon to indicate a unique or special use of the language; or complex, refined, and manipulative use of words can operate in an individual's best interests and significantly affect others' understanding and action. Language games are the most frequent tools used by those who have need for control or wish to express their own personal agendas at the expense of the relationship with their colleagues in the organization. The leader must address these activities as soon as they appear so that their legitimacy never gets initially established.

> **Managing Word Games**
>
> - Make effective communication a clear expectation of team relationships.
> - Create a continuing dialogue around clear and effective communication.
> - Directly and immediately confront individuals who frequently use language as a weapon or personal tool.
> - Help staff develop techniques of validation using clear and effective communication.
> - Clarify meaning in all questionable communication or information that is ambiguous or unclear.

> **Gem**
>
> Either locating or laying blame has absolutely no value in the action of problem solving. Undertaking blame-based processes always guarantees that staff will avoid confronting legitimate issues and problems with an attitude open to obtaining meaningful solutions and sustainable problem resolution.

Eliminating Blame

The presence of blame is always an indicator of the lack of accountability and the clarity necessary for responsibility to be ascertained and appropriately expressed. Blame is always a sign of ineffective valuing of contributions and roles in the organization. Furthermore, it is an indicator of the lack of accountability embedded in the organization's values. Locating blame rarely leads to or sustains effective problem-solving processes. In the presence of blame, individuals flee from problem identification, solution seeking, and corrective action. The good leader recognizes there is no value in blame and works diligently to remove blame strategies from the organization's patterns of working behavior. Here again, the leader eliminates blame-based activities and responses as quickly as he or she sees them.

THE VALUE OF EFFECTIVE LISTENING

Listening is a fundamental and essential tool of good leadership and conflict management. The listening demeanor, which essentially encapsulates the leadership role in active listening, is one of the most effective leadership devices to incorporate as a conflict skill set. However, listening is frequently more difficult than most leaders realize.

Rather than a passive function, listening is actually an active process. It is a discipline. Listening requires a level of openness and awareness that is critical to effective communication. Most people treat listening as a passive exercise, more receptive than active. Effective listening is reflected in the ability to take in the full expression of communication that comes from another individual, recognizing that listening has a visual as well as aural capacity. The active listener is constantly screening the full expression of communication. Looking at gestures, body language, verbal cues, and intensity and method of expression is all part of effective listening. Managing conflict is, perhaps, more precisely specified in this facility for effective and active listening.

Often the single greatest problem with regard to listening is also its simplest—most people simply don't want to listen. Talking is often perceived as a much better experience than listening. However, the

> **Effective Listening Tips**
>
> - Keep focused on the facts.
> - Look for both the meaning and the feeling of the words you're hearing.
> - Inhibit your desire to immediately respond.
> - Clarify quickly when you don't understand.
> - Don't allow eyes to wander; stay focused on the subject.
> - Lean into the conversation; body language is important.
> - Make no judgments, just listen.
> - Take notes if you find it helpful.

good listener plays a much more powerful role in the management of information and the circumstances of communication.

The leader should be listening at least 50% of the active time in a leadership role. While this is a minimum, it does give the leader an opportunity to evaluate the degree of listening that she or he brings to the role. There are some measures that can help with delineating awareness related to the leader's level of listening effectiveness, including:

- *Note your interruption quotient.* Frequent interruptions are an indicator that effective listening is not occurring. Usually high-level interrupters are more interested in what they have to say than to what they have to hear. Assessing and measuring the interruption level or intensity in the individual leader's self-expression can be a clear indicator of listening effectiveness.
- *Ask others about your own listening skills.* The good leader will ask someone he or she trusts about specific personal listening skills. It is important that the leader be specific when asking about listening skills. It might even be wise for the leader to ask a friend to call or watch the leader listen and to make evaluative comments related to the style of the leader's listening and suggest improvements or changes that could occur in the personal listening style.
- *Develop self-awareness regarding your listening process.* Periodically the leader should undertake a self-assessment regarding the listening approach. Self-monitoring body language, level of understanding, awareness of the other person's style of communication, and the ability to effectively condense and articulate what is being heard are all tools to help the leader assess listening skills. In this process, it is often helpful for the leader to ask the person communicating for information about her or his own assessment of the leader's presence, awareness, and responses to the individual's effectiveness of communication.

There are a number of listening mechanisms that, when left unexamined, create some real problems in assuring communication effectiveness (Kossgard, Schweiger, & Sappienze, 1995). The leader must examine these challenges to communication in her or his own behavior and also the behavior of staff. Effective listening communication behaviors are simply the first line of defense in managing conflict effectively. The following should be red flags:

- Clearly not wanting to hear what someone is sharing and actively defending oneself against what one is hearing can impede the availability to and willingness to listen effectively.
- The method of communicating that one is listening to may be personally irritating or uncomfortable. This generates a desire to be nonresponsive and not present to the message or the messenger.
- Feelings of being overwhelmed and tired can make the listener not available to the message. Increased levels of response or energy may not be readily available in a particular moment of communication.
- Anticipating one's own answers while listening to the message is a great impediment to effective communication and listening. Getting ready to give an answer before listening completely is one of the most frequent barriers to effective listening.
- Past practice or past habits of listening that have been unaddressed for a long period of time (past listening rituals) can be one of the great barriers to developing healthier, more effective mechanisms for listening.

Quantum Tip

Like most things in life, timing is important when effective listening is required. Make sure that important messages are not delivered in the midst of chaos or intense business. Find a place that is quiet enough to enable concentration and conversation.

Barriers to Effective Listening

- External stimuli like sound, light, people who interrupt with their opinions, mannerisms, inflections, and movement
- Mind-sets, the listeners' emotional and mental characteristics, and responses
- Unclear language, ambiguity, and misinterpretation contributing to level of understanding
- Feedback elements such as premature responses or comments, early listener evaluation, feeling responses (resentment, defensiveness, suspicion, etc.)

Good Listening

1. Stop talking—listen.
2. Put the communicator at ease.
3. Make sure you want to hear the message.
4. Limit distractions.
5. Focus on the other person.
6. Patiently hear.
7. Assess your emotions.
8. Don't judge.
9. Ask questions for clarity.
10. Count to 3 before you respond.

Listening

Donna is trying to let Marie know that she is going to need some help in understanding her patient's diagnosis. She has been attempting to explain her understanding to Donna at the nurses' desk. While Donna is talking, Marie has been doing her charting, answering a call bell, sending off a lab request, and checking a medication request. Marie has been shaking her head as Donna speaks, but keeps on with her activities.

1. How do you feel about Marie's listening posture?
2. Is Donna's message likely getting through to Marie?
3. What is a better approach to Donna and Marie's interaction?

Conflict and Listening

- Seek to clearly understand.
- Clarify for a real meaning.
- Look for the deeper message.
- Always listen between the lines.
- Listen from your heart as well as your head.
- Distinguish between facts and feelings.
- Empathize, not sympathize.
- Make sure your listening is goal directed.
- Remember, conflict involves more than one person; listen to all messages.

Note Taking in Active Listening

- Assess intensity or emotions in the situation.
- Keep notes short and point based.
- Reflect back to the individual what you have written.
- Review notes taken between parties to validate critical points.

- Preconceived notions about what is being heard or about the person communicating can limit availability to hearing what is really being said. Judgments made about the person can impede the value of his or her message.
- Diminishing the value of the messenger can often limit how one listens and how much one hears. Devaluing the communicator always diminishes the value of that person's message.

Conflict resolution is embedded in the ability to really hear and understand the messages that underlie any element of conflict. In order to respond well, the manager dealing with conflict must be able to hear and understand a multitude of messages that indicate the underlying issues or concerns between and among people. Being available to others, open to their needs, positioned carefully to hear what it is they have to say, and clear that the messages heard are important considerations in effective conflict management.

Body language and perceptive availability are critical elements and signs of readiness to listen. Paying attention to whether arms are crossed or relaxed; whether posture is slouched or the listener is sitting up straight or leaning into the conversation, facing the speaker directly and closely; and whether the listener is making continuous and focused eye contact are all indicators to the communicator as to whether the listener is fully available and listening to the message.

Some leaders who are active listeners always carry a small notebook in their pocket for such purposes. These people recognize that not everything that is said can be heard and remembered over time. While the context of the conversation and the needs of the communicator must be taken into consideration when taking notes, note taking is a valid way of exemplifying your presence and your willingness to hear. Simply because note taking does not occur frequently enough reduces others' perceptions and expectations that it is either permissible or viable. The leader makes it clear and safe for listener and communicator to use whatever mechanisms better assure that communication has been properly heard and noted.

It is appropriate for the listener to consciously and infrequently ask questions to clarify the content of the message. The infrequency and precision of questions is a clear indicator of whether the mechanism is successful in expanding and validating what is being communicated. It also serves as an exemplar with regard to the level of intensity of listening and of clarifying what is being heard. Rather than asking open-ended questions, the leader should be precise and specific, using questioning as a way of clarifying and understanding the specifics of the message. As always, questioning joins with awareness, presence, focus, availability, body language, and openness as the foundation and framework for effective listening. Without having refined the tool of effective listening to a high degree, the ability to undertake meaningful conflict resolution is measurably limited.

IDENTIFYING THE CYCLE OF CONFLICT

Like any other human dynamic, conflict has content, particular elements, and specific processes. Kinds of conflict generally fall into relationship-based, value-based, structural-based, data-based, and interest-based categories (Moore, 1996). Each one has its own characteristics and elements that mark it as unique. The leader becomes skilled at identifying the kinds and characteristics of conflict being dealt with and the responses that best address them.

Since the leader is always looking for specific conflicts, it is wise to become skilled in identifying the particular characteristics of conflict that most often appear within the culture of the service or department. Each setting is unique with regard to the makeup of the staff and the stressors on them and the work that they do. The good leader makes a conflict potential assessment as a part of delineating which strategies are going to be most helpful in dealing with conflict. In this assessment, the leader is attempting to get a handle on those specific potentials for conflict that will most often be a concern in the ordinary management of the service.

The leader looks at the makeup of the staff, the demographics (both cultural and age related), the breadth of the work, and the skill level of the staff. Embedded within these factors is the potential for specific kinds of conflict that may recur. In this manner, the leader makes the potential for conflict a normal and usual part of her or his organizational and resource planning. This leader knows that the greater the awareness of the circumstances and characteristics of conflict, the earlier it can be addressed appropriately.

Relationship-Based Conflicts

In any work environment, there are a number of personalities and situations whose vagaries create conditions that can lead to conflict. Differences between people always provide a source for a variety of relationship-driven crises or conflicts. Differences in personality create problems in interaction and communication and often lead to misunderstandings. These differences can frequently lead to specific altercations reflecting emotional involvement and personal animosity. Left unaddressed, these differences can escalate and create real polarization between the involved parties and those who relate to them. Relationship conflict is the most frequently experienced conflict in most organizations. Communication irregularities emerge and miscommunication becomes common. Negative behavior becomes repetitive and, if not resolved, becomes a way to sabotage and offend the opposing party, which can affect the work, workers, and those they serve.

The good leader recognizes the potential for this conflict early in the process. Usually unkind words, snide comments, asides, negative comments to others, and avoiding behaviors are the early signs that a relational conflict is present. Since the leader always expects some level of conflict to exist, she or he is able to see these signs and begin to take action right away.

The leader will first want to get at the originating source for the conflict. Confronting both parties separately with regard to the behaviors expressed is the critical path to getting at the root problem underlying the behaviors. Beginning the questioning with an open-ended approach is best. The leader might say one of the following:

I'm noticing that . . .
Can you tell me . . .
I'm wondering if I'm seeing . . .
Help me if I'm perceiving this right . . .

At this stage, the leader is just trying to get a level of understanding about the existence of a problem and the basic perceptions of what the problem might be through the words of each party. Through this process, the leader is simply validating whether a problem exists and the underlying nature of the concern. The leader is also ascertaining the degree of perceptive agreement that exists between the parties regarding their issues.

Cycle of Positive Conflict Process

1. Underlying issues exist in the person or his or her values.
2. Differences emerge between persons.
3. Differences are manifested in behavior.
4. Conflict emerges and escalates.
5. Conflict affects relationships or processes.
6. The need to address conflict arises.
7. The conflict is mediated.
8. Solutions are explored.
9. New directions or patterns are established.
10. Evaluation indicates change effectiveness and indication of next steps or further actions.

Assessing for Conflict

- Define cultural and age demographics of staff.
- Determine level of work intensity.
- Look at range of staff skills.
- Review staff longevity.
- Assess amount and rate of changes occurring in the service or department.

Look for Early Signs of Conflict

To identify the potential for conflict, look for:

- Negative behavior
- Secret conversations
- Exclusion from groups
- Whispering
- Open fighting
- Snide comments
- Sarcasm
- Strong language
- Changed body language

Look for How People Are Expressing Emotions and Feelings

Important emotions to look for:

- Passive feelings
- Crying
- Anger
- Fear
- Threats
- Silence
- Sarcasm
- Physical tension
- Running away

Rules of Engagement

- Open dialogue
- *I* statements only
- Ownership of own feelings
- Openness to differences
- Hearing the other
- Continued presence
- Truthfulness
- Equity in relationships

The leader initially responds to emotions and feelings. It is impossible to get at the problem without first going through the emotional content of each party's issues. In relationship conflict, the parties are reacting to their own feelings and impressions of what has happened to them and how they are feeling about it, rather than to the real issue that may be the causative factor. If the leader tries to get to the causative issues too soon, the parties may block and refuse to move there since they have not had an appropriate opportunity to work through the emotional content related to the issue.

Sometimes the leader might need to carefully move individuals through their feelings by validating and supporting the person while clarifying the underlying issues along the way. The leader attempts to get the individual to a more reality-oriented place from which some rational work might be done as the individual moves through the conflict. At some point, the parties must be in the same place in order to move the conflict closer to resolution. The leader attempts to prepare each to understand where both individuals are in relation to feelings and content. The leader, acting as a neutral, will seek to have each party express his or her feelings with a language that accurately expresses feelings without further polarization, energizing a new level of emotional intensity.

As the process moves toward engagement, the leader seeks to focus on expression and rules of engagement as well as to remind each party of the expectations regarding communication and conflict management in the service or the department. Having created an appropriate milieu for conflict management, the leader wants to ensure that the parties are aware of the expectations and of the need to resolve issues that impede the ability of the staff to communicate and deal with differences. The leader identifies the conflict resolution process as one of the mechanisms that exemplify the components of communication within which the unit operates. It is only at this point that the leader begins to bring the parties together to a dialogue and to work through their differences.

Values-Based Conflicts

Perhaps one of the most difficult classes of conflict to resolve is one that represents differences in values. Every person brings different experiences and beliefs to the expression of their human journey. Cultural, social, religious, moral, and personal values are all part of what defines an individual. In a multicultural society such as that reflected in the American experience, cultural and personal differences are a common experience. Yet with the richness of these differences comes the inevitable conflicts that arise when individual values come in conflict with the values of others.

Creating a Culture of Acceptance

- Evidence of fairness
- Ownership of feelings
- A level playing field
- No favoritism
- Balanced exchange of views
- Safe place for expressing feelings
- Good conflict processes
- Focus on solution seeking

The leader creates a culture of acceptance and openness to differences and to the vagaries of response they reflect. In anticipation of the potential for conflict, the leader sees to it that cultural and value awareness is inculcated into the educational and developmental activities of the service. Everyone should be expected to participate in activities that teach them about the value and practice of acceptance and about the behaviors that are forbidden between and among different ethnic, cultural, national, and religious groups.

Because values-based conflict is so difficult to resolve late in the cycle of conflict management, it is wise to confront it at the earliest possible moment. A breach in the code of conduct or expectations of behavior should be addressed as soon as it happens. The absolute unacceptability of such patterns of behavior should be clear to everyone at the outset. Refusal to conform one's personal behavior to these rules of good relationship should be grounds for the strongest disciplinary action.

Ethnic irregularities have no room for dialogue or debate. Any discrimination based on color or disparaging remarks that reflect on ethnic origins have no room for misunderstanding. In a world of many colors and ethnic backgrounds reflecting the broadest array of human beings, any conflict based on this has no room for negotiation and misunderstanding. In the human experience, there are some a priori considerations that operate beyond question. Race is one of them. The only room for conflict in this arena is where a misunderstanding or misrepresentation of one's remarks or behavior has occurred and needs clarification and restating between the parties. Cultural or language difficulties or misrepresentations can create a perception that simply may not have been intended. The process of continuous cultural and values education for staff should keep such misunderstanding to a minimum.

Religious and values differences can create significant problems. There are a number of problems that can come out of religious differences related to beliefs, practices, and accommodation. Special considerations to religious and values practices can create negative feelings in others who do not hold the same beliefs. Resentments and feelings of preference can emerge, creating conflict. Here again, being clear in advance about what the expectations are regarding the presence of staff with different practices and the impact of those on the staff relationship is a critical obligation of the leader. Adjustments required in the schedule and even assignments and role adjustments need to be clear to all staff members with attention paid to how equity is maintained between and among staff members. Achieving equity between and among staff members with different religious or values needs is challenging for the leader and the staff. Dialogue and negotiation regarding these adjustments must be delineated up front with the staff. This approach keeps the issue before the staff, makes it a part of their ongoing work experience, and creates an expectation that such accommodations are always a part of the work environment.

When accommodations to the expression of particular religious practices is especially difficult or verges on creating resentment, the leader must reanimate dialogue around the differences in light of reinvigorating acceptance and undertaking creative ways of addressing the related issues and resolving the conflicts these issues generate. If the leader has been successful in the aggressive creation of an environment of acceptance and openness, the expectation is that such problems can be dealt with and ultimately resolved.

In cases where there is intractable religious-based conflict, it is often wise for the leader to expand the dialogue and include experts from outside the service to guide the discussion and advance resolution. It is often helpful to involve pastoral assistance from representatives from the religious traditions at issue and have them help the participants find some common ground and define areas of resolution or accommodation. The leader always acts as a resource purveyor when resolution processes require an alternative mechanism for resolution.

In values-based conflicts, it is also helpful for the leader to expand the dialogue to values that can be shared by all participants. Those values that operate in the broader human context and reflect common human needs and interests can help refocus the issue to one that engages human experience, regardless of value tradition or expression. Attempting to find common areas of value (such as family, home, nation, loyalty, sentiment, children, etc.) can change the emotional and relational content of the conflict and create a common frame of reference for its resolution that might not have been originally anticipated.

Scenario

Marie, the nurse manager, is working to create an atmosphere for resolving conflict between two of her staff members. She is getting the room ready for the mediation dialogue. Marie will facilitate the mediation; she is busy thinking about the process and how to make it favorable for dialogue and solution seeking. She is a little tense about the process but realizes that her recent certification in workplace mediation will be helpful in facilitating this process. She has made the room comfortable with chairs facing each other, and she will sit in the middle seat to guide the interaction. Marie has thought about each step of the process and reminded herself not to take either party's position and to stay focused on managing the dialogue and keeping faithful to the step-by-step process of dialogue and movement to resolution.

Key elements for Marie to address include the following:
- Comfort of participants
- Peacefulness of the space
- Use of the conflict process
- Keeping the discussion focused on the issues
- Exploration of alternatives to original positions
- Expression of feelings
- Support of participants as they move through the process
- Clarification of issues and enumeration of progress
- Definition of a solution, expectations, and follow-up on actions

---

Dealing with Religious Values and Language in Conflict Situations

1. Set the language boundaries.
2. Don't allow one participant to hold others hostage to particular beliefs.
3. Focus on issues, not beliefs.
4. Stay centered on tangible issues.
5. Keep dialogue directed to how the issue will be resolved.

Dealing with Values-Based Conflicts

1. Look at the *why* and *who* issues.
2. Discuss tangible solutions that can be seen clearly by all parties.
3. Find common issues and values.
4. Link common values where they can be found.
5. Keep dialogue centered on core causes and drivers.

Finally, it is important for the leader to know that it is sometimes necessary to allow people to agree to disagree. Values are sacred to the individual who holds them; they can't easily be surrendered to others. The leader may have to get the parties to determine how they will live with their differences and make the necessary accommodations to those differences as a part of their relationship. Respect is critical to effectiveness of this process. If each can respect the position of the other, common ground can be found and progress can be made with regard to the quality of the work relationship.

Structure-Driven Conflicts

Structure-driven conflicts recognize inequities inherent in the system or structure of work. These can be classified as inadequate or unfair policies, processes, rules, behaviors, and practices, as well as contextual and organizational factors that inhibit cooperative relationships.

The leader recognizes that no workplace is free of structural and operational challenges to the ability to do work and to build relationships in the system. Differences in pay grades, benefits policies, reward systems, job and role status all contribute to perceptions of structural inequity. Even if there is a rational basis for these practices, the inherent inequity needs to be addressed as a possible source of unresolved conflict.

Gem

Everyone shares some common value with others. The good mediator is always looking for something that ties the parties' experiences together so it can help anchor further dialogue and assist in identifying common ground.

The leader recognizes that there must be openness with regard to people's specific concerns regarding any particular structural inequity. The leader acknowledges its presence and clearly enumerates the logic behind the apparent inequity. Understanding the value of implementing a particular advantage by one group in relationship to others is a valuable first step. In those places where the inequity established is sufficiently egregious, mechanisms and efforts at self-correction must address the structural element. Where such inequities can be changed or struck down in the organization, they should be, as soon as possible, with a solution that can be implemented.

There is a perceived inequity and imbalance at the professional level of a number of organizations. These perceived imbalances generally indicate that one profession or work group is preferred or treated favorably compared with another profession or work group. This perceived inequity often creates much internal conflict in the organization that may not always be directly expressed. Its hidden conflict operates as an organizational subtext or frequently lies just below the surface. In this specific set of circumstances, the leader must recognize the foundations of the perceived inequity early and clearly. If it is status inequity evidenced by differentiation and role or reward, the justifications and support for these differentiations must be clear enough to make sense to the group that feels disadvantaged. While these inequities cannot always be changed or altered, they can be understood. The role of the leader is to generate such understanding.

Confronting Imbalances

- Eliminate favoritism.
- Balance dialogue.
- Remove status barriers.
- Find a common language.
- Keep the issue centered.
- Limit unrelated dialogue.
- Call parties by their first or last names.
- Remove any status symbols.
- Reword for increased understanding.

Hidden Conflict

- Favoritism
- Class levels of employeeism
- Status barriers
- Differentiated benefits
- Professional cliques
- Management secrets
- Management control
- Exclusionary behaviors
- Extreme executive perks

Where there are more challenges in justifying the inequity and it does not appear to be legitimate or functional, the leader must support individuals in undertaking a process in which the inequity can be actively addressed and pursued further. In such circumstances, advocacy for a particular approach or solution, communication with the appropriate leadership individuals, or structural or organizational approaches to finding solutions must be determined by the stakeholders in the conflict. Without the leader advocating for a specific process for problem resolution, the structural problem will continue to frustrate and challenge the effectiveness and integrity of the work group.

Additional structural challenges that can generate conflict relate to the environmental or the architectural construct within which work unfolds. In many clinical organizations, the structures of the organizations themselves impede the effectiveness of the work. Where the structures can be altered, they should be. Where the architectural and structural elements of work cannot be altered or adjusted, mechanisms and methods for accommodation or modification must be explored by those affected by the structural impediments. In addition, continuing leadership attention and focus must be centered on addressing the structural barrier in a way that ultimately removes it. This emphasis indicates that the leader is committed to supporting the clinical work. The leader also represents in this activity an understanding that these issues are part of her or his role in continuously challenging those structural elements that do not support the clinical work of the organization. Whether the architectural modifications or structural adjustments can be undertaken is not as important as the commitment of the leader to continuous support of the staff by challenging organizational leadership to modify structural impediments as evidence of leadership's commitment to the clinical work of the organization.

> **Structural Conflict**
>
> - Inadequate architectural design
> - Bad policy requisites
> - Inadequate procedures
> - No guidance for action
> - Bad management practices
> - Poor support services
> - Inadequate communication
> - No electronic clinical record
> - Poor problem-solving processes

Interest-Based Conflicts

Conflicts that reflect an interest foundation are generally caused by a mutual commitment, yet conflicting relationship, to a shared interest. In health care, each interest-based conflict can take on the mantle of professional boundaries and turf protection. Each practice profession attempts to advance its interests in undertaking the work of patient care. In so doing, the boundaries between the professions become clouded or at least uncertain. As these boundaries become less firm, the potential for conflict begins to emerge. Because all the professions are interested in advancing their own role in rendering effective patient care, their interests can frequently conflict. Adding to this significant concern is a long history of hierarchical relationships between and among the disciplines in a very structured health delivery system. Such controls were originally designed to protect the interests of physicians in undertaking their clinical work. Physicians historically have operated at the apex of the clinical hierarchy, based on the assumption that by virtue of education and role they are clearly most advantaged in managing and controlling the clinical activities of the patient. However, over the years, as care has broadened and become more complex, the hierarchical model and unilateral locus of control by the physician is no longer adequate in meeting the needs of the patient. More interactive-based approaches to delineating and delivering patient care are now requisites for practice. Having failed to resolve boundary conflicts at earlier levels of the relationship, contemporary conflicts accelerate in intensity and passion as the issues become critical to the practice roles of the individual professions. Professional capacity, competence, and ability to perform the work are now limited by the various professions' availability to each other and the lack of technologies and methodologies for resolving these role-based interest conflicts.

> **Resolving Interest Conflict**
>
> - Identify interests.
> - Have all parties own their issues.
> - Give feelings ample play.
> - Clarify each party's role in the conflict.
> - Find common themes.
> - Use the parties' language.
> - Identify critical event(s).
> - Anticipate personality clashes.
> - Enumerate new work demands.
> - Give everyone time to express their loss(es).

The leader has a special set of challenges in bringing together disparate groups in an effort to resolve boundary and relational issues between them. However, this work must be considered as fundamental to the role of the leader in every clinical setting. Furthermore, the leader must help the professional groups supply time and commitment to addressing the specifics of the conflict that may impede their ability to relate and impact patient care. The leader must have the groups focused on their common interests, such as advancing patient care efficiency or effectiveness, rather than allow them to continue to focus on their positions. This

> **Working with Disparate Groups**
>
> - Name their frame of reference.
> - Identify needed "gets" early.
> - Balance feeling issues.
> - Name the boundary issues.
> - Enumerate common themes.
> - Find common language.
> - Look for conflict triggers.
> - Reduce personality clashes.
> - List expectations of each party of themselves and of others.

Interdisciplinary Conflict Considerations

Each discipline has its own content and contextual boundaries that define it. The leader recognizes the real value members have for their intradisciplinary identities and relationships. Members will bring these parameters to the conflict table and will hold onto these identities. The leader looks for the boundary issues early so that dialogue around interfacing at the boundary and reestablishing new intersections or roles there can be discussed and resolved. This is especially true as practice changes are challenging what professionals do and is changing their interactions and relationships almost daily. The leader will need to be especially adept at anticipating these conflicts and get to them as early (before, if possible) as possible. Late engagement of these conflicts can result in high "noise," extended conflict, and challenging resolution.

Continuous Dialogue

1. Have regular meetings with staff.
2. Make differences OK.
3. Create a safe space for dialogue.
4. Mix the disciplines in dialogue.
5. Use a flip chart to record processes.
6. Use effective/proven processes.
7. Have staff lead discussions.
8. Set priorities for problem solving.
9. Meet with dialogue leaders before formal meeting with others.
10. Always make conflict normative.

Gem

The great conflict leader is always aware of the power of effective information. No conflict dialogue should progress without the most accurate information necessary to validate process and progress. Information is the most powerful tool in the conflict process. The leader seeks it, gathers it, presents it at the right time, clarifies it when it is ambiguous or seeks more of it when it is inadequate. Resolution is a truth-seeking process. There is nothing more devastating than resolving a conflict on a false premise—for process must always begin again. The opportunity to recover the energy of the first resolution is difficult, if not impossible to regain.

creates some common ground upon which solution can be sought. In addition, the leader must help the groups deal with their resolution by using objective data. This translates passion and feeling derived from an experiential or perceived framework into a framework reflecting data-driven evidence regarding actual activity and its impact. Building a data-generating process (research) helps create the objective framework around which differing groups or professions can converge. In health care, the generation and use of objective data can provide a strong framework for common action in the resolution of interest-based conflicts.

In interest-based conflict management, the leader focuses on solutions that address the broad needs of all the parties, based around their common interests such as patient care. Calling the stakeholders back to those issues and keeping them focused on their mutual impact can help the leader in moving the parties to common resolution. In undertaking this approach, the leader will need to recognize that the offering and management of trade-offs, options, and alternatives will be a necessary part of the conflict interaction between groups that express differing or conflicting professional interests. While keeping the groups broad based and focused on impact and outcome, each will reflect on what will have to be sacrificed or traded in order to find common ground. Groups keep score, and the leader should too. Any inequity in the number and kinds or significance of trade-offs will be noted by the parties and will dramatically affect the ability of the leader to move them to common ground and conflict resolution.

The leader must always recognize that these conflicts are dynamic; that is, they are continuous, and one level of resolution always leads to a higher level of dialogue and more intensive conflicts. As the complexity of care and service becomes more intensive, so do the conflicts associated with them. The leader, therefore, establishes an ongoing mechanism or format for continuous dialogue and interface between the involved disciplines as a mechanism for assuring that the normative conflicts of multidisciplinary practice are addressed as an ordinary and usual part of doing the business of the clinical organization.

Data-Based Conflicts

Conflicts related to data are generally driven by either limited access to information or lack of information. Information is critical to the effectiveness of organizations in today's clinical workplace. Without appropriate information in a useful configuration, clinical work cannot be successfully undertaken. In fact, the complex of information necessary to do the work now makes the work completely information dependent. This information is critical to the ability of any of the disciplines to fulfill their obligations in rendering clinical service throughout the healthcare system. Furthermore, business, clinical, support, and material information must interface in order to create a sufficient data foundation upon which effective clinical choices can be made. It is this generation and interface of information that creates some of the most difficult and intractable problems and conflicts.

Information is resource intensive. As a result, there are wide variabilities related to the distribution and quality of hardware and software across the healthcare system. Emphasis has historically been placed on building a business infrastructure and information system, and much business sophistication has emerged as a result. Clinical information infrastructures are just now being expanded and linked to business infrastructure in ways that can have an impact on resource use and clinical decision making. However, information priorities, mechanisms for generating information, distribution of resources in building information infrastructures, and the quality and kind of information generated all have an impact on organizational effectiveness and integrity. Therein lies the source for the emergence of conflict. Each of these issues can generate its own internally fixed sources of conflict from access, availability, accuracy, quality, efficacy, and utility of information.

The leader must recognize that a fit is necessary between resource allocation and information usefulness. Since there are intersecting groups, all requiring various components of the information complex, some level of agreement must be achieved as to what information is necessary, important, and vital to clinical decision making. Agreements between organization-established priorities and clinically useful data processes and information must be interfaced in a way that is resource wise and reflects service utility. In addition, the leader must ensure that there are structural and process formats, within which these priorities and elements should reflect the useful and common set of criteria to which all stakeholders have contributed. The leader's role is to reduce the structural opportunities for conflict by assuring that appropriate processes and interfacing regarding information collection, management, and generation have been effectively delineated and structured within the organization. The leader makes sure that the right stakeholders are at the appropriate table so that deliberations include those upon whom decisions will impact. When issues have been overlooked or forgotten, the leader, recognizing the process is fluid, brings the stakeholders together again to deliberate and reassess with the intent of establishing a process that works successfully. Where there are challengers to the skill set and ability of the stakeholders, the leader assures that appropriate experts and expertise is available in order to guide the team to correctly delineate needs and resolutions with regard to information management solutions. Through this complex of activities and systems approaches to handling the information infrastructure, the leader creates an ongoing mechanism that embeds conflict resolution in the information system utilization process.

Information Systems' Value in Conflict
1. Creates opportunity for access
2. Links and integrates information
3. Is a vehicle for common problem responses
4. Is data rich
5. A common tool, useful to all participants
6. Can make data conflicts clearer
7. Supporting source for objective information
8. Immediate implementation of many solutions
9. Reduces ambiguity of inputs or responses
10. Useful for evaluation of outcomes/effectiveness

In each of these arenas are specific and unique activities related to resolving the conflict. While this workbook certainly introduces some of the steps that can be undertaken by leaders to address conflict, it isn't a comprehensive reflection. The leader must recognize that conflict management is a significant skill set and obtain as much development and education as necessary to build conflict management skills. Facility in conflict management comes with discipline, practice, and time. The leader, recognizing how important conflict management is to successful group interchange and group dynamics, therefore commits considerable time and energy to understanding and developing those skills.

REFRAMING CONFLICT WITH AN APPRECIATIVE APPROACH

New work in appreciative inquiry leads to some additional thoughts associated with the process of conflict resolution. Through the use of the four dimensions of appreciative inquiry, the traditional problem-solving approach to conflict resolution can be transformed into an appreciative approach that more effectively creates a positive context for conflict processes. In appreciative inquiry, the contextual framework for questions related to any process reflect the following four generative questions: (1) What gives life? (2) What might be? (3) What should be? and (4) What will be?

In appreciative inquiry, effective communication deals with emotions first and data second. The leader is listening first to understand as a way of gaining the experience of the conflict from the perspective of the individual and only then follows up with facts. After the elements of the conflict are identified, the leader asks the individuals to tell about a time when they worked together well; this frames the approach of moving the individuals toward the ideal. The attempt of the leader is to help respondents focus on what is possible by having them idealize what a positive situation looks like, what it feels like, and what it sounds like. In this way a positive context and personal affirmation is identified, and the conflict situation can be compared to it and specific elements of achievement can be identified. With the basic elements of the preferable clearly articulated, the leader can move the conflict toward creating the ideal. At this time, the effort is directed toward obtaining effective long-range and mutually beneficial outcomes. The leader helps the individuals establish the relationship between mutual outcomes and personal benefit. In this way the frame is drawn out of a conflict context and moves toward an ideal relational context providing a more desirable and positive mutual benefit as a goal rather than simply resolving a particular conflict.

In the appreciative approach, the focus on the process is to diminish emphasis on the negative and to raise the positive potential embedded in the conflict. The approach emphasizes collaboration and integration of individual needs, values, and outcomes in a way that emphasizes a future state and how one might best live in it. The goal is to create a sustainable framework for interaction that consistently and constantly focuses on the positive potentials, creating an ongoing living image of how individuals work and relate together over the long term. While the appreciative approach is an emergent concept, its focus on mutuality and positive imaging of a future state creates the potential for a strong and effective approach to the continuous management of conflict.

THE LEADER CREATES SUSTAINABLE SOLUTIONS

The leader is committed to creating an environment where solution seeking is the normative pattern of work behavior. The leader seeks to maintain a healthy environment for the conflict process to be integrated into the business practices of every service or department. When all is said and done, an ongoing dynamic of development and skill building in conflict processes is a normal part of the function and learning activities of the organization. At a minimum, the leader assures that the following should always occur:

- Staff remains skilled in conflict identification.
- Managers maintain expectations and processes for conflict resolution.
- The department remains a safe place for addressing differences.
- Actions are followed up.
- Continuing education includes conflict skill development.
- Shared decision making works.
- Role/performance expectations are continuously negotiated.
- Manager–staff interaction occurs frequently.

Gem

Leaders engage and embrace conflict as a regular component of the array of leadership tasks. Building the dynamic or conflict resolution into the practices of the department or unit creates the milieu for staff that makes conflict safe and expects that it will be dealt with as a regular part of the function and operation of doing business.

CONFLICT SCENARIO—ORGANIZATIONAL CONFLICT

Sam had been on the critical care unit for 3 years and had just received his advanced certification in cardiac critical care. He was excited by the opportunity to move to the cardiac care center after reading a personnel posting of a new position for an advanced cardiac nurse within the cardiac care center. Sam immediately submitted his credentials and his application for the position. He was interviewed by the nursing staff from the cardiac care center and by their management team. At the completion of the interview by the management team, Sam was assured that the position was his and that he could count on hearing from them shortly about his having obtained the position.

Two weeks passed and Sam still had not heard any news with regard to his application. He called the human resources department and was informed by them that someone else had been selected for the position. Sam was hurt and upset by the news. He informed the human resources officer that he'd been assured after his interview with the nursing management team that the position was his. Since that time he had merely been waiting to hear confirmation as to when he might begin his new position in the cardiac care center. The human resources officer assured Sam that unless he'd received formal confirmation from the human resources office he should not have reason to believe that the promise of a position had been made. This news caused Sam to be further upset and concerned with regard to the potential for this new position.

The more Sam thought about this the angrier he became. His hopes had been high, he'd obviously interviewed well and been well received, and yet still did not obtain the position. Furthermore, he felt that he had been promised the position based on his interview performance. What made him even angrier was that no one bothered to communicate either positively or negatively with regard to his application for the position before it had been offered to someone else. Upset with this set of circumstances and concerned about his future, Sam petitioned for a formal mediation in an effort to resolve his conflicting concerns.

Scenario Exploration

Clearly there are a number of issues involved in Sam's experience that raised the potential for conflict. Spend some time discussing the issues and circumstances related to this scenario and the places where the potential for conflicts is embedded.

1. What was the first moment that indicated a potential for conflict?
2. What was missing in the interview process that facilitated the potential for conflict?
3. What actions in the interview process helped create subsequent conflict?
4. What did Sam do/not do to participate in creating the conditions for conflict?
5. What are the critical elements resolving this conflict?

Undertake a role-play process in relationship to this conflict. There should be three members of the role play (Sam, the human resources department representative, and the mediator), and each role should be rotated among the members of your group. Initiate a formal conflict resolution process using the principles identified in this chapter. Follow the process template contained at the end of the chapter. Discuss both the process and the outcome of the mediator role play.

Fran's Story

Fran had been an exceptionally competent charge nurse on the neurosurgery unit for 10 years. She had never had any problems with new staff. There had been plenty of them over the years, many coming and orienting to the nurse role fresh out of school and, after a year or 2, leaving for other positions. Fran did not lament the movement but saw it as a normal part of developing a nursing career. She saw herself as a mentor for these new nurses and was hopeful that her role modeling was well received and that those she coached operated at a skill higher level after their experience with her.

(continues)

CONFLICT SCENARIO—RELATIONSHIP CONFLICT *(continued)*

Debbie was a different case. Since she had shown up, she created nothing but stress for Fran and the rest of the staff on the unit. Fran thought Debbie had a chip on her shoulder the size of a redwood. Many staff members commented that Debbie took no counsel from any of them. Some thought Debbie acted as though she were better than everyone and could do no wrong. Every time Fran approached Debbie to advise her of some issue of practice or new opportunity for learning, Debbie appeared distracted and acted as though she wanted to run. Debbie would speak out during clinical rounds declaring everything she knew about the diagnosis or care needs of the patient being discussed. She constantly interrupted and corrected other staff when she thought they were wrong. Whenever Fran tried to talk about Debbie's behavior, Debbie would tell her to mind her own business and suggested that she might want to attend to her own practice instead of critiquing others' work all the time. Fran thought Debbie had better adopt a different attitude or she would not last long in the unit. Fran felt she would blow up at Debbie if Debbie made one more disparaging remark. Fran felt that such a blowup toward Debbie was long overdue.

Debbie's Story

Debbie was in her first role as a registered nurse in primary care. She had graduated at the top of her class and had always been under the gun to perform well and to be the best nurse she could be. Her mother always insisted that Debbie be the best and do the best in everything she attempted. And Debbie had been the best from the first grade all the way through college. She felt she must continue to hold that status in this new job, especially when so many counted on her doing the best clinical work she could muster. This first job was her foundation year in the profession and it was very important for her to prove herself.

Debbie wished Fran would leave her alone. It seemed to her that Fran was always looking over her shoulder snooping around for trouble. Fran always seemed to find out what Debbie was doing wrong and seemed happy to point it out to her. Debbie felt that even when she contributed to the clinical rounds, Fran would have something negative to say. Debbie wondered what Fran knew that Debbie didn't know. Debbie wished Fran would stop spying on her and simply leave her alone. Fran seemed to be just trouble and kept wanting to make trouble for Debbie. What was Debbie going to do about Fran?

Scenario Exploration

Take a look at this scenario and discuss its implications from the perspectives of both Fran and Debbie. As a group, explore the following questions:

1. Describe how each person sees herself in her role.
2. How does each person view the other's role? Is it accurate? In what way do they differ?
3. What are the errors each has in the perception of the other?
4. How do the misperceptions drive the behavior each has toward the other?
5. What are the real underlying issues affecting their relationship?
6. How might you suggest the mediation process to each of these nurses?
7. Break up in groups and take turns doing a role-play mediation of this scenario. Evaluate each other as you follow the mediation process and apply it to this case. Please note: there is no right answer to this case, just one that works for the participants. Share your perspectives on the case and the mediation process at the completion of the exercise.

REFERENCES

Kossgard, M., Schweiger, D., & Sappienze, H. (1995). Building commitment, attachment, and trust in strategic decision-making teams: The role of procedural justice. *Academy of Management Journal, 38*(1), 60–85.

Moore, C. (1996). *The mediation process: Practical strategies for resolving conflict.* San Francisco: Jossey-Bass.

SUGGESTED READINGS

Cooperrider, D., Whitney, D., & Stavros, J. (2008). *The appreciative inquiry handbook: For leaders of change.* San Francisco: Barrett-Koehler Publishers.

Deutsch, M., & Coleman, P. T. (2000). *The handbook of conflict resolution: Theory and practice.* San Francisco: Jossey-Bass.

Diehl, P. F., & Lepgold, J. (2003). *Regional conflict management.* Lanham, MA: Rowman & Littlefield.

Drafke, M., & Kossen, S. (2002). *The human side of organizations.* Upper Saddle River, NJ: Prentice Hall.

Fenn, P., & Gameson, R. (1992). *Construction conflict management and resolution.* New York: E & FN Spon.

Fredrick, C., & Atkinson, C. (1997). *Women, ethics and the workplace.* Westport, CT: Praeger.

Fujishin, R. (2001). *Creating effective groups: The art of small group communication.* San Francisco: Acada Books.

Gorden, M. (1972). *Comparative political systems: Managing conflict.* New York: Macmillan.

Green, R. L. (2001). *Practicing the art of leadership: A problem-based approach to implementing the ISLLC standards.* Upper Saddle River, NJ: Merrill.

Gudykunst, W. B. (1978). *Bridging differences: Effective intergroup communication* (3rd ed.). Thousand Oaks, CA: Sage Publications.

Hare, A. P. (1992). *Groups, teams, and social interaction: Theories and applications.* New York: Praeger.

Honeycutt, J. M. (2003). *Imagined interactions: Daydreaming about communication. Interpersonal communication.* Cresskill, NJ: Hampton Press.

Jones, T. E. (1999). *If it's broken, you can fix it: Overcoming dysfunction in the workplace.* New York: Amacom.

Kalbfleisch, P. J., & Cody, M. J. (1995). *Gender, power, and communication in human relationships.* Hillsdale, NJ: Erlbaum.

Kellett, P. M., & Dalton, D. G. (2001). *Managing conflict in a negotiated world: A narrative approach to achieving dialogue and change.* Thousand Oaks, CA: Sage Publications.

Levi, D. (2001). *Group dynamics for teams.* Thousand Oaks, CA: Sage Publications.

Linstead, S., Fulop, L., & Lilley, S. (2004). *Management and organization: A critical text.* New York: Palgrave Macmillan.

Rahim, M. A. (2001). *Managing conflict in organizations* (3rd ed.). Westport, CT: Quorum Books.

Richman, L. (2002). *Project management step-by-step.* New York: Amacom.

Stewart, J. R. (2002). *Bridges not walls: A book about interpersonal communication* (8th ed.). Boston: McGraw-Hill.

Tojo, J., & Dilpreet, C. (2007). *Appreciative inquiry and knowledge management.* Northhampton, UK: Edward Elgar Publishers.

Watkins, M., & Rosegrant, S. (2001). *Breakthrough international negotiation: How great negotiators transformed the world's toughest post-Cold War conflicts.* San Francisco: Jossey-Bass.

A P P E N D I X

Workbook Conflict Template 1

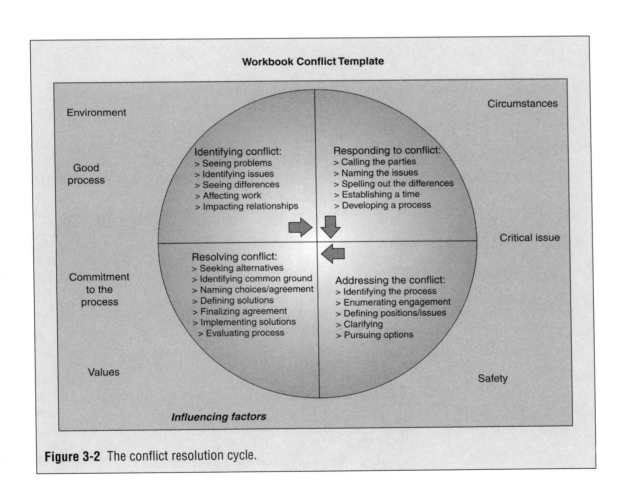

Workbook Conflict Template

Environment

Circumstances

Good process

Identifying conflict:
> Seeing problems
> Identifying issues
> Seeing differences
> Affecting work
> Impacting relationships

Responding to conflict:
> Calling the parties
> Naming the issues
> Spelling out the differences
> Establishing a time
> Developing a process

Critical issue

Commitment to the process

Resolving conflict:
> Seeking alternatives
> Identifying common ground
> Naming choices/agreement
> Defining solutions
> Finalizing agreement
> Implementing solutions
> Evaluating process

Addressing the conflict:
> Identifying the process
> Enumerating engagement
> Defining positions/issues
> Clarifying
> Pursuing options

Values

Safety

Influencing factors

Figure 3-2 The conflict resolution cycle.

Workbook Conflict Template 2:
Follow a Process for Conflict Resolution

Eight Steps to Conflict Resolution

1. Make a safe space for the conflict resolution process.
   - Comfortable
   - Quiet
   - Caring
   - Open
   - Prepared
2. Get a basic understanding of the issues.
   - Issues
   - Feelings
   - Elements and details
   - Reality base and clarity
3. Name individual needs.
   - Needs identified in parties' own words
   - Needs parties have of each other
   - Perceptions of meeting needs
   - Clear up misperceptions
4. Identify expectations from each other.
   - Name the "gets" each wants.
   - Sort through the differences.
   - Identify resource issues.
5. Clarify alternatives.
   - Identify critical issues.
   - Name the alternatives.
   - List the remaining issues.
   - Check off the differences.
6. Bridge the issues.
   - Finding common themes/ground
   - Hidden gems of agreement
   - Affirmations of common interests
7. Define agreements.
   - Generation of alternatives
   - Selection of alternatives
   - Determination of priorities for action
8. Finalize an agreement to action.
   - Finalizing agreements
   - Determining parties' actions
   - Acting on agreement
   - Evaluating process
   - Follow-up on agreement actions

CHAPTER ⬤ 4

Confronting Crisis:
The Leadership of Constant Change

CHAPTER OBJECTIVES:

Upon completion of this chapter, the reader will:

1. Understand the characteristics of crisis and change and the appropriate processes and responses to them.

2. Discuss the elements of *crisis and change*, indicating the appropriate leadership behaviors in helping people respond to them.

3. Apply the concepts and skills of predictive and adaptive capacity within the role of the function of the leader as a practical aspect of adaptation to change.

4. Apply systems model approach to change and crisis management as an effective way of getting people and organizations through crisis and in adapting to it.

INTRODUCTION

Complexity and chaos science has now revealed that change is a constant and dominant force operating at every place in the universe (Gharajedaghi, 1999). Interestingly enough, probability, variability, and the unexpected vagaries of chance are increasingly seen even at the most significant nanolevels of matter. In short, the continuous presence and action of change in every dynamic of human experience continuously changes the way we see that dynamic and we respond to it as people both personally and organizationally. Our historic approaches to change as a linear and iterative process that demonstrates both a beginning and an end represents inaccurate and inadequate thinking about the action and process of change. In this mental model, change is seen as a continuous line of forces and actions with specific and clear stages that can be planned for and anticipated.

> ### Crisis and Change
>
> Change is constant and the potential for continuous and dynamic crisis is always present. A systematic approach to crisis can be undertaken but all crisis can be undertaken, but all crisis cannot be anticipated. Proactive insight and skills related to crisis management is critical to thriving through crisis events.

Reality, however, is quite different. Change is often random, unanticipated, and comes at times where individuals and groups are unprepared or unaware (Bridges, 2002). Often change comes through "the side door" in a way that could not be seen or planned for regardless of the degree of insight and predictive capacity. Managing

---

Gem

You might not be able to anticipate a particular crisis but you can manage it if you have the right tools and processes in place. Crisis always occurs, so the only variable that counts is readiness and preparedness for appropriately addressing it.

Unanticipated Crisis Scenario

Community Hospital had been the major health resource for a growing community of 50,000 people for the last 60 years. This hospital provided the full range of healthcare services directed to meeting community needs and had become identified as the community's healthcare resource. Over the years the community had come to depend on Community Hospital with the belief that it would remain its primary healthcare resource for the foreseeable future. However, a large hospital corporation had been looking at the local market for the past year to determine whether there was market viability for a second hospital and medical center for the fast-growing community. Major assessment activities were undertaken related to market analysis, demographic studies, service demands, and the potential for profitability and market viability activities over the past 8 months. Community Hospital was aware of the activities and had been watching them with interest as they were reported in the local newspaper over that same period of time. However, because Community Hospital had developed such a strong presence and clear identification with its community, it did not fear or anticipate many changes in its existing status or relationship in the community.

It was not long, however, before the major hospital corporation decided to establish its presence in the community and build a second major medical and hospital presence in the high-growth area of the city. Major television commercials and community initiatives were undertaken to raise questions about current adequacy of service and the need for more vibrant, contemporary, futuristic, and technologically advanced health service within the community. Promises of quality, service, and the best and most advanced clinical and technological services piqued the interest of the community, which began to dramatically change the practice and business characteristics of the local business enterprises and medical staff arrangements and agreements. Before long, physicians, patients, and business relationships were dramatically altered in the community and Community Hospital began to suffer major service and financial challenges.

Questions for Discussion:

1. Should this crisis have been anticipated, and if so, when?
2. What kinds of early response activities could Community Hospital have undertaken?
3. When is it best to anticipate a crisis, and what are some early indicators?

---

crisis and dramatic change is a relatively new field of study of applied management. Skills in this new arena reflect the leader's ability to forecast and anticipate potential crises, respond to them, help others deal with them, and to develop the ability to accommodate and to adjust to systems failures. Today, with the intensity related to globalization and increasing social and cultural interaction, the potential for change and crisis management accelerates, and the need for skills that systematically address such realities becomes more critical (Hamson & Holder, 2002).

In today's world it's very difficult to avoid crisis. However, crisis management is a systematic approach to addressing the issues of crisis, its origins, and its impact on people and organizations. Crises are generally unpredictable, yet not unexpected. Every person and organization can expect crisis events to unfold as a part of their life experience. The challenge is not so much that crisis occurs but that we are all so surprised by it and unprepared for its impact. So little of organizational constructs and infrastructure is directed and designed in a way that helps individuals and organizations anticipate the occurrence of crisis, accommodate its impact, and adjust organizational structures and behaviors to accommodate the vagaries of crisis and change and to continue to thrive. The notion of thriving in a crisis is often considered foreign to the notion of crisis and the perception of pain and the negative impact it has on persons and organizations.

EARLY WARNING

Crises very rarely occur without some level of early warning (Weick, 2001). The critical factor in early engagement of crisis is the development and presence of tools and mechanisms, which provides an ongoing leadership and organizational mechanism for becoming aware of the potential for crisis in advance of crises actually occurring. The first step of any early warning systematic process is the leaders' understanding and acceptance that crisis occurrences are a normative part of the human experience and they are to be anticipated rather than being surprising. It is this understanding of the inevitability and normative circumstances related to the potential of the onset of a crisis that best conditions organizational leadership to create a programmatic and systematic approach to confronting crisis. In short, a systematic framework—a model—needs to be incorporated into the operational and structural characteristics of the organization as a way of assuring that well-planned mechanisms for addressing the onset of a crisis event is in place long before crises actually arise.

Hospitals and health systems are very good at anticipating clinical crises as well as community and natural disasters. Their capacity for disaster planning is unparalleled and can usually be compared with the most well-prepared plans for such crises as exist in any organization. However, these crises tend to be the least common occurrences affecting the viability and stability of the hospital or health system. It is usually other major significant crises that place the hospital or health system at greater risk than those natural or clinical disasters. Crises related to finance, management, market, competition, environment, and operations create more significant risks for the organization than do natural or clinical disasters.

Much of the reason for the impact of this kind of risk is the lack of systems that predict and anticipate changes in current conditions and challenges threatening the status quo (Argenti, 2002). The ability to develop the skills requires in all leaders a deep understanding of social and organizational complexity and the processes associated with facilitating human dynamics within the context of complex systems. The ability to comprehend the action of complexity and the human response to immediate and dramatic change is an important set of leadership skills that are required as a basic foundation for the expression of leadership competencies related to the management of crisis. Complexity theory and science have provided leaders with major new insights regarding predictive and adaptive capacity and the need to incorporate particular dynamics and applications into the ordinary and usual management practices of organizations (Kelly & Allison, 1999).

The ability to understand both the complexities and applications essential to a positive response to crisis demands an understanding of the cybernetic nature of all action and human experience. This demand represents a clear need for recognizing the cyclical nature of all action, including human action, recognizing the inevitability and eventuality of major and dramatic shifts in both experience and reality. Because of this inevitability, all human organizations must reflect a strong capacity for adaptation and change. Since change is the only constant in the universe, structuring organizations to be continuously adaptive and mobile is a critical requisite for long-term viability. The need for an organization to continue to thrive calls for its leadership to be ever vigilant with regard to the continuous and unrelenting risks embedded in change dynamics operating both internally and externally and having both negative and positive implications for the organization's health and life (Heifetz & Linsky, 2002).

> ### Gem
> Since change is the only constant, the onset of a crisis might truly indicate a leader's failure to see the signals of crisis either through the lack of an effective scanning system or through failure of personal diligence.

A PREDICTIVE AND ADAPTIVE MODEL FOR CRISIS AND CHANGE

The organization's ability to adequately respond to crisis depends strongly on its capacity to anticipate and plan for it. It is now increasingly a requisite of the leader's role to be able to incorporate a deep and full understanding of the necessary components of a responsive process that adequately prepares, anticipates, and plans for successful response to inevitable crisis. Recognizing the elements of building such a plan, the leader constantly incorporates the mechanisms for crisis management into the usual and ordinary operational processes and mechanics of managing the organization from strategy to application. The use of a systematic approach to the management of the crisis dynamic calls for a model or approach that deeply incorporates essential elements of each stage of the planning and adaptation process into the ongoing activities of systematic and organizational leadership.

Whatever models are created, leaders must understand that crises can come from both within and outside the organization. While many leaders anticipate that the majority of significant crisis is generated by changes in the external environment, the truth is, many crises and adversity with regard to the organization's viability come from challenges arising from within the organization. Clearly recognizing internal and external sources of crises helps leaders plan for appropriate activities and strategies related to the origins and sources of conflict or crises in a way that can more directly and realistically address the issues they raise.

Anticipating and planning for crises requires more than good leadership. A systematic approach to addressing issues of crises calls for structural, process, and leadership capacities that work in conjunction with each other and represent the organization's overall commitment to incorporating crisis events into the usual and ordinary operational activities of the organization (Millar & Heath, 2004). A comprehensive model or systems approach first addresses the external and internal conditions and elements necessary to make crisis awareness a functional part of the organization and then creates an organized and structured approach to adequately and accurately address the potential and conditions associated with the onset of crisis. Tying all of these elements and processes within the context of good management process and leadership skills creates a comprehensive frame within which anticipating and planning for crisis can move from a critical event to the ordinary and usual process of good management.

All of the elements of good management, beginning with mission, purpose, meaning (values), and leadership are the essential first steps for assuring integration of crises processes with the core values and related infrastructures of the organization. At every level of the organization, from the board of directors to service and productivity, the continuous and dynamic external and internal environmental scanning processes must represent a cybernetic (continuous) loop of interacting activities that act in concert to assure that organizational awareness and response is incorporated into the ongoing activities of both leadership and work. The model should reflect all the components and elements that will assure their convergence around appropriate anticipation and planning for inevitable crisis (see **Figure 4-1**).

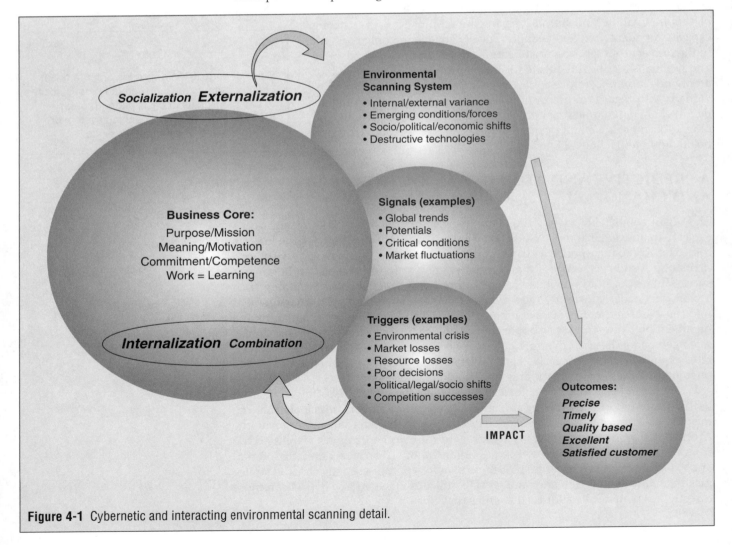

Figure 4-1 Cybernetic and interacting environmental scanning detail.

CORE ELEMENTS: EXTERNALIZATION–INTERNALIZATION

Organizations are constantly influenced by their relationships to both the external and internal environments (Stabor & Sydow, 2002). Indeed, the convergence of both external and internal forces frequently reflect the character and content of the continuous, dynamic, and cybernetic dance between an organization's interaction with the external environment and the fit of the internal infrastructure with the organization's ability to thrive. This goodness of fit is perhaps the most critical factor in ensuring and advancing the viability of the organization, its efficacy, and its sustainability. Frontline healthcare providers often either are not aware of this reality or fail to recognize its impact on the applicability and viability of their own work. One of the major tasks of leaders, in this circumstance, is to constantly keep this awareness in front of the clinical service providers, assuring that it plays some role in influencing and impacting decisions they make and actions they take.

> **External Forces**
>
> 1. Social, political, economic, market, community, human, and environmental.
> 2. Critical shifts in the competitive marketplace.
> 3. Innovation in technology or service.
> 4. Introduction of new factors resulting from radical change.
> 5. Natural or human generated disaster.
> 6. Convergence of seemingly unrelated forces.
> 7. Change in demand or community/individual needs.

The external forces constantly influencing the integrity of the organization and the broader social context generally relates to social, political, economic, market, and community concerns that have a continuous and constant influence on the design of the organization, the structuring of its clinical work, the activities of its various services and functions, and the actions of its multivariant clinical professionals. These forces are constantly dynamic, ever changing, and continuously reflective of the changing circumstances in the broader social arena. Financial, policy, political, environmental, and social shifts, even if they are subtle, can have tremendous influence on the structure and operations of the health system, agency, service, or institution. At the governance and administrative levels of the organization, mechanisms must be in place that alert people in those levels of shifts that are occurring in the broader social context that can intersect or converge in a way that results in significant impact on the organization. The critical factor in this set of circumstances is the force of convergence of seemingly unrelated factors. It is the confluence of these distinct circumstances that create the conditions that ultimately become crises. The failure to recognize the relationship between seemingly nonrelated elements or events can be the first sign of a potential crisis or conflict. Often failure to see this emerging reality at the earliest possible moment can usher in significant reaction a later stage of conflict, sometimes too late to avoid a negative impact on the organization.

ENVIRONMENTAL SCANNING

External sociopolitical forces have a greater impact on governance leadership and executive decision making. The impact of these forces on mission, vision, purpose, and values are significant with regard to the decision making occurring at the executive level of the organization. Often these external social forces impact on what the organization is, how it behaves, and what it does as a system. The internal forces that converge with external influences reflect in the organization's behavior; how, what, and who the organization is translates into decisions and actions. Everything related to the character of the organization reflects its positioning in the broader social context and represents to its community its value and contribution to the life and needs of that community.

Environmental scanning (see **Figure 4-2**) provides information for the organization with regard to those external forces that reflect the dynamic of change and its impact on the life cycle of the organization (Stabor & Sydow, 2002). Structures and leadership action in the organization within the context of environmental scanning relates to the tools and skills available to leaders that can help them interpret and apply external dynamics and changes to the operating reality of the organization. Whatever formal processes exist in the organization, executive leaders can use these processes as tools to help interpret the impact and force of change and to translate that into language

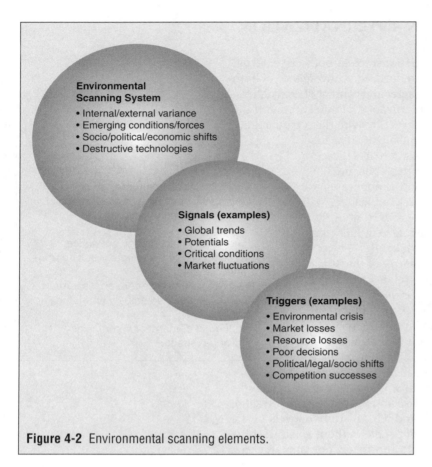

Figure 4-2 Environmental scanning elements.

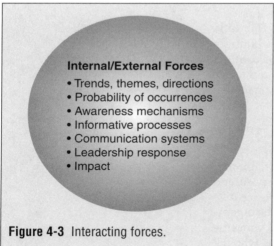

Figure 4-3 Interacting forces.

Gem

You might not be able to anticipate a particular crisis but you can manage it if you have the right tools and processes in place. Crisis always occurs, so the only variable that counts is readiness and preparedness for appropriately addressing it.

---

that departmental and first-line leaders within the organization can reflect upon and, if necessary, respond to.

EXTERNAL AND INTERNAL FORCES

The ability of the organization to have and demonstrate insight with regard to the forces impacting strategic and critical action is a fundamental skill set of good leadership. Interacting forces, whether external or internal, are constant and can serve to inform the leadership of the organization about conditions and circumstances that may affect decisions and actions and ultimately impact the sustainability of the organization. In quantum reality, many of the interacting forces affecting decisions and actions are unknown and operate as a backdrop to the perceived issues and concerns of formal leadership. It is an element of predictive capacity in quantum leadership that themes, trends, or directions that operate individually or collectively tell the leader about the probability of certain occurrences rather than simply and precisely enumerate them (see **Figure 4-3**). For the leader, it is important that an in-place mechanism functions continuously as a subset of the leader's role to inform and alert the leader regarding internal and external realities, their changes, and the potential (probable) impact on both the function and trajectory of the organization.

PROBABILITY

The contemporary quantum leader recognizes the significance and value of determining the probability of an action. It is more important to be able to focus on issues of probability than it is to be able to predict current or future events with absolute certainty. By aggregating data from various sources having an impact on the organization and synthesizing the information that was gathered, the leader exercises the best indices of probability in informing judgments and decisions upon which subsequent action will be based (Snyder & Duarte, 2003).

Without being overly complicated, the leader uses probability to indicate the likelihood of an event, occurrence, or situation. It should be noted, however, that gathering more information ad infinitum does not increase the probability of the correctness of decisions. What is more likely to facilitate the probability of an occurrence is both the veracity and accuracy of the data and the intensity of its relationship, such that when it converges, the composite of information provides the data that most likely is an indicator of probability.

- The leader attempts to assess the likelihood (probability) of an event(s).
- Leaders look at the number of similar events, look for the common elements of those events, and assess the likelihood of their reoccurrence.

- Since the sum of all possible events is 100%, the leader looks for the percentage of probability of any given event occurring in any given situation as an indicator of the predictive value of that event.
- Leaders calculate the probability of an event as a way of clarifying and specifying the likelihood of its occurrence (see **Figure 4-4**).
- Leaders become aware and develop skills in calculating complex probability relationships such as:
  - *Independent versus dependent events*—The outcome of two events are independent if the fact that one event happens, it does not affect the probability of a second event happening.
  - *Contingent probabilities*—A contingent probability exists when determining the probability of a second event given that a first event happened. If the outcome of two events are independent, the contingent probability is the same as the regular probability (as in Figure 4-4).
  - *Disjointed events*—A disjointed event occurs if at most only one of the events can happen; e.g.: Nancy winning a raffle and a bowling tournament: not disjointed—she can win both; Ann and Sue competing against each other in a poker game and both winning: disjointed—only one of them can win.
    - In disjointed events, the probability of at least one happening is equal to the sum of the probabilities of either event happening.
    - When the events are not disjointed, the probability of at least one event happening is equal to the sum of the probabilities of either event happening less the probability of both happening.
  - *Multiple events*—In multiple events, the expected number of successful events is equal to the probability of a successful event times the number of occurrences or attempts.
  - *Probability of a successful event*—The probability of at least one successful event is generally less than the probability of a successful event times the number of occurrences or attempts. The lower the probability of a successful event, the closer to the probability of at least one successful event is to the product.
  - *Probability of effectiveness*—Probability of effectiveness is influenced by the ability of the leader to accurately read the data, predict probability, make judgments about current circumstances or variants affecting the probability, and take appropriate action (Hassett, 2007).

1. Determine the total of equally likely events. (**N**)
2. Determine the number of successful events. (**S**)
3. Probability of success = **S** ÷ **N**.

Example:

What is the probability of rolling a 1 on a die?
- Ordinary 6 sided die:
- 6 equally likely possible events, (1,2,3,4,5,6)
- 1 successful event (1)
- $Pr(1) = 1 \div 6 = 16.7\%$

What is the probability of rolling a 1 or 2 on a die?
- Ordinary 6 sided die:
- 6 equally likely possible events, (1,2,3,4,5,6)
- 2 successful events (2)
- $Pr(1) = Pr(2) = 16.7\% + 16.7\% = 33.3\%$

Figure 4-4 Calculating probability.

The use of probability tools is increasing in effective management decision making, especially that related to developing predictive and adaptive capacities in the leader's role. While there is also increasing focus on innovations related to intuitive leadership, it is not yet well developed, and the use of statistical and mathematical approaches to assessing the value and veracity of probability thinking is still the predominant skill set that helps the leader synthesize data and make decisions with a high probability of success. While probability can certainly be used for other operational and management processes, it is especially useful in looking at predictive processes and determining their degree of significance and impact on decisions that occur within the organization. Since the effort of a leader is to help manage and possibly minimize crisis, the use of predictive tools is most helpful in limiting the potential for unanticipated crisis.

Probability tools can also be used for predicting the potential of internal crises as well. However, good management, financial, and operational systems internally provide the most appropriate array of useful tools in advancing the ability to predict

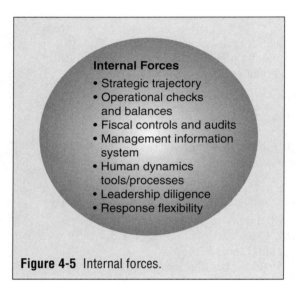

Internal Forces
- Strategic trajectory
- Operational checks and balances
- Fiscal controls and audits
- Management information system
- Human dynamics tools/processes
- Leadership diligence
- Response flexibility

Figure 4-5 Internal forces.

Unanticipated Crisis Scenario

Community Hospital had for the past 15 years, been the major coronary artery bypass surgery (CABG) center for the local region. It had met the cardiac needs of its population and had been very successful with the surgical procedure with great deal of positive clinical outcomes and a low level of negative clinical safety and risk issues. Recently, however, the cardiac surgeon's number of CABG's had been increasingly negatively affected by the growth in invasive cardiology services development and use of angiography and stenting for coronary occlusion. In fact, the increase in the invasive cardiology service had been dramatic and the need to expand the service required additional space for the use of the interventional cardiologists.

The chief of the interventional cardiologists had recently spoken to the chief of cardiac surgery and had suggested to him that, in the interests of the expanding cardiology service and of the patients they served, it would be appropriate for the surgeons to make a couple of operating suites available on regular basis to the invasive cardiologist for their procedure. The cardiac surgeons were furious with the cardiology request on top of the financial and service pain they were feeling in the reduction of number of CABGs being done in the surgical suite. Extreme conflict and crisis arose between the two services and much emotional pain and aggression began to exist between the two departments. The chief executive officer and chief nursing officer were caught in the middle of a significant organizational and service crisis that appeared to be growing in intensity.

Questions:

1. Could this crisis have been predicted?
2. What would be the most effective tools in identifying the signals indicating change?
3. What now? And what inclusive processes need to be in place to help all stakeholders recognize the signals of change collectively and sooner?

and manage organizational crisis (**Figure 4-5**). The application of good management principles and operational tools helps not only facilitate the potential for diagnosing and addressing internally generated conflict but can also help avoid or limit that potential. Most organizational crisis refers to (1) strategic misjudgments, (2) operational or financial malfeasance, and (3) the failure of positive human dynamics in the organization. Developing and using ongoing internal tools and checks and balances and continually assessing, implementing, and evaluating programs of effective organizational stewardship helps limit and control the vagaries of internal conflict potential.

READING SIGNALS

An essential component of good environmental scanning is evidenced in the leader's ability to recognize the signals as they become critical indicators of the potential for crisis and change impacting people and organizations. A good, strong operational and data core that provides information, tools, and systems that help keep the organization aware of its internal and external environments works to anticipate and avoid crisis, it is not sufficient. Scanning skills also include devices that help recognize specific signals that alert the leader to particular circumstances, indicators, and events that have the potential for significant impact or change with regard to the organization. Signals may be deeply embedded in a complex array of data to which the leader responds. These signals may be embedded in the trends, advantage of new technology and therapeutics, introduction of new devices or clinical processes, or simply a change in process or methodology. For example, the introduction of cardiac stents slowly yet inexorably has altered the percentage of patients using coronary artery bypass graft procedures as a way of clinically addressing the narrowing of cardiac vessels. Cardiac stents are easier to insert and are less invasive, with fewer physiologic accommodations and symptoms than those associated with coronary artery bypass grafts. A radical shift in clinical therapeutics is the result of the introduction of this new technology. The leader must have a depth of insight, access to expertise, and an ability to synthesize data within the context of existing circumstances and potential impact on current methodologies and ways of doing business.

Signals are often either clearly visible or are obscure in their availability in the data the quantum leader reviews (**Figure 4-6**). Signals are frequently embedded in both the individual elements of data or through the synthesis of data and the concluding story that data reveals. Sometimes it is a single technological innovation that serves as a signal of the potential for significant change. Other times it can be found in what the leader discerns after aggregating a series of data elements that converge to reveal indications of a major shift or dramatic emerging new reality. Either way, the leader is constantly aware of the potential of change embedded in the usual and ordinary processes of reviewing and using information and data sources in a way that affects thinking and acting within the context of a constantly shifting reality.

The greatest element of skill with regard to scanning for signals is the leader's internal awareness of the constantly shifting landscape and the elements deeply embedded in the chief indicators or drivers of change. In order to maintain that awareness, several things are important in the activity set of the leader, including:

- *Reading broadly.* The leader is constantly aware of trends and issues affecting her or his scope of responsibilities and analyzing the content for obvious, subtle, and sometimes obtuse indicators of a shift.
- *Reading outside one's field.* The leader is aware that a multitude of changes are going on just outside one's own field of vision, and this requires the leader to tap into data sources that are not a usual and ordinary part of the leader's experience. Reading at this level of breadth develops a keener awareness on the part of the leader and also exposes the leader to new frames of thinking. Doing this reading can directly or tangentially affect the organization.
- *Accessing information on the creative fringe.* It is important for the leader to be aware of thinkers, ideas, processes, and the inventions that reflect the level of innovation and creativity ahead of the field. Being available to what may sometimes appear outrageous or marginal can prepare the leader to better anticipate those moments when something outrageous, ridiculous, or innovative sets a new direction for the world (just think about Apple, Microsoft, and Google).
- *Sharing ideas and innovative information.* Making such sharing a normative part of meetings, dialogue with colleagues and coworkers, and interdisciplinary interaction gives leaders the opportunity to explore new thinking or potential change.

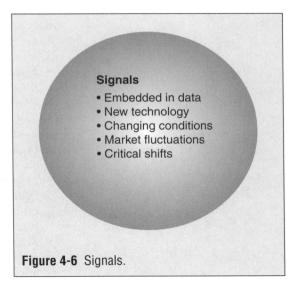

Figure 4-6 Signals.

TRIGGERS

The skills necessary to read signals are also indicated in response to trigger events. Trigger events are critical moments that serve to challenge awareness of an organization or its leadership with regard to direct, immediate, or dire circumstances. Trigger events are those critical actions occurring either contextually, peripherally, or in the midst of the work environment in a way that creates the immediate need for response. Usually, trigger events are the last line of response occurring late in the cycle of predictive and adaptive circumstances and have been usually preceded by either long-standing or clearly enumerated signals.

Triggers often result from the confluence of forces, action, or nonaction in relationship to specific signals that are indicators of a major shift in an organization's or individual's reality (**Figure 4-7**). While signals suggest the introduction of a major condition or circumstance of change, triggers represent the specific and significant impact of that change. Still, trigger events can often be missed by an organization. When that happens, organizations are frequently driven into a reactive state attempting to reconfigure to contemporary or ongoing symptoms evidenced by the change having already occurred. The ability to respond appropriately is significantly diminished since trigger events suggest that the impact of change indicated by prior signals has initially been missed or ignored and is now operating to directly affect the integrity and functions of the organization and its people.

Trigger events tend to increase in number and intensity to the extent that they are ignored or their recognition has been delayed. If they are ignored long enough or if response has been delayed over a sufficiently long period of time, the organization becomes more reactive and catch-up time between the demand for change indicated by the trigger

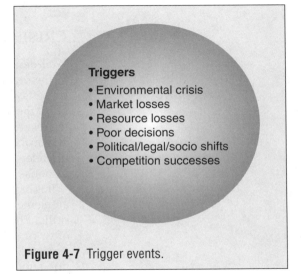

Figure 4-7 Trigger events.

events and the organization's actual response to change extends dramatically. There are several things the quantum leader needs to consider in addressing trigger events:

- *Specific signals to which the trigger event relates.* These signals can serve as a way of measuring the impact of the signals on a strategy and function of the organization and its people.
- *The number of trigger events.* Trigger events rarely occur as single entities. Usually a number of trigger events converge to indicate a serious gap between where the organization and its people are and where they need to be if they were responsive to the demands of any particular signal.
- *Response time to triggers.* Frequently, triggers, like signals, are ignored or missed by organizations, putting leadership in a tenuous position. Requiring a relatively quick turnaround time is a means of appropriately configuring the demand for change.
- *Response to missed opportunities.* Frank evaluation of the missed opportunity is a requisite of strong leadership in order to help leaders avoid blame, punishment, and recidivistic activities that keep the organization from focusing on its issues, diagnosing its response to signals and trigger events, and reconfiguring infrastructure and strategic process to be better responsive to signals in the future.

CRISIS PREPAREDNESS

Much work has been done and literature published related to direct crisis intervention and crisis response. There are many references to that, some of which can be found in the references in this chapter. However, the truth is that much crisis could be more effectively managed if it was linked into the ongoing operational activities of the leadership and staff of the organization. The predictive skills and processes present in an organization and covered in this chapter are critical to assuring the organization's and leader's effectiveness. An effective environmental scanning system and processes managed by senior leaders in the organization and demanded of first-line departmental or service leaders can do much to help the organization anticipate the inevitable transformations that impact all living systems (see **Figure 4-8**). Still, identifying conditions, circumstances, signals, and triggers are not sufficient to adequately prepare the organization for its proactive response to the potential for crisis. Crisis preparedness planning must be built into the operating infrastructure and management processes of the organization as much as any other management processes or ongoing part of doing business in response to customer or patient needs. The wise leader knows that building an operating framework for successfully accommodating the inevitable impact of change is as necessary as good policy and effective budgeting.

CRISIS PLANNING

Well-designed crisis plans reflect the character and content that give life and direction to the organization (**Figure 4-9**). All organizations are at one time or another affected by crisis. Good leaders recognize this as an operating given. Therefore, the only way to offset the inevitability of crisis is both information and preparation. Information gathering relates to the work discussed above reflected in an effective environmental scanning system. Nothing affects crisis preparedness more than clarity and readiness. Expectations of leadership performance include the obligation for systematic and organized planning response to anticipating, predicting, and adapting to the impact of crisis.

It is important for the leader to recognize that crisis management skills are as much an element of performance value as are human resource management or budgeting skills. Recognizing that crisis potential is constant and therefore an expected part of work demands helps to support the tenet that crisis management capacity is an expected skill set embedded in the work of management. Therefore, the organization should clearly state that policy, performance, and role evaluation will include

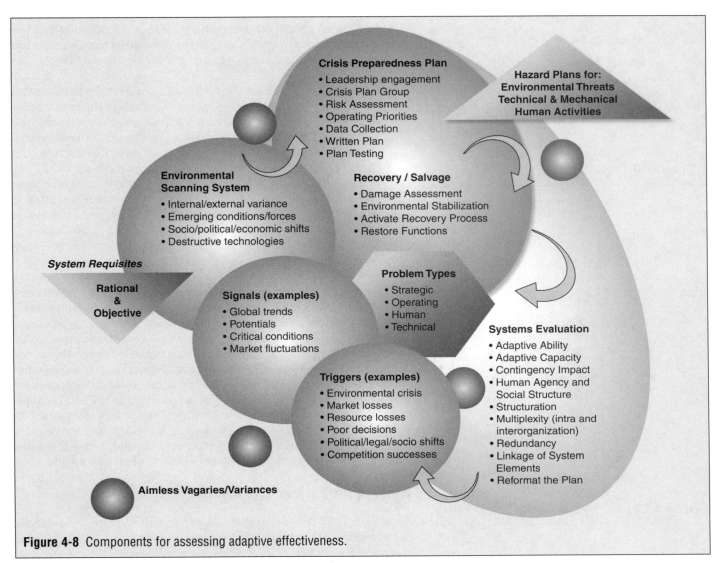

Figure 4-8 Components for assessing adaptive effectiveness.

the organization's expectations for comprehending and applying environmental scanning skills, interpreting and implementing crisis prediction and planning processes, and acting in concert with the crisis plan. Crisis planning elements should include:

- The role and performance expectation of leaders in constructing and acting consistently with the requisites of crisis management activities.
- Full participation in crisis plan construction activities as well as the development, application, and evaluation of all crisis plans, including those hazard plans for environmental, technical, mechanical, and human threats.
- Processes for recognizing both signal changes and trigger events (or their potential) and the probability of their impact on the strategy, priorities, and operating activities of the organization and its people.
- The design, construction, and application of specific plans for particular crisis potentials or hazards.

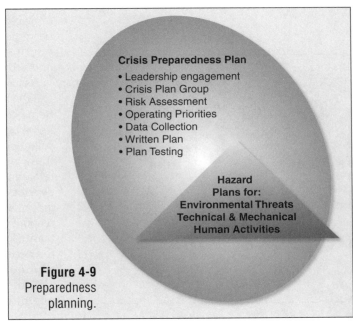

Figure 4-9
Preparedness
planning.

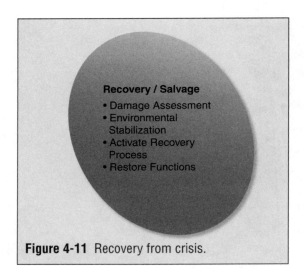

Sensitivity Focus

- Specific field of endeavor
- Market particulars
- Service uniqueness
- Technology arena
- Region or locality

Figure 4-10 Sensitivity.

- The skills, checks, and responses built into leadership process, including crisis activities as a part of the regular management and leadership performance dynamic at every leadership level of the organization.
- Enumeration of areas of sensitivity obtained from the field, context, environment, or particularly unique situations of the organization and its people as a part of developing a risk assessment framework. This helps define the arenas of risk and focus the activities associated with identifying its potential in those areas directly related to the functions and activities of the organization (Rike, 2003).
- Mechanisms for the organization and its people to include requirements for response to signal and trigger recognition regardless of where it might occur in the organization. Use of good information systems and data algorithms for getting to this information in a timely fashion and responding to it appropriately are critical tools of ongoing crisis awareness, prediction, and response.

Preparedness simply means awareness and response. Awareness should not be an accidental or involuntary mechanism, but rather, it should be included in the normative expectation of leadership practice at all levels of the organization. Mechanisms, processes, and an information system infrastructure should make it possible for predictive and adaptive strategies to be seen as a functional component of the effective work of management. If this is so, less idealization of crisis intervention and accommodation skills will occur, a reduction in the total number of crisis events will be noted, and better skills will be developed for preparing the organization and its people for addressing the ongoing vagaries and dynamics of the change process and, indeed, making change a normative part of the work experience (see **Figure 4-10**).

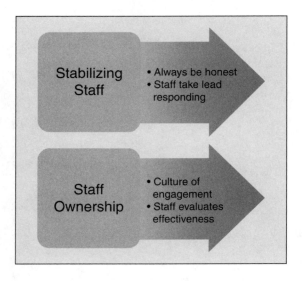

Recovery / Salvage
- Damage Assessment
- Environmental Stabilization
- Activate Recovery Process
- Restore Functions

Figure 4-11 Recovery from crisis.

RECOVERY AND SALVAGE

Even with all of the preparedness mechanisms in place, crises occur. Leadership demonstrates awareness of crisis reality by assuring that the response strategies to a crisis are appropriate and specific and, more importantly, assure success and thriving. Mechanisms must be in place to assist leaders in responding to the crisis and undertaking the best, most proactive responses necessary to address the conflict and to return the organization to its continuing focus on its purposes, goals, and activities.

Assessing the level of impact and damage to the organization is usually the first line of response to the impact of a crisis (see **Figure 4-11**). Being clear about the crisis situation and its effect on the organization helps position leaders in the most enlightened framework for appropriate planned response. Also, the assessment phase helps establish a framework of comparison between the actual crisis and the planning related to it in order to evaluate the veracity of the crisis response plan developed at an earlier time. It gives leadership an opportunity to make judgments about the goodness of fit between crisis planning and crisis response. This has two benefits—the first to address the adequacy of planning activities in preparation for the crisis and the second to make the necessary revisions in the plan in order to more adequately address a future conflict.

At the earliest stages of crisis response, the leader must be willing to inform and stabilize staff in order to maximize their capacity to respond

Stabilizing Staff
- Always be honest
- Staff take lead responding

Staff Ownership
- Culture of engagement
- Staff evaluates effectiveness

appropriately to the crisis situation. The crisis event must be placed in the context of a larger reality so that a broader perspective may be developed for staff response and a calm and organized approach may be undertaken in order to address it. The systematic, organized, and balanced response from leadership creates the context for staff response and provides a frame of confidence and rationality to staff engagement of activities that can lead to appropriate and successful crisis response. Staff engagement and involvement in crisis response activities is a critical indicator of success. Furthermore, it represents a level of trust and inclusion and suggests ownership investment on the part of the staff not only in the work of the organization but in its culture.

Each crisis recovery will have a crisis recovery plan that relates specifically to proactive and effective issues of addressing the crisis in a meaningful way. All crisis recovery plans should at least have the elements listed in **Figure 4-12** as a way of assuring or checking off that all appropriate responses to the crisis and to its potential for recurrence have been adequately addressed.

- Establish the command center for crisis response based on nature of the crisis.
- Identify and assist first responders and their work.
- Express confidence and control.
- Communication and information management.
- Adequate command center and resources for immediate action.
- Identify and engage all partners in recovery process.
- Reconfigure normalcy ASAP.
- Assess progress, make changes, note impact on plan, change plan.
- Coordinate action plans and initiative to assure comprehensive response.
- Evaluate process and progress, adjusting in operation and planning for strategy changes.

Figure 4-12 Response activities.

CORRECTING DISCONTINUITY

Crisis certainly means different things to different people. What might appear as a financial crisis to the business office may only appear as an irritant to the clinical services. Crisis therefore demands both definition and the establishment of a hierarchy of impact. This process enables the organization to rate crisis and to adjust the intensity of response based on the degree of crisis and its ultimate impact on the organization. When we see crisis more as a discontinuity than as a singular seminal event, it is easier to put it in context and to assure that its parameters don't widen beyond the real frame of the crisis. In addition, it is wise to keep crisis as compartmentalized as it demands so it does not impact or upset more components of the system than it needs. Since the crisis is often a continuous discrepancy between a particular critical event and the operating function of the system, it is important to relate the specific crisis to a specific systems component that is directly affected by the critical events (Mitroff, 2004). Good leaders will make sure that the crisis does not spill out into other aspects of the organization not directly affected nor necessarily involved in directly addressing the crisis.

Of course, preparing for a crisis can be safely compared to preparing for the unknown. Demonstrated in this chapter, however, is the value of integrating both predictive and adaptive capacity within the context of the role of the leader. In so doing, the quantum considerations of the impact of probability can be utilized to their maximum potential as a way of both anticipating normative crisis and of addressing it in his earliest possible stages. A very large element of predictive capacity is the leadership determination and management of internal operating risk related to not seeing crisis in its potential stage, or failing to recognize it as a potential and not responding to it early enough to be able to manage the organization and participant response in a timely fashion (Ranadive, 2005). Through the process of environmental scanning and within the dynamic of predictive strategies, enabling the organization and adapting responsive strategies creates an increasing level for continued success and long-term thriving for the organization. Since all these factors are predominantly a human function, some critical assessment of the human capacity and human activities associated with predictive and adaptive crisis management must be explored.

Controlling the Crisis Scenario

Joel had been manager of the medical surgical unit of Community Hospital for 12 years. Never in his career had he ever experienced a serious clinical crisis. However he and his staff were in the midst of one now for all of the 22 patients on his unit had contacted Methicillin resistant Staphylococcus aureus (MRSA). The infection had moved quickly through the unit and now every patient on the unit was at risk for the spread of the infection. Joel had just received a confirmation of the information and had not yet undertaken any action.

All had been well on the unit when he came in on Monday morning, yet, here it was Thursday afternoon and a serious problem had clearly emerged. In assessing the records he noted that all was well on the units until a young man, wounded in a gunfight, was placed on this unit and was the first case of MRSA. The staff had isolated this young man quickly and, as far as he knew everyone had been consistent with Universal Precautions. Still, on this Thursday afternoon MRSA had spread and unless something significant was undertaken shortly it would be a major crisis not only for his unit and his patients but also for the hospital.

Questions:

1. As Joel is thinking about the data that he's received, what are the implications of the data and how does it inform his first steps?
2. What mechanisms should already be in place in the organization and which controls should be operating and into which Joel should be able to tap as a part of his planned response?
3. What are the three first steps Joel should undertake in response to his MRSA crisis?
4. With whom should Joel be collaborating as he initiates the first stages of response to his MRSA crisis?
5. Does Joel compartmentalize the crisis or does he expand in order to access systems resources?
6. What might be the potential signals and subsequent trigger events that could have indicated the ultimate presence of the MRSA crisis?
7. What key elements would you suggest Joel include in his evaluation of response to this crisis as a way of informing future activities related to the potential for a similar crisis?

Human Dynamics of Crisis

Clearly, one of the most important elements of crisis management is the coordination and integration of the needs of people throughout the crisis process. Both from the perspective of anticipatory and predictive skills as well as intervention competence, leaders and staff need a level of continuous support. In addition, specific skills must be available in the organization and are an expected part of the competence of individuals if there is to be any level of guarantee that crisis management will occur in an effective and appropriate manner. It is expected that specific skill sets be available in particular roles in order to assure that the right cascade of expectations and performance in relationship to crisis is both enumerated and properly exercised. Specific role expectations must be clear and well defined as they are undertaken in the organization (Mittelstaedt, 2005).

Board

The board is perhaps the first major link in the organizational response change within the crisis process. From the perspective of establishing strategic clarity by assuring that the strategic plan is consistent with the mission purposes and objectives of the organization comes the first step in a series of steps necessary to assure full board engagement (see **Figure 4-13**). The awareness of the obligation of the organization to have an operational frame for predictive and adaptive strategies in crisis planning begins with the board's creation of a scanning framework. Within this framework is the overall environmental scanning plan and the subordinating crisis intervention plans related to strategic, operational, clinical, or environmental crisis. The scanning plan is both broad in its expectations regarding external awareness and even internal challenges all the way through specific delineations that indicate explicit responses to specific particular crisis. In addition, the board specifies with clarity where accountability exists all along the crisis management process and what roles are played out at the various levels and positions in the organization, especially in relationship to leadership roles. The roles of specific managers and clinical leaders in the organization have within them the expressed delineation of functions and activities related not only to responding to the crisis, but also in support of staff and patients as they address critical issues affecting their role in the crisis process.

It is also important for the board to clearly define the reporting expectations they have with regard to environmental scanning and the particular signals that may indicate the need for strategic readjustment, direction change, or technological reconfiguration. This reporting and communication expectation is critical to the board's continuing engagement and the immediacy of their response measured against the critical degree and impact of the signal or potential change. The convergence of signals and data that suggests the need for strategic or directional realignment is effective only insofar as it provides sufficient support and timeliness so that appropriate engagement can be positively enacted at the highest levels of the organization. It is at this point that strategic, policy, direction, and service changes can be undertaken in a way that maintains the stability and viability of the organization. The more seamless this process is at the governance level, the more fluid and flexible the adjustments to critical change can be at the operational level.

Senior Executives

It is at the executive level where translational activities that drive crisis responsive activities take form. The C suite of the organization is responsible for translating planned activities into tactical and applied actions in the organization in a way that ensures appropriate performance in both anticipating the potential for crisis and managing the system through it (see **Figure 4-14**). It is the obligation of the senior executives of the organization to take the appropriate action related to the particular stage addressed in the environmental scanning and crisis management process. Since the executives are responsible for the management and translation of the strategic plan in the organization, anything having to do with a challenge or threat to the integrity of the strategic plan falls within the purview and auspices of executive leadership. The design of the plan and successful implementation of it throughout the organization becomes a major obligation of the functional activities of executive leadership. It is at this level of the organization where synthesis of data, communication, and other sources of information converge to indicate new understanding, impact on strategy, a shift in direction, or adjustments in the internal environment suggested by changes in the external reality.

Accountability for the effectiveness of the environmental scanning process, as well as the system of crisis management, rests with the senior executives. The integrity and efficacy of the environmental scanning and crisis plan along with its various subcomponents become the critical tools for executive effectiveness. They are also responsible for the appropriate locus of control for specific accountability with regard to various components and functions of crisis management; e.g., specific delineation of departmental managers' roles in scanning technology related to their specific clinical services.

Along with the assignment of accountability to departmental leadership go the essential tools for action in order to give them both the competencies and the requisite resources for success in both environmental scanning activities and signal and trigger identification. Expectation for performance should be accompanied with a methodology and a set of tools that can assist the department manager in undertaking that work. Since the focus of environmental scanning at the departmental level will be on the technical and clinical forces specific to the function or service characteristics of the department, the tools must be just as specific. Access to appropriate external and internal data, journals, technical monographs, trends, policy, and practices provide an appropriate framework for the kinds of tools necessary to the expectation by the executive for the departmental manager (see **Figure 4-15**). Within the context of the environmental scanning and crisis identification process outlined by the board and the senior executive team, the role of the departmental manager must be such that the specific kinds of information relevant to that individual's role must be made available with the cost of such resources borne as a part of the operating reality of the department.

In addition to providing tools for department directors, it is also important to make sure that internal reporting mechanisms provide an opportunity to generate information from all levels of the organization that impact the external and internal circumstances influencing strategy, tactics, or operational judgment. Building communication mechanisms between critical positions in the organization that express accountability

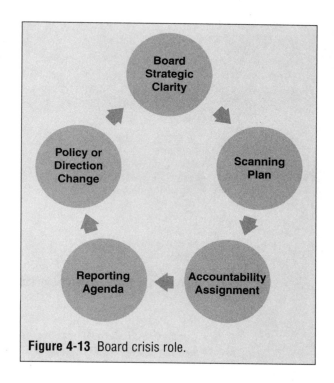

Figure 4-13 Board crisis role.

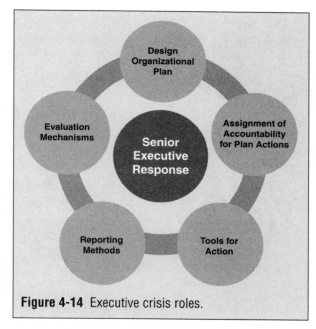

Figure 4-14 Executive crisis roles.

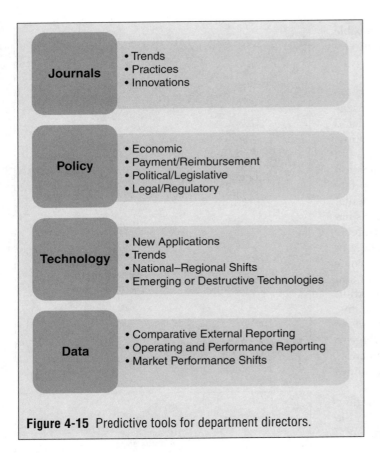

Figure 4-15 Predictive tools for department directors.

for specific scanning and predictive activities is a critical element that assures the success of the developed crisis management model.

Communication strategies and reporting mechanisms should focus on translating and demonstrating the clarity of the signals and the potential impact they have on the work of the organization (see **Figure 4-16**). The veracity and effectiveness of these reporting mechanisms and their ability to generate data early in the cycle of communication has a significant impact on the organization's viability and on addressing those factors that will impact it early enough to make a discernible difference (Argenti, 2002). If staff or department directors are generating information that indicates trigger events are in play, evidence of late-stage activities becomes very apparent and accelerates the chance that reactive strategies related to corrective action or accommodation may be the next step the organization is forced to take. Reporting mechanisms must be incorporated into a cycle of management accountability in the communication and interaction between departmental directors and senior executives in the organization. Ongoing and regular interactions around environmental factors, technological changes, or other social and political implications should be considered a regular reporting activity within the management structure. It is incongruous in most organizations that exceptionally detailed plans related to financial and budget management are required at all levels of leadership, yet little attention is paid to the environmental and contextual issues that have a more dramatic impact on long-term financial viability than does regular budget management and variance analysis.

No strategy or mechanism can be deemed viable and effective if there aren't ongoing evaluation processes that look at both the structure of the model and the effectiveness of actions within it. An organization needs to attest to the veracity of this crisis management process through internal analysis and comparative assessment related to its ability to anticipate, predict, and accommodate the potential for crisis (Millar & Heath, 2004). Failure to do so effectively may not simply be an indication of poor response. Failure to anticipate and predict might be a stronger indication of the effectiveness of the model than of the skills of the leadership.

Evaluation systems that are relevant both in assessing the veracity of the model and the effectiveness of leadership activities provide significant indicators of organizational effectiveness and sustainability (see **Figure 4-17**). A regular board-generated assessment of the environmental scanning model as well as the crisis-planning activities and the related plans is the first place to generate an assessment of effectiveness. The board has the overall accountability for assuring that the operational functions within the organization demonstrate what is necessary to ensure the vitality of the organization, the integrity of its strategic activities, and the success of its tactical and operating choices in ensuring the continued thriving of the organization.

The ability to thrive depends on the goodness of fit between the model and plans in place for anticipating, predicting, and accommodating change and crisis and the

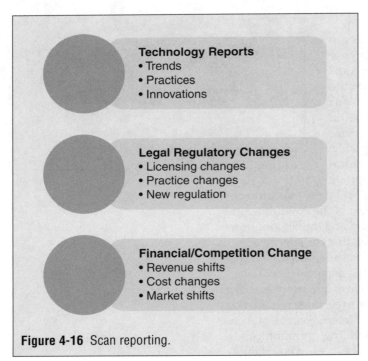

Figure 4-16 Scan reporting.

ongoing operations and functions of the organization in advancing its interests. The senior executive team evaluates the environmental scanning model, demonstrates its efficacy, and presents data with regard to its effectiveness to board leadership. It is the obligation of the board to assure the effectiveness of the overall environmental scanning model and make whatever adjustments are necessary to make it more valuable. The context of environmental scanning includes the crisis and disaster plans that relate to the specific service requirements and social obligations of the institution as an accountable member of the larger community. Senior executives need to demonstrate to the board that all of the crisis-related plans operate effectively and accomplish the ends that meet the board's intent. In addition, senior executives must assure the board that the testing and response activities related to assuring the effectiveness of the plans have proven successful. Whatever accommodations need to be made to reflect adjustments in the planning activities, the improved responses need also be noted and communicated to the board in order to assure them that the model operates consistent with its need and demonstrates an effective and meaningful response.

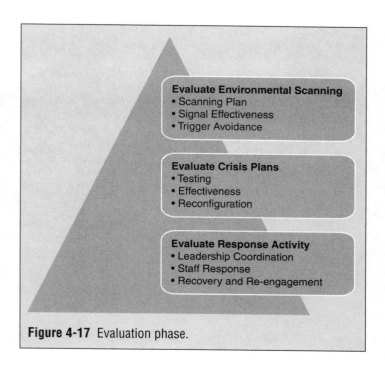

Figure 4-17 Evaluation phase.

Departmental Managers and Staff

The effective implementation and application of an environmental scanning model and crisis plan depends entirely on how first-line management and staff will articulate a plan with their own activities and successfully implement its requisites. Crisis plans should always be developed in conjunction with first-line staff in order to assure that the realities of decision making in practice in the service arena are the key driving force for the implementation plan. It stands to reason that staff closest to the realities of impact and implementation are the critical variable in ensuring the success of implementing crisis plans.

Staff also has value with regard to the environmental scanning activities, especially when those activities directly relate to issues of service and practice. Professional workers especially have a critical relationship to issues and circumstances that affect practice activities and potentially serve to challenge or change the conditions and circumstances that govern or influence practice activities. Wise organizational leaders always seek to engage their professional colleagues in scanning activities and in participating in dialogue and decisions related to the impact of change driven by both external and internal circumstances. Frequently, a change in professional requisites, practice models, or the technology related to service can have a dramatic impact on the functions and activities of the organization. Changes in professional standards of practice, education, ethics, and values can have a radical effect on the priorities, choices, and actions of the organization and its leadership team. Integrating the professional roles in environmental scanning and crisis planning activities assures inclusion of potential shifts in practice, priorities, and financial realities as they affect the mission and strategic activities of the organization. Failure to incorporate professional staff in these leadership activities occurs at the organization's own peril. Therefore critical inclusive and functional activities associated with staff involvement and participation must be well enumerated as a part of the organization's application of its environmental scanning and crisis planning process (see **Figure 4-18**).

> ### Quantum Leadership Gem
>
> Not including professional staff in decisions that relate specifically to environmental scanning and crisis planning threatens the integrity of the organization and almost certainly advances a serious potential for crisis. Professional staff is closest to the point of service and often has the most incisive access to emerging potential for crisis. Engaging them is critical to ensuring organizational success.

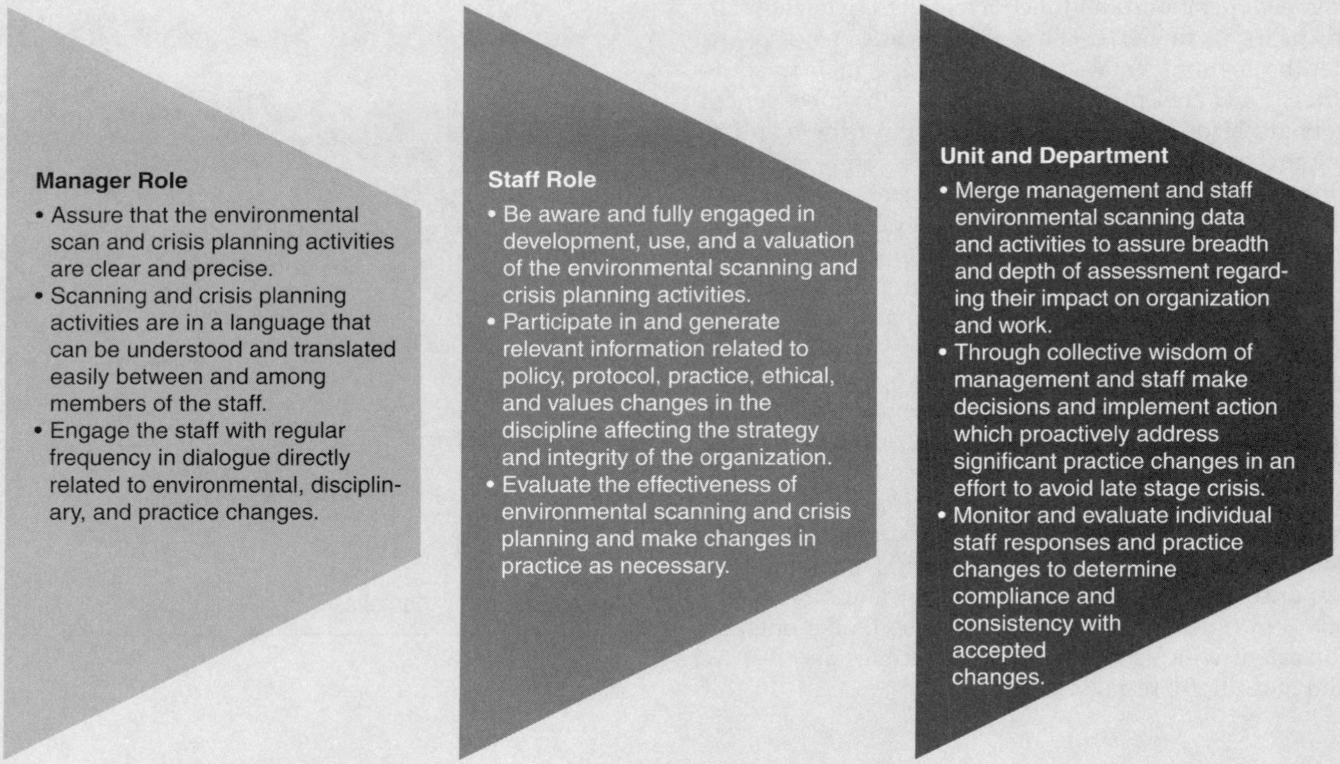

Manager Role
- Assure that the environmental scan and crisis planning activities are clear and precise.
- Scanning and crisis planning activities are in a language that can be understood and translated easily between and among members of the staff.
- Engage the staff with regular frequency in dialogue directly related to environmental, disciplinary, and practice changes.

Staff Role
- Be aware and fully engaged in development, use, and a valuation of the environmental scanning and crisis planning activities.
- Participate in and generate relevant information related to policy, protocol, practice, ethical, and values changes in the discipline affecting the strategy and integrity of the organization.
- Evaluate the effectiveness of environmental scanning and crisis planning and make changes in practice as necessary.

Unit and Department
- Merge management and staff environmental scanning data and activities to assure breadth and depth of assessment regarding their impact on organization and work.
- Through collective wisdom of management and staff make decisions and implement action which proactively address significant practice changes in an effort to avoid late stage crisis.
- Monitor and evaluate individual staff responses and practice changes to determine compliance and consistency with accepted changes.

Figure 4-18 Departmental response.

1. At the unit or departmental level, leaders should assure that regular meeting and discussion time is devoted to particular professional policy, protocol, practices, and values. These are reviewed with attention to their implications and impact for changing practices.

2. The unit or departmental manager should review with professional staff the broader environmental and contextual changes leadership has discerned that may affect the organization's priority and the work of the professional staff. Dialogue should reveal issues of impact, accommodation, adjustments, or change in clinical practice.

3. Staff-generated insights with regard to environmental, market, discipline-specific, and rule changes should be given as much weight to the impact on organizational integrity and strategic choices as any other scanning insight occurring at the management level.

4. Honest and open communication and transparency of environmental scanning and crisis-related data must be as available to staff leadership as it is to the management team in order to assure and maintain levels of trust and full engagement between management and staff.

5. Staff investment in the evaluation processes helps assure the relevance of those activities and to specify with a high level of clarity the point-of-service changes and adjustments necessary to increase the effectiveness related to implementing plan activities.

SYSTEMS EVALUATION

Environmental scanning and crisis planning is a dynamic exercise. While the constructs and elements of the scanning and planning processes may remain relatively constant, the content and elements are forever changing; just as the social, contextual, and environmental characteristics influencing the dynamics of an organization are in constant flow in shift, so must also be the elements of the plan. The organization can only be as adaptive as the information and tools it has to undertake adaptation. Therefore it is critical that an evaluation mechanism be embedded in the environmental scanning and crisis planning process so that it may be viewed as a functional element of the dynamics of environmental scanning and crisis planning (Rike, 2003).

Embedded in the governance activities of the board related to environmental scanning and crisis planning are factors that indicate how relevant and adaptive the scanning model and crisis plans have been (see **Figure 4-19**). Using continuous evaluation processes identified in this chapter, the board and senior executives assess the viability and adaptability of the plan and the veracity and integrity of its adaptation to both successfully predicting the potential for crisis and providing tools for adapting, changing, or accommodating the impact of crisis on the organization. Clearly, the adaptive capacity of the organization includes its ability to change course and to make internal adjustments to external and operating realities in real time. The turnaround time an organization undertakes to adjust to changes in its reality is a significant driver represented in cost and resource use. The later this stage of engagement, and the higher the intensity of the response to the signals or triggers that indicate the strength and immediacy of change, the higher the cost and more incisive the impact.

The fluidity and flexibility of the scanning model and crisis plan are good testament to the viability and effectiveness of both. If the organization can evidence its ability to engage the potential for crisis early in the cycle of its impact, sufficient evidence is provided that both the model and crisis plans are valid and viable. However, if the organization finds itself responding at the same level of reactivity and intensity as occurred before the development of the environmental scanning model and crisis plans, strong evidence suggests their lack of vitality. Certainly, the board does not want to have in place mechanisms that make no difference or that have no impact on the organization's effectiveness.

A number of elements are essential to ensure multilevel participation in the evaluation of the effectiveness of either model or crisis plans, as shown in **Figure 4-20**.

Evaluating systems effectiveness is as critical a process as any other element of use for the environmental scanning model and for crisis plans. If a model is not flexible and easily adjusted, then its viability and applicability are in question. From board to staff, an organization must find that the models it develops and within which it operates have great utility, fluidity, and flexibility, and that they can be applied in a wide variety of circumstances. Adjusting and implementing the model and creating viability is the work of all leadership. The ability to address, anticipate, and predict a crisis is the sign of effective and enlightened leadership. Both the organization and the professionals who serve within it should expect no less of their leaders.

This chapter has focused on articulating and using a model for the application of predictive and adaptive capacity in leadership and in organizations. While predictive and adaptive capacity is certainly an element of the skill set of the leader, it is also a construct of the organization. The effectiveness of the organization depends on the systems that are constructed and whether they are utilized in a way that helps

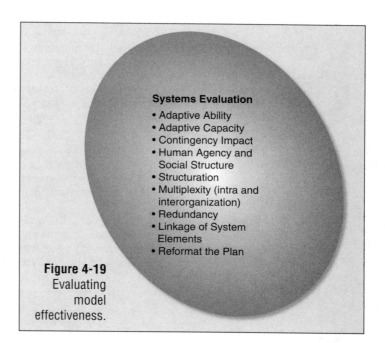

Systems Evaluation
- Adaptive Ability
- Adaptive Capacity
- Contingency Impact
- Human Agency and Social Structure
- Structuration
- Multiplexity (intra and interorganization)
- Redundancy
- Linkage of System Elements
- Reformat the Plan

Figure 4-19
Evaluating model effectiveness.

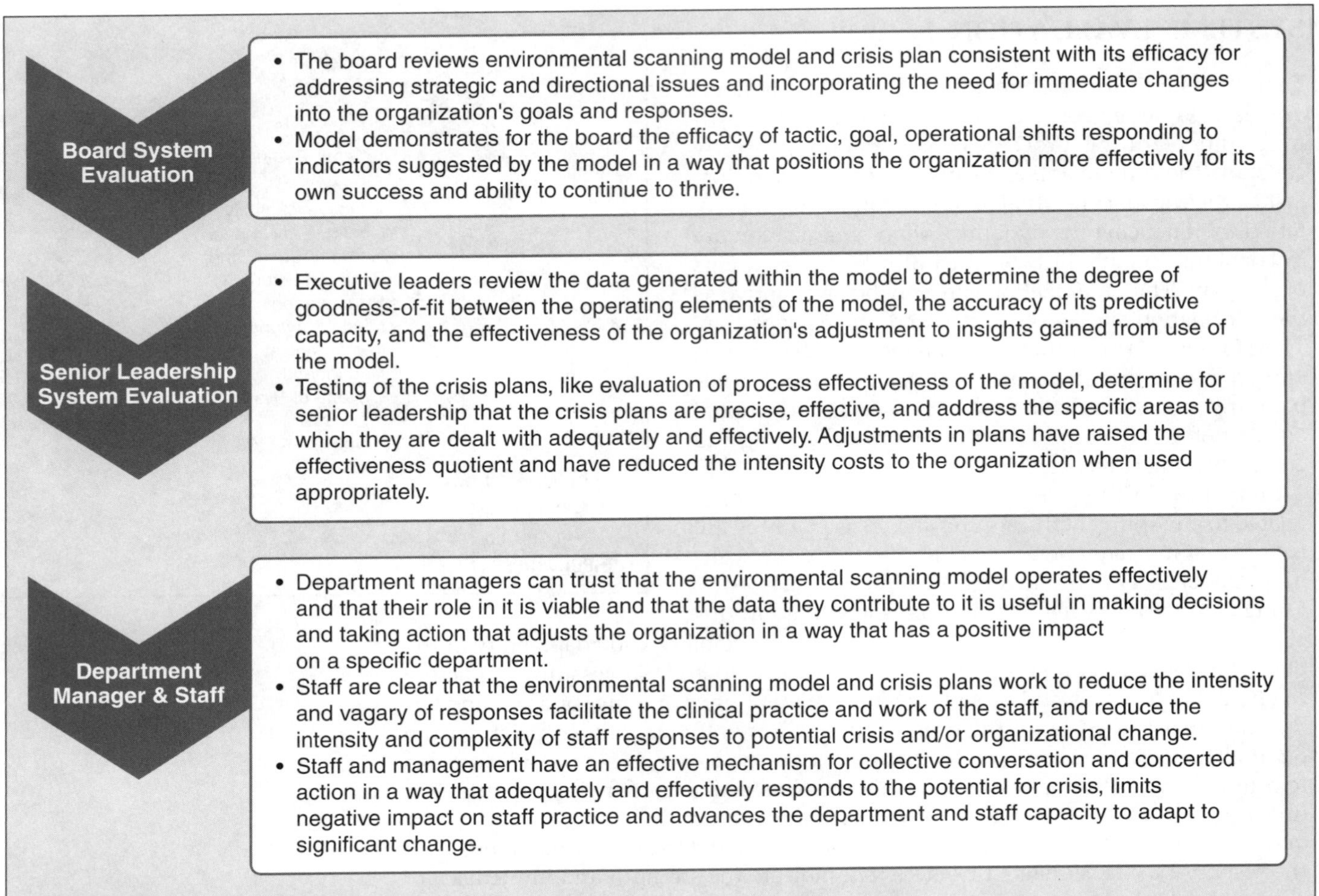

Figure 4-20 System evaluation.

Board System Evaluation
- The board reviews environmental scanning model and crisis plan consistent with its efficacy for addressing strategic and directional issues and incorporating the need for immediate changes into the organization's goals and responses.
- Model demonstrates for the board the efficacy of tactic, goal, operational shifts responding to indicators suggested by the model in a way that positions the organization more effectively for its own success and ability to continue to thrive.

Senior Leadership System Evaluation
- Executive leaders review the data generated within the model to determine the degree of goodness-of-fit between the operating elements of the model, the accuracy of its predictive capacity, and the effectiveness of the organization's adjustment to insights gained from use of the model.
- Testing of the crisis plans, like evaluation of process effectiveness of the model, determine for senior leadership that the crisis plans are precise, effective, and address the specific areas to which they are dealt with adequately and effectively. Adjustments in plans have raised the effectiveness quotient and have reduced the intensity costs to the organization when used appropriately.

Department Manager & Staff
- Department managers can trust that the environmental scanning model operates effectively and that their role in it is viable and that the data they contribute to it is useful in making decisions and taking action that adjusts the organization in a way that has a positive impact on a specific department.
- Staff are clear that the environmental scanning model and crisis plans work to reduce the intensity and vagary of responses facilitate the clinical practice and work of the staff, and reduce the intensity and complexity of staff responses to potential crisis and/or organizational change.
- Staff and management have an effective mechanism for collective conversation and concerted action in a way that adequately and effectively responds to the potential for crisis, limits negative impact on staff practice and advances the department and staff capacity to adapt to significant change.

the organization deal with highly probabilistic circumstances and occurrences that affect its life and its future. Crises need not be accidental, interruptive, or critical in their impact on the organization. Only late-stage crisis response creates such negative forces for the organization and its people. Through the use of a model, such as suggested in this chapter, a framework for building probability-based management strategies into the operating structure of the organization can be constructed in a way that has a positive impact on success and sustainability. Making the application of just such a model a part of the operating life and activity of the organization is itself a great predictor for successfully anticipating, handling, and harnessing the energy of probability and the potential for crisis in a way that advances and strengthens the organization and its people.

REFERENCES

Argenti, P. (2002). Crisis communication. *Harvard Business Review, 80* (12), 20–28.

Bridges, W. (2002). *Way of transition.* New York: Perseus Books.

Gharajedaghi, J. (1999). *Systems thinking: Managing chaos and complexity—a platform for designing business architecture.* Boston, MA: Butterworth-Heinemann.

Hamson, N., & Holder, R. (2002). *Global innovation.* Oxford: Capstone.

Hassett, M. (2007). *Probability for risk management.* Winsted, CT: Actex Publishers.

Heifetz, R., & Linsky, M. (2002). *Leadership on the line.* Boston: Harvard Business School Press.

Kelly, S., & Allison, M.A. (1999). *The complexity advantage.* New York: McGraw-Hill Publishers.

Millar, D.P., & Heath, R.L. (2004). *Responding to crisis: A rhetorical approach to crisis communication.* Mahwah, NJ: Lawrence Erlbaum.

Mitroff, I. (2004). *Crisis leadership: Planning for the unthinkable.* New York: Wiley.

Mittelstaedt, R.E. (2005). *Will your next mistake be fatal? Avoiding the chain of mistakes that can destroy.* Upper Saddle River, N.J.: Wharton School.

Ranadive, V. (2005). *Power to predict: How real-time businesses anticipate customer needs, create opportunities, and beat the competition.* New York: McGraw-Hill.

Rike, B. (2003). Prepared or not . . . that is the vital question. *Information Management Journal, 37* (3), 25–35.

Snyder, N.T., & Duarte, D.L. (2003). *Strategic innovation: Embedding innovation as a core competency in your organization.* San Francisco: Jossey-Bass.

Stabor, U., & Sydow, J. (2002). Organizational and adaptive capacity: A structural perspective. *Journal of Management Inquiry, 11* (4), 408–424.

Weick, K.E. (2001). *Making sense of the organization.* Malden, MA: Blackwell Business.

SUGGESTED READINGS

Dana, J. (2006). *Complexity.* Frederick, MD: PublishAmerica.

Fink, S. (2000). *Crisis management: Planning for the inevitable.* New York: Backinprint.

Hassett, M. (2007). *Probability for risk management.* Winsted, CT: Actex Publishers.

Porter-O'Grady, T., & Malloch, M. (2007). *Quantum leadership: A resource for healthcare innovation.* Boston: Jones and Bartlett.

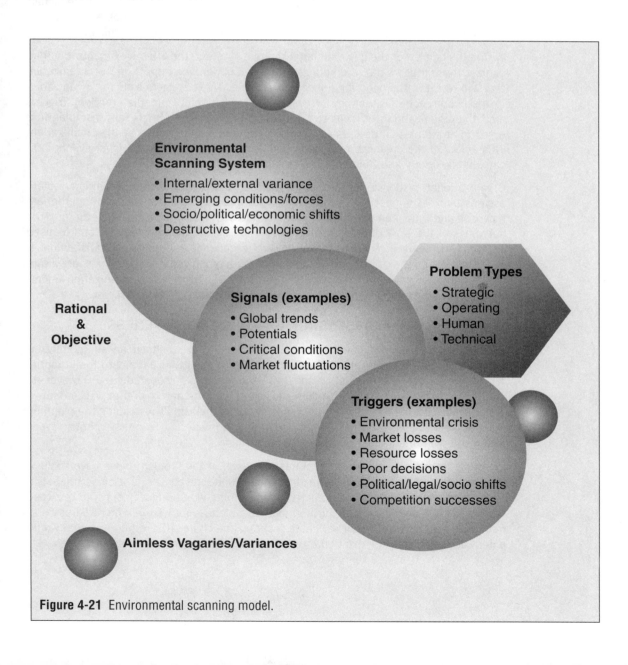

Figure 4-21 Environmental scanning model.

ENVIRONMENTAL SCANNING AND CRISIS PLANNING

In the interest and effort to assure that an organization is able to carry out its mission, purposes, and objectives in a sustainable way, it must be able to assess its place in an ever-changing world and in shifting conditions that affect its competitiveness and viability in its market. To do this, it must have an effective environmental scanning process that helps it anticipate, predict, and act on forces that affect its existence and viability. Therefore, an environmental scanning model helps focus objectively and deliberatively in a way that frames an organization's ability to predict and adapt to environmental and circumstantial shifts and changes.

Those who use an effective environmental scanning system are able to predict and anticipate critical events regardless of where they occur through the system's ability to identify signals that alert the organization to potential or impending circumstances or occurrences having an impact on the organization. The scanning processes that constantly send these signals to the organization provide a continuous flow of information about broad-based global, environmental, market, technological, and human potentials having a direct impact on the organization's ability to do its business (Weick & Sutcliffe, 2001). These signals represent to the organization those issues and concerns as well as trends and potentials that directly affect the mission, purpose, and work objectives of the organization.

Within the context of the environmental scanning system, the effective organization recognizes those triggers that exemplify a direct and impending impact on the organization that will result in the need for a specific response. These triggers alert the organization to the occurrence of situations or events that will require immediate action. Triggers alert the organization's officials to the need to implement its crisis response plan in a way and at a time that assures appropriate response is undertaken by the organization. This ability of the organization's leaders to immediately respond to trigger events indicates its flexibility and fluidity in the face of crisis.

Organizational response to the application of the environmental scanning system assures that the impact of crisis is minimized, and the organization, given appropriate response and time, can maintain its viability and continue to do its work. Therefore, the outcomes of the work of the organization, while necessarily adjusted, are still focused on quality, timeliness, service, and/or product excellence and customer satisfaction. It is implied within the context of the model that both employees and customers are aware of the action of environmental scanning and of the activities the organization undertakes to respond to crisis and continue to meet the needs of those it serves.

COMPONENTS FOR ASSESSING ADAPTIVE EFFECTIVENESS

Establishing a framework for environmental scanning is not itself an adequate context for addressing inevitable crisis. The ability to predict and anticipate the potential for crisis provides the foundation for organizational crisis preparedness. However, to assure that appropriate action is taken consistent with the nature of the crisis, adaptive effectiveness demands a specific crisis-planning mechanism. Those doing the planning must be able to confront the strategic, operating, human, and technical problem types that result from the impact of crisis events.

Planning for crisis preparedness requires that each of the problem types have specific planning processes that enumerate the organization's responses to a crisis impact in all problem areas. Good crisis preparedness planning would identify specific response plans for each problem type. Furthermore, the plans would sufficiently address particular kinds of threats—environmental, technical/mechanical, and human—that would potentially affect the organization through one or all of its potential problem types.

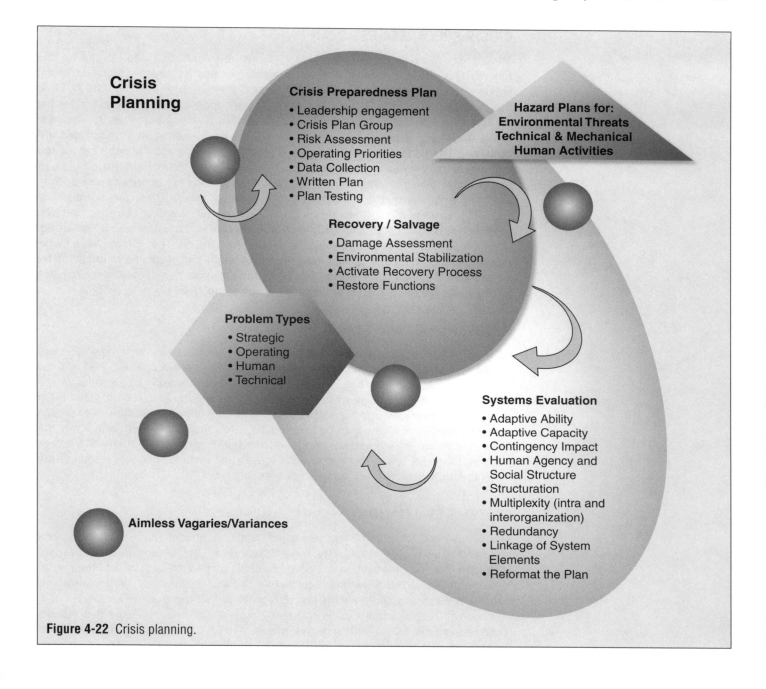

Figure 4-22 Crisis planning.

CRISIS PREPAREDNESS PLAN

The composite crisis preparedness plan includes elements that address the specific functional priorities of the organization in each of its problem areas. The structure and elements of crisis preparedness planning can be credited to B. Rike (Rike, 2003). Effective planning would include the specific engagement and expectations of leadership and the role they would play in implementing designated planning activities. A crisis plan group should also be identified, with specific tasks and responsibilities associated with each role. Tying crisis to the environmental scanning system and the potential for specific response requires a well-refined mechanism of risk potential and the assessment of risk impact on the organization. A good planning process ascertains risk-specific operating priorities that best respond to the potential crisis. These are clarified with appropriate outlined responses. From the environmental scanning activities and data collection related to potential signals and likely trigger events, a database is established to inform particular crisis response steps (McCrackan, 2005). The written plan includes all of these elements and is detailed and clear enough that it can be mutually understood by all the stakeholders and effectively implemented. A mechanism for regularly testing (6 months to 1 year) is included as a part of the crisis planning process.

RECOVERY/SALVAGE STAGE

As a part of the cycle of crisis preparedness, the organization must have adequate means and processes for immediate recovery from a crisis event (Rike, 2003). Crisis preparedness anticipates that, given time, a crisis will inevitably occur. Adequacy of operational, matériel and process responses that lead to organizational stabilization should be incorporated into the recovery plan. The goal of crisis modeling is to prepare sufficient predictive capacity to be able to adequately respond to a crisis in a way that restores effective work processes and maintains the integrity and viability of the organization. Plans related to recovery and salvage should include adequate resources and matériel for damage recovery and normal work processes.

SYSTEMS EVALUATION

An effective predictive and adaptive system needs continuous monitoring and assessment to assure sufficient capacity and a goodness of fit between the organization's environmental scanning system (including its crisis preparedness plan) and the prevailing external and internal realities, constantly in flux, which affect the organization's viability. Anticipating and planning for crisis requires that the adaptive conditions of an ever-changing set of influences be constantly assessed in order to assure that planned responses are consistent with potential crises. A model for assessing adaptive effectiveness must include focus on the system's adaptive ability and capacity to address prevailing or potential conditions or circumstances that might negatively affect it.

Systems evaluation should include the elements related to human response to critical events and the ability of leadership, management, work, and the social infrastructure to adequately adapt and respond to a crisis event. Much of the effectiveness of the organization hinges on the ability of human and social systems to act consistent with planned responses and to adapt processes and behaviors appropriate to the situation. This structuration ensures that the actors in a crisis can consistently reproduce and change work and social practices in the face of a specific crisis. This means appropriate preparation with regard to legitimacy of authority, interaction and communication, control, and the morality and ethics of response.

A good systems assessment includes the review of multiplexity (the diversity of interactions and relationships between organizational networks) and redundancy (the presence of sufficient slack in the organization contrasted with efficiency in resources, processes, information, and adequate human dynamics). The linkage between essential networks of resources, supplies, supports, and systems ensures that the various affected units and related activities are sufficiently interdependent yet coupled in a way that facilitates effective crisis response and the return to normalization. Finally, good systems evaluation results in a reformatted crisis preparedness plan that reflects the adjustment to the new realities. Further enabling the assurance of an effective and systematic response strategy is the question tool set (tool for assessing adaptive effectiveness, see below). The focus of this set of questions is on the relationship to each element of the organization's adaptive capacity to effectively address a potential or real-time crisis.

Sample Question Tool for the Model for Assessing Adaptive Effectiveness

Crisis Preparedness Plan

The plan should provide clarity around the three major threats—natural or environmental threats, technical or mechanical hazards, and human activities—by identifying the specific threat influencing crisis preparedness.

Step 1: Leadership support and commitment. Is there clear evidence of leadership responsibility and accountability for coordinating, integrating, and linking disaster preparedness and a recovery plan as well as managing it, evaluating it, and updating it?

Step 2: Establishing the crisis planning group. Is there a designated group of diverse participants accountable for disaster identification, impact assessment, cost estimation, replacement issues, risk, and response to the identified crisis potentials for the organization?

Step 3: Performing the risk assessments. Is there a data-driven identification of the risk for the previously identified disasters, the consequences and impact of the disasters, cost assessments of damaging impact, replacement and recovery costs, and likelihood and risk of worst-case scenarios?

Step 4: Establishing processing and operating priorities. Are there elements that include equipment needs, communication devices, policies, procedures and steps of response, human resource needs, vital records needs, and contingencies necessary to establish an operational response?

Step 5: Performing data collection. Is there a mechanism for detailing and locating contracts and agreements, backup information systems, staffing information, inventory management, master lists, policies and procedures, security systems, backup sites, and command posts?

Step 6: Writing the plan. Do appropriate internal teams share a role in writing components of the plan related to administrative action, facilities, crisis logistics, support systems, computers and information systems, system restoration, and individual department operations?

Step 7: Testing that plan. Is there a regular plan testing process (at least annually) that undertakes testing the plan to determine the following: need for modification, reliability and compatibility of systems, facilities, and planned procedures, the presence of adequate procedures and processes, appropriate team training, organizational responsiveness demonstration, and mechanisms for updating and adjusting the plan?

Recovery and Salvage Processes

Step 1: Damage assessment. Is there a mechanism in place for assessing how much damage has occurred, the nature of the damage, the effect of the damage, records and communication systems damage, and insurance carrier responsiveness?

Step 2: Environmental stabilization. Are portable services available for electricity, water, air circulation, work environment management, and architectural and operational facilities within which recovery can be managed?

Step 3: Recovery team activation. Are work crews, processes, and mechanisms under way with clear understandings of responsibility and contribution and with adequate support to accomplish the task?

Step 4: Restoration of function. Have the environmental, operational, and process elements been integrated with structural and support processes and sufficiently recovered in order to assure ongoing normal operations at previous levels or within a new definition of performance capacity?

Systems Evaluation

Adaptive Ability

Is there an intra- and interorganizational process of adaptation that represents a dynamic process of continuing learning and adjustment that addresses ambiguity and complexity in the system?

Adaptive Capacity

Does learning in the organization take place at a faster rate than the rate of change in the conditions required to dismantle old routines and create new processes?

Contingency Impact

Are there systematic mechanisms in place that assist the organization in anticipating and planning for the impact of a variety of contingencies affecting its ability to operate (see Crisis Preparedness Plan)?

Human Agency and Social Structure

Can the human behaviors and responses aggregate sufficiently well to indicate a cohesive and collective response to critical events and contingencies?

Structuration

Are structure and human interaction linked dynamically with good integration of communication, power, sanctioning, and the forces necessary to facilitate and constrain legitimate action?

Multiplexity

Are the number and kind of interorganizational networks and interfaces sufficiently mature, complex, and linked to adequately respond to crisis across systems, including the full variety of stakeholders?

Redundancy

Is there sufficient slack (employees, productive capacity, overlaps, jobs, mistake tolerance, communication channels, and information capacity) to meet the dramatic impact of any major crisis or contingent event?

Linkage of System Elements

Do all systems link in a seamless connection demonstrating a network of responses at every level of the system, representing a comprehensive synthesis of organizational response to crisis?

Reformat the Plan

Do the revised plan and contingency format represent the adjustments, changes, updates, and enhancements necessary to assure as effective a plan for crisis in contingency as possible?

REFERENCES

McCrackan, A. (2005). *Practical guide to business continuity assurance.* Boston: Artech House, Inc.

Rike, B. (2003). Prepared or not…that is the vital question. *Information Management Journal, 37* (3), 25–35.

Weick, K. E., & Sutcliffe, K. M. (2001). *Managing the unexpected: Assuring high performance in an age of complexity.* San Francisco: Jossey-Bass.

CHAPTER 5

The Vulnerable Leader

CHAPTER OBJECTIVES:

Upon completion of this chapter, the reader will:

1. Develop an understanding of the value of leadership vulnerability as it relates to current healthcare organizations.

2. Apply skills in becoming more vulnerable and open to risk taking, using focused leadership scenarios.

3. Learn new techniques of information management, overcoming silence, assuring an ethical climate, and recognizing cosmology episodes to mediate leader risk.

4. Reinforce the value of the characteristics of high-reliability organizations as essential quantum leader tools.

INTRODUCTION

I don't have all the answers; am I a failure? Traditional organizations hold leaders to standards of rationality, clarity, and foresight—yet most leaders cannot meet these standards because they are human and face an incredible amount of unpredictability and fallible analyses of data. To be able to prosper and thrive in the current millennium, the leader must shift from the somewhat comfortable position of control to one of great uncertainty and vulnerability. In reality, uncertainty and need for vulnerability has always existed for leaders. With the current explosion of information technology and availability of information, the choice to lead using command and control behaviors is no longer an option. To be sure, no leader is alone in this journey. Colleagues, patients, and the community are aware of the plethora of data, data sources, and lack of clear pathways.

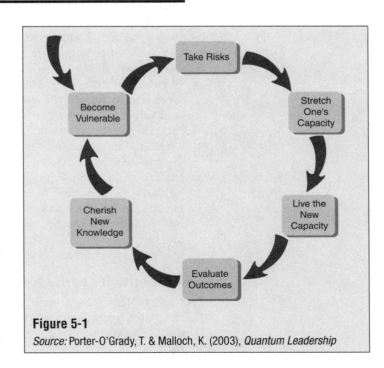

Figure 5-1
Source: Porter-O'Grady, T. & Malloch, K. (2003), *Quantum Leadership*

Vulnerability
Traditional Characteristics
• Weakness
• Open to or defenseless against criticism
• Susceptible to being wounded or hurt physically
• Susceptible to temptation or corrupt influence
Quantum Characteristics
• Openness to others
• Openness to new ideas
• Aware of limitations

Vulnerability and Transformational Leadership
Adherence to inspectional and fault-finding supervision under the guise of standards-based practice has serious negative consequences on goal achievement. Excellence is achieved when the emphasis is on approaching work so that vulnerability turns into possibilities and stagnation becomes transformation.
Jeffrey Glanz, Chairman, Wagner College, Staten Island, New York

A NEW LENS FOR LEADERS

Openness to new ideas requires skills embedded in the acceptance of vulnerability and all of the emerging realities that are encompassed in the cycle of vulnerability (Porter-O'Grady & Malloch, 2007). Yet most leaders believe that others expect them to have answers, to know the needs of the future, and, of course, to make money! When faced with the reality of the uncertain marketplace, most consumers are seeking honest and authentic leaders, not clairvoyants or charismatic magicians. Consumers recognize the uncertainty and, given the probable impact on their personal future, want to be a part of making decisions that impact their health. Consumers do not want to be mere recipients of healthcare plans created for them without their input.

The phases of the vulnerability cycle are presented as distinct entities for the purposes of discussion only. In reality, they are more often seamlessly linked. The six phases in the cycle are: becoming vulnerable, taking risks, stretching one's capacity, living the reality, evaluating the outcomes, and cherishing the new reality. Then the cycle begins again. The vulnerability cycle offers a new lens through which leaders can examine and evaluate leadership behaviors of both themselves and members of their team. Each phase will again occur with new situations and new strategies for the quantum leader to thrive on (Porter-O'Grady & Malloch, 2007).

VULNERABILITY

Vulnerability and Bad Leadership

While traditional leadership views vulnerability as a weakness, the new age of leadership embraces vulnerability as an essential competency. The notion of the vulnerable leader does not equate with bad leadership. The vulnerable leader of the quantum age is open to all realities, is collaborative, and is aware of limitations. In contrast, the bad leader, or bad leadership, is characterized by the power wielding of Richard Nixon; the master communications manipulation of Adolph Hitler; the tyranny of Howell Raines of the New York Times; those who do not address known dishonesty of their employees; or Dennis Kozlowski of Tyco, whose impudence, greed, and tax evasion resulted in criminal indictments (Kellerman, 2004). These leaders could have benefited from a greater understanding of vulnerability as a key leadership trait, evidenced by openness to others or to new ideas and by recognition of limitations. Vulnerability is a more appropriate way to lead, rather than through manipulation to protect one's reputation, dishonest communication to deceive others, arrogance, believed invincibility, and outright greed.

Of great importance is the reality that leadership is not a moral concept; leaders are trustworthy and deceitful, brave and cowardly, generous and greedy. To assume that all good leaders are good people is to be willfully blind to the reality of the human condition; such an assumption also limits our opportunity for becoming more effective at leadership (Kellerman, 2004). Further, leaders must remember that just because they are leaders, they are not necessarily trustworthy, brave, and generous and never deceitful, cowardly, or greedy. The recognition of fallibility allows leaders to manage the human condition and ultimately achieve greatness.

Authenticity Is the Key

Leadership styles, among them autocratic, democratic, and situational, provide templates for behavior. None, however, are absolute or appropriate for all situations. This plethora of leader styles can be daunting for the emerging leader. Formal monitoring programs provide guidance and recommendations to support role development. Yet, conforming to the normative leadership style of the organization or the recent literature recommendation can spell disaster for the leader. According to George (2004), great world leaders all had very different leadership styles—George Washington, Winston Churchill, Margaret Thatcher, Mother Teresa, and John F. Kennedy all led in their own unique way.

In reality, the success of the leader is more closely linked to personal authenticity than it is to a particular leadership style. It is your authenticity—not your leadership style—that really matters. Attempting to emulate another's leadership style can be disastrous. New leaders may desire a model of shared leadership but must understand and live the basic values in their personal lives in order to make shared leadership a reality. A lack of congruence between personal and professional values creates a reality gap that is obvious to team members. This gap compromises leader authenticity, as the leader talks the talk of shared leadership but is unable to fully live the values consistently.

The values of the authentic leader are shaped by personal beliefs and developed through study, reflection, and dialogue with others. These values create a moral compass for the leader and provide guidance in determining the right thing to do rather than blindly attempting to emulate the style of another leader.

A broad understanding of leadership styles serves merely as background information to understanding behavior options. Being one's own person is the key to developing an authentic leadership style that is consistent with one's personality and character. Ongoing development of one's personal leadership style continues as different situations and different people are encountered.

The authentic leader accepts personal faults as well as strengths and avoids attempting to win approval of others by covering up shortcomings and thus sacrificing authenticity to gain respect from others. There is no way a leader can do everything, be on top of the incoming mail, read the most recent literature, and be responsive to everything and everyone; attempting to be such a leader is only fooling oneself. According to Lencioni (1998), vulnerability is essential for building trust and requires behaviors that reflect caring about others and their success. The authentic, vulnerable leader knows what he or she knows, what he or she does not know, and is content with the limits of his or her capacity.

Integrity is closely linked to authenticity for the effective leader. In addition to personal authenticity, the vulnerable leader emulates integrity, a characteristic that is not just the absence of lying but the presence of telling the whole truth, no matter how difficult it might be. Leadership integrity is the uncompromising adherence to moral and ethical principles. From authenticity and integrity, trusting relationships emerge.

The next section of this chapter presents specific leader vulnerability behaviors that will further enhance vulnerability as a very positive characteristic.

Gem
If they can't trust you, why would they ever follow you?

Gem
Information voids will be filled by rumors and speculation unless they are preempted by open, credible and trustworthy communication. Pull no punches. When you know an answer, give it. When you don't, say no. When you're guessing, admit it. But don't stop communication.
Jean B. Keffeler

Dimensions of Authentic Leaders
• Understand their purpose
• Practice solid values
• Lead with heart
• Establish connected relationships
• Demonstrate self-discipline
Bill George, 2004, "The Journey to Authenticity"

LEADER BEHAVIORS

Vulnerability: Mindfulness for the Right Signs

Every signpost or red flag in health care does not require attention and action. One unhappy patient or disgruntled employee should be noted; whole systems analyses should not be undertaken when other processes are working well. For example, if one visitor of 10,000 complains about parking proximity, a full-scale analysis of parking conditions is not needed. The complaint is data to be considered and then be aware of for new complaints about parking. In contrast, one patient who is injured in a fall in the bathroom creates a situation that should be analyzed and promptly addressed to assure the highest degree of patient safety.

Discussion

Soap/Alcohol Dispenser Placement

The placement of soap/alcohol hand-washing dispensers within the direct line of vision between the patient and the caregiver has been identified by staff as the best way to assure frequent hand washing.

1. How should this be resolved?
2. Who should be involved in the discussions?
3. What rationale/principles should guide the decision making?

Learning to identify those critical, differentiating signs requires mindfulness for specific events. Creating focus among the plethora of issues and work to be done in any healthcare organization begins with awareness and attention to the point of service—the point of patient care where the fundamental work of the organization occurs. The critical interactions and outcomes of health care occur primarily at the patient–caregiver interaction. Not only must the leader focus on the point of service and be cognizant of the work of caregivers, the leader must follow the recommendations of direct caregivers. Traditionally, leaders have sought opinions and advice from bedside caregivers, but they have not always deferred to them as the ultimate authority. Deferring to the expertise of the provider is much more than recognizing and valuing the opinions of providers, and it is essential for the best processes and solutions.

THE REALITY OF UNCERTAINTY

Vulnerability necessarily leads to uncertainty. There is no road map for the future. While the adage, "history repeats itself" may be true in some situations and in a rather general way, the reality is that there are no guidelines for the transition from the industrial age to the information age. Some leaders desire an organization in which employees can be programmed to plod along monotonously and follow established policies, but the events and complexities of patient care render this approach unrealistic. Continuing to work to keep employees in line is futile and frustrating.

Gem

If you face a delicate situation, don't go into it wearing your spurs or you'll rip it apart. Instead, dress for the occasion. Cloak yourself in diplomacy. Vest yourself with wisdom, and wear a smile.

Ann McKay Thompson

Theories within complexity science can assist leaders in creating meaning and understanding of the world as it is, thus mediating some uncertainty. The creation of new pathways for resource use, creation of effective teams, and evaluation of progress become the norm for leaders rather than uncommon events. Specifically, work of complex systems is reflecting the complexity principle that identifies complex systems as being characterized by nonsequential processes that contain many common mode interactions (Zimmerman, Lindberg, & Plsek, 1998). Simple cause and effect is rare indeed. Leaders should expect the unexpected and become wary when the sequence of events becomes predictable.

Mediating Uncertainty: High-Reliability Organizations

The common occurrence of unpredictable challenges places significant demands on leader creativity and imagination. Striving to understand and mediate uncertainty is the most appropriate and logical approach for leaders, rather than working to eliminate variety and hope for stability. Working to achieve stability is irrational given the complex nature of healthcare work.

According to Weick and Sutcliffe (2001), recognizing the complex nature of organizations, detecting incredibly weak warning signs, and taking strong decisive action when appropriate are the hallmarks of a high-reliability organization (HRO). HROs have gained credence for their ability to become highly reliable in minimizing errors and thereby increasing patient safety. In addition, HROs have achieved greater stakeholder motivation, time savings, and cost efficiency. These organizations demonstrate the ability to build effective practices and identify unexpected events early on and then respond to these unexpected events in ways that are adaptive rather than destructive. Leaders of HROs thrive in vulnerability, identify different approaches to issues, and take risks in addressing situations in nontraditional ways.

The following five characteristics define the high-reliability organization and have direct application to the healthcare industry:

High-Reliability Organizations' Defining Characteristics

1. Preoccupation with failure
2. Reluctance to simplify work
3. Sensitivity to operations
4. Commitment to resilience
5. Deference to expertise

Weick & Sutcliffe, 2001

1. *Preoccupation with failure.* The first characteristic of an HRO is preoccupation with failure. In a high-reliability organization, the leader is preoccupied with failure as a means to identify those critical warning signs that signal the need for more examination and quick response. This includes mindfulness to little things, continual scrutiny of the status quo, reviewing expectations, and changing expectations when new information is gained. Minor occurrences are believed to be the precursors of larger, more damaging events.

   In many situations, it is not about how much data is collected or how many questions are asked, but rather what questions are asked about the real-time data that is produced (McGee, 2004). Creating organizational mindfulness to the right signals is about using resources and data effectively. Asking questions that will provide precise and minimum information rather than general aggregated data will avoid an overload of data that must be examined. Leaders need data that will cause them to change a judgment or course of action. For example, if patient feedback data indicates an issue with perceptions of nurses initiating intravenous lines, the issue has specificity and can be quickly investigated and addressed.

   All failures provide insight about the workings of the system. Elaborate screening programs and data-collection processes are in place in most facilities and are intended to probe the vulnerabilities of the organization and provide lessons in preventing repetition of costly mistakes. Quality management programs are highly developed, yet these programs are often criticized for failing to identify and address significant errors or sentinel events in a timely manner.

   Further, organizations are challenged to create cultures of safety that support no-blame approaches to managing error. Encouraging employees to report even small and inconsequential incidents to facilitate a rapid response for learning and correction can be confused with witch hunting, which focuses on isolating the failure, assigning blame, and never discussing it again. Few failures can be traced to a single individual.

   Interestingly, Weick (Coutu, 2003) tells us that newcomers to an organization are able to identify potential problems and early warning signs more often than experienced, long-term employees. However, new employees are often reluctant to point out problems lest they be identified as troublemakers. Much can be learned from new employees if leaders are able to create cultural expectations that all new employees are required to share such observations at a designated time and without threat of becoming outcasts.

2. *Reluctance to simplify interpretations.* This trait emanates from the tendency to disconfirm evidence that does not meet our expectations. Rather than surrendering to the simplification and standardization of processes, HROs focus on the interactions between people with differing expectations and abilities, which result in different views of the same event. This behavior supports the creation of a safe and respectful environment that allows each person's perspective to be considered and integrated into the work.

   The large volume of procedures performed in healthcare organizations necessitates standardized formats and procedures. Yet, caregivers most likely follow the 80/20 Pareto rule: 80% of patient care can be managed within the standard template while the remaining 20% are anything but routine processes. Simplification of patient care processes using clinical protocols and pathways as

---

Discussion

Creating Mindfulness

1. How mindful is your organization to weak signals?
2. What weak signals have been identified and quickly corrected?
3. What weak signals were missed and resulted in an adverse outcome?
4. Identify new processes to avoid missing a similar signal.

Data Questions in HROs

Ask these questions:

1. What is the level of patient satisfaction this month?
2. What specific complaints were received this month about specific services?
3. How many new patients used our facilities this month?
4. Are there any supply issues? Has there been a change in product or shortage of needed items?

Avoid these questions:

1. What real-time information will allow us to detect critical events as quickly as possible—within 1 hour, 2 hours, 24 hours, etc.?
2. How can we react faster to negative results?

New Employee Scrutiny

As part of the completion of new orientation, request new members to make three suggestions specific to their ability to do their work based on their initial impressions of the organization.

Discuss the ideas with other members of the team and identify both the advantages and disadvantages of the suggestions.

1. Should changes be made?
2. Is it possible to change?
3. Who will support the changes?
4. Who will oppose the changes?
5. What will you do with this information?

the sole determiner of care is potentially dangerous because it limits the precautions individuals take, as well as their ability to envision other deviations that could be harmful.

3. *Sensitivity to operations.* With this trait, leaders believe that expertise resides in those who provide care at the point of service rather than in the executive role. Less bureaucracy, high interaction with caregivers, and sensitivity to the big picture reinforce this sensitivity. This emphasis results in early problem identification and early action.

   Organizational policies are often so well established and followed that the basic work or operations of the facility are compromised. Nearly every valid and well-established policy should be overridden or modified in certain circumstances. The principles of systems theory, in which there are multiple inputs into system operations that use many resources resulting in many differing outputs, can assist individuals in understanding these dynamics.

   Consider the patient with diabetes. The diabetic patient may be an emergency patient, an outpatient, an inpatient, or a surgical patient. Standards of care for diabetic patients are clearly identified for medications, blood glucose monitoring, and skin care. However, in each of the aforementioned settings, these standards must be applied within the context of the service in order to achieve the desired outcomes. The standards for blood glucose monitoring instrumentation are applied to the process in each setting using different personnel, different documentation formats, and different feedback mechanisms. Each context requires attention to ensure that standards are met and that the care is individualized to the needs and location of the patient and the standards are met.

   Further, this sensitivity to operations within each setting is expected to support high-reliability organizations. Assuring that blood glucose monitoring is performed accurately and efficiently is an ongoing accountability, no matter how routine the process appears.

4. *Commitment to resilience.* The processes of the healthcare system necessarily result in error, due to the human factors of both patients and those providing the care. The expectation for resilience requires new systems and processes to detect and manage errors at the earliest possible stage. According to Weick and Sutcliffe (2001), resilience requires mindfulness about errors that have already occurred and correcting them before they worsen and cause serious harm.

   The notion of error or mistake has resulted in behaviors that seek out the individual responsible for the error and lay blame on the individual. Focusing on resilience begins with a reconceptualization of the concept of error, from a negative event to a reality-based event that did not achieve the intended goals.

   Increasing one's capacity to cope with unanticipated events requires not only a reconceptualization of errors but also preparation for the inevitable surprises by expanding knowledge of new processes of resilience. Creating expectations for thorough and honest evaluation of processes that did not achieve desired goals should become the norm rather than the exception.

5. *Deference to expertise.* HROs develop the ability to alter the traditional deference to status and rank for making decisions in favor of those who have the expertise to make the decision. The decision makers in HROs are found throughout the ranks of the organization, depending on the issue, accountability, responsibility, uniqueness of the problem, and environmental characteristics.

   Traditionally, the executive team has made decisions without the benefit of a clinical perspective, which often results in hindering or delaying patient care. Efforts to minimize such decisions and shift to decisions by experts will necessarily include the complexities of judgment, timing, and team processes and result in more optimal outcomes.

Risk Taking: The Leader's Reputation

Can you afford to make mistakes? Can your organization afford to make mistakes? When is a mistake tolerable? How many mistakes or messages can you make without an impact on your effectiveness? Attention should first be given to the language of mistakes and errors and the existing negative connotations of these words. In order to value information from an unsuccessful attempt, language that is less negative should be considered. Rather than "The organization cannot afford to have you make a mistake," questions that are more appropriate for the desired culture of accountability could be used, such as:

- Can you afford to rework your work?
- Can you afford not to rework your work?
- Can the organization afford or expect to rework processes?
- Is it the right thing to do?

Given that life is dynamic and continually evolving, reworking the work and correcting missteps is a responsible leadership behavior. Thus, the answer to these questions is a resounding "Yes!" Rework is essential for progress to be made.

When risk taking is spontaneous and haphazard, rather than a systematic process of assessing the situation, weighing alternatives, and taking responsive action based on existing knowledge of the organization and the social, economic, and political context in which it exists, the potential for less-than-satisfactory outcomes and unnecessary rework increases dramatically. When the leader embraces systematic risk taking, there are no limitations, only expectations for better results.

MEDIATING RISK TAKING

Strategy: Information Management

As organizations adopt more and more computerized management and clinical information systems, data about care proliferates. These technology advances for collecting and managing information bring significant challenges for the leader. Real-time availability of data brings the expectation that leaders will interpret and respond to the data, which is an overwhelming task. The more open the leader is to information, the greater is the expectation for action.

Withholding information in order to sustain power or avoid conflicts is an age-old organizational problem. Criticisms of corporate board/CEO-compromised relationships in which CEOs have usurped control from boards through the withholding of information and strong-willed actions are not isolated (George, 2002). Such behaviors are also present throughout the ranks of the healthcare organization, from staff nurse to manager to director to executive. Selective information sharing between members of the organization results in less-than-optimal decision making, decreased trust, and poor outcomes.

According to George (2002), creating open communication pathways is about more than good leadership; it is about the legal and fiduciary responsibilities of members of the organization to share the essential information with those accountable for the overall work. Leaders necessarily must be vulnerable in sharing information once believed to be sensitive and must be more open to hearing information that is not positive. Leaders who are not prepared to take the steps to be more open to sharing and receiving all of the pertinent information with the organization should consider leaving the leadership role if they cannot change, rather than compromise the expected governance authority of the organization. All employees are accountable for sharing information

---

Gem

The difference between what the most and the least learned people know is inexpressibly trivial in relation to that which is unknown.

Albert Einstein

Withholding Information Discussion

Identify a situation in which a member of the organization withheld information that you believe should have been shared to improve patient care. Consider each of the following roles:

- Housekeeper
- Nursing assistant
- Registered nurse
- Pharmacist
- Respiratory therapist
- Director
- Shift leader
- Vice president, patient care services
- CEO

1. Why do you think the information was withheld?
2. What steps could be taken to encourage communication of information?

Information Sharing Guidelines

1. Share all data with immediate supervisor specific to:
   - Clinical outcomes specific to achievement of goals
   - Adverse outcomes
   - Patient feedback
   - Employee feedback
   - Physician feedback
   - Cost of care: labor and supplies
2. Provide information in a timely manner—ASAP, daily, weekly, monthly.
3. Present data/information in an objective and straightforward manner. Do not attempt to bury negative information.

Gem

Timing Is Everything

Implementing the second-best idea now is a better strategy than doing the best thing a week from now. It is a bigger risk to delay making decisions than to make marginal ones.

Executive Leadership, National Institute of Business Management

---

about activities that occur, regardless of the perceptions of negativity. Sharing information appropriately is the essence of vulnerability, of openness to others, new ideas, and awareness of limitations.

To shift the power imbalance, clear expectations for communication should be included in job descriptions, as should a defined review process to ensure objectives are achieved. Once the expectations for information sharing are identified and understood, the next challenge is to ensure that the review process is not a rubber stamp but rather an open, honest, and accurate examination of activities that includes a free flow of ideas and willingness to challenge assumptions and make changes when services can be improved.

Strategy: Embracing Risk

Given that risk taking is an essential behavior in organizations, strategies to thrive as a risk taker are needed. One strategy is to understand and articulate the intangible assets of the organization as a means to guide leaders in determining when and why to take risks. As a result, risk taking can become calculated and focused when consideration is given to three specific types of information: the nature of existing customer relationships, networks of influence, and the information cache within the organization.

Customer relationships include a large number of community members who have frequent and meaningful interactions with the organization, whether through the media, patients, or employees. Healthcare organizations also possess detailed knowledge about the community, patients, former patients, and employees and their perceptions of the service provided. Finally, these groups see the healthcare organization as the source of expertise. It is respected and trusted.

Networks of relationships exist with key stakeholders such as supply vendors and consultants, who provide valuable insight into the organization. The group of former patients could also be considered as the organization's user group, the group of individuals who use the service and know what works and what does not work for them.

The information owned by a healthcare organization is more than the documented patient care information or strategic plan for the future. Knowledge of marketplace activity, technical know-how, financial resources, and by-product information all contribute to the information available to the leaders.

As the leader engages in risk taking, using the available resources about the community, the relationships and internal information can greatly assist in providing data as to the feasibility of ideas, groups from which to seek input, timing within marketplace activities, and overall perceptions of services from multiple stakeholders.

Strategy: Overcoming Silence

Too often leaders are reluctant to express ideas for fear of retaliation or rejection. Past experiences and assumptions about the potential reactions of others render the healthcare professional immobile and ineffective.

Leaders must become open and honest in three key situations: sharing opinions and assessments during interview processes, communicating with the media, and providing feedback when negative events occur. Leaders must not only develop competence in these three areas, they must become experts and resources for those with whom they work. Efforts by quantum leaders to reverse the practices of institutionally imposed powerlessness, which expects nurses to not assert themselves individually or collectively, will continue the journey to optimal authenticity. As greater personal and professional authenticity emerges, feelings of low self-esteem, powerlessness, and lack of collegial support can only decrease.

Overcoming this silence leads to increased personal authenticity and greater public awareness of the importance of the role of nurses and all other healthcare professionals. Reversing the spiral of silence begins with regular discussions of situations within these three situations, identifying specific events in which silence negatively impacts open and honest communication.

Strategy: Avoiding Risk

In some situations, taking risks is not appropriate, no matter how enticing the idea may be. Any risk that does not support core values, deprioritizes the essential responsibilities of the discipline or organization, or provides little return on investment for organizational initiatives should be avoided. Holding to the truth of the work of the healer can only be reflected in unwavering support of value-based quality care that is appropriate to the context of the care and the needs of the patient. When challenging issues are presented, such as the importance of fairness and ethical practices specific to resource allocation, personnel issues, and conflict resolution, the leader must respond with integrity that reflects the authentic self.

Strategy: Reducing Fear

Great decisions bring out the best in teams and further reinforce their ability to achieve greater goals. Yet, typical decision-making team processes often set people against each other. When groups face tough issues, team members with the best of intentions may find themselves locked in divisive and destructive debates. Rather than energizing the processes of teams, this serves to polarize members. Fear, according to Maruska (2004), is the reason. Fear-driven group processes continue because results are generated in many situations. Leaders who have been successful with bullying, threatening tactics do not consider this approach unacceptable; rather, such leaders believe the approach is appropriate because it generates results. Unfortunately, while short-term results may be achieved, it is often at the cost of long-term results. Fear-induced behaviors marginalize performance and discourage employees from further meaningful participation in power struggles that are predestined to support the intimidator.

Overcoming the use of fear and shifting to a more collegial environment in which risk taking is valued requires transformation of processes, from motivation by fear to a focus on shared visions, hopes, and dreams. Shifting the focus to shared visions rather than fearful expectations requires a mental model that is much more palatable for teamwork. New behaviors include letting go of personal agendas, a willingness to explore new options that will benefit the team, finding common ground, and creating new, hopeful goals, rather than fear-laden acquiescence to an unsupported solution.

Strategy: Assuring an Ethical Climate

The influence of the workplace on ethical or principled practices is significant, as it may render the leader vulnerable to conflicting peer opinion, loss of colleague approval, physician conflict, and patient dissatisfaction. More often than not, leaders risk changing their relationships and reputation in creating and sustaining an ethical climate.

Many organizational cultures discourage employees from challenging or disagreeing with others and label such behaviors as negative and disruptive. A culture of trust and openness, in which employees are encouraged and expected to identify and confront ethical dilemmas as

---

Discussion

Reversing the Spiral of Silence

Consider the following situations:

- You supported hiring a long-time employee from another department who has a reputation of being very negative.
- Your CEO reacted negatively and aggressively to the press regarding local competition. When asked by the CEO if the communication was distasteful, you respond that it was okay.

1. What different responses could or should be made to these situations?
2. What are the risks to you/the organization? The benefits to you/the organization?

Gem

There is no sin punished more implacably by nature than the sin of resistance to change.

Anne Morrow Lindbergh

The Cycle of Fear Outcomes

1. People get left out of decision making.
2. Participants lose sight of what they really want.
3. Real issues get ignored.
4. Information gathering is biased.
5. Participants are personally attached to preset positions.
6. Decisions don't last.
7. Conflict ensures.

Maruska, 2004

Gem

Only those who attempt the absurd will achieve the impossible.

Albert Einstein

a team, often requires risk taking in order to make the best decisions and simultaneously value employees.

Employees who participate in decision making and have access to the information necessary to make informed decisions are empowered and contribute significantly to organizational performance. A culture that fosters and reinforces the value of risk-taking behaviors is an essential characteristic of a high-performing organization. The following questions should be considered to ensure ethical decisions:

- Is the action under consideration legal?
- Is the action consistent with organizational policies and guidelines? If not, should a policy be developed or modified?
- Is the action consistent with organizational values?
- Am I personally okay with the proposed action?
- Would I be satisfied if someone took this action with me?
- Would the most ethical person I know do the same thing?

The diversity of values and beliefs creates a world in which a systematic reflection and analysis of what is right and what is wrong as well as what ought to be done is essential. Ethical issues abound in healthcare organizations. The influences of the work setting, demands for greater profits, expectations of safety, and individual motivations require that good and fair decisions are made on a daily basis.

According to Olson (1998), how ethical dilemmas are addressed and the conditions that allow employees to engage in ethical reflection are determinants of the organization's ethical climate. The ethical climate of the organization can either serve to reinforce good and just decisions or to avoid addressing ethical dilemmas, thus blocking healthy dialogue and effective decision making.

While employees should be free to say what is needed about an issue and free to disagree with each other as a means to better understand situations and other perspectives, the organizational culture often does not support or encourage such behaviors. Olson (1998) also suggests that nurses experience the ethical climate through their perceptions of organizational conditions and that practices should be present to support the management of difficult patient situations that have ethical implications. How these issues are resolved, whether openly or not at all, reflects the culture support of vulnerable behaviors. Examples of supportive behaviors are listed in Key Elements of an Ethical Climate (left).

Group Discussion

Consider recent ethical dilemmas that occurred with a peer, manager, physician, or patient.

1. How was the issue discussed?
2. When was the issue discussed—shortly after the event, later, or never?
3. What should you do in the future to improve the ethical climate of the organization if a similar issue arises?

Key Elements of an Ethical Climate

1. Team members listen to each other.
2. Patients know what to expect.
3. Patients have access to information.
4. Employees believe their manager listens to them.
5. The organization's policies help employees.
6. Nurses believe they practice nursing the way it should be practiced.
7. Conflict is dealt with openly.
8. Nurses and physicians trust one another.
9. Nurses and physicians respect others' decisions.
10. There is a sense of the need for questioning and learning in the organization.

Strategy: Managing Turnover

The uncertainty of availability of the right individuals to do the work of health care continues to be one of the most significant challenges for the leader. Having the right people to do the job and to do it well is a fundamental expectation for effective leadership. Unfortunately, the rapidly changing environment, cultural mandates, and labor regulations often result in individuals in positions who no longer have the necessary skills for the work of the organization.

To compound the problem, mixed messages are sent to leaders: minimize turnover, maximize productivity, and assure high employee satisfaction. The expectations to be productive and have competent employees become impossible to achieve when some employees have failed to upgrade knowledge and skills and are not competent to meet the new demands.

According to Waldman, Kelly, Arora and Smith (2004), the average costs to hire and train new employees varies from $3,926 for administrative assistants to $125,543 for attending physicians. The cost for registered nurse turnover ranges from $22,000 to $64,000 or one to three times the salary of the departing nurse (Jones & Gates,

2007). These costs associated with turnover raise concerns as to how to manage and decrease the majority of turnover as a cost-savings measure. Two types of turnover are identified in these calculations: healthy turnover and avoidable turnover. It is the avoidable turnover that the leader can positively impact.

Healthy turnover includes a certain number of individuals who are highly mobile and focused on development of skills in a variety of settings, as well as those no longer committed to or supportive of the organization. This turnover is unavoidable and an essential part of organizational life. It is especially true for the individuals of generations X and Y, who are generally focused on skill acquisition and personal development rather than loyalty to an organization.

> **The Cost of Turnover**
>
> The annual cost of turnover (hiring, training, and reduced productivity) represents about 5% of the annual operating budget. Stated differently according to Bland and Gates (2007), it would be revenue neutral to offer each departing nurse (who chose to stay) a staying bonus equal to 86 percent of his or her annual salary or give every nurse on staff a 33% retention supplement every year!

Avoidable turnover results from issues related to healthcare policy and practices. Professional disillusionment with the quality of patient care, control over practice, work assignment and schedules, and wage levels can all fuel turnover that may in fact not be necessary. Excessively high rates of turnover of experienced clinicians is more than the cost of doing business. Quality patient care is compromised, the risk of errors increases, morale deteriorates, and overall productivity declines. The quantum leader develops skill in distinguishing avoidable turnover from healthy turnover and focuses on the former.

Strategy: Increasing Involvement

The power struggles between all healthcare providers, physicians, nurses, therapists, dietitians, social workers, and housekeepers continue to displace the goals of a community of healthcare providers learning to live in an age of complexity where goals transcend power struggles. It is ironic that the nursing profession continues to work to empower nursing and to gain autonomy, and yet one of the greatest challenges in health care is to develop collaborative processes as the means to better patient care. Indeed, it is possible to create and sustain relationships in which the members are both empowered and collaborative.

Leading others is out of date and incongruent with the modern organizational life in the current marketplace. Complexity science proposes a new and better approach rather than one steeped in autocracy and omniscience. Authority rests in the ability of the leader to see the entirety of the organization and the potential of its people. Quantum leaders cultivate the conditions for the organization to change and grow through the interconnections among people, not through specific individuals using command and control behaviors.

One such way to achieve the new age of leadership is through the leaderless organization concept. The leaderless organization makes sense for many reasons, especially since the Internet has dramatically increased the volume and accessibility of information that is available both horizontally and vertically. No longer is information controlled and meted out as the information holder deems appropriate. Allowing or expecting employees to manage themselves can be a significant challenge for the leader. Managing systems and structures of the work context and expecting employees to own the work processes theoretically should lead to better outcomes. Making it a reality requires much more than a declaration of a shared leadership culture.

First, the leader must stop owning every problem and making every decision and must expect that employees are capable—not incapable—of being self-starters, are problem solvers, are responsible, and are independent thinkers. Not only believing that one can trust colleagues but also living this belief is essential.

The second strategy in the leaderless organization is to recognize and value the role of the middle manager as an innovator and source of point-of-service information. While this role has indeed evolved considerably over the last 10 years, the quantum middle manager is much different from the traditional manager. This role has emerged to be one of both leader and manager, one in which the characteristics of thoroughness, persistence, discretion, persuasiveness, and comfort with change are foundational. Quantum managers' skills are not in being contrary or revolutionary; rather, they are able to work through existing networks, to uncover opportunities, build coalitions, and make change happen. The integration of these skills and competencies into the role of the middle manager serves to further deemphasize command and control while reinforcing openness and valuing of the collective wisdom of the team. The quantum leader is liberated through this complexity approach to leadership and also thrives in the notion that one cannot know or control everything.

MEDIATING RISK

Strategy: Recognizing a Cosmology Episode— The Ultimate Vulnerability

Leaders are often faced with situations in which they believe the universe is no longer a rational, orderly system. Events defy explanation. A cosmology episode, according to Weick (Coutu, 2003), is the opposite of déjà vu, in which everything suddenly seems familiar and recognizable. In contrast, a state of panic ensues in a cosmology episode and anxiety abounds.

An example of a cosmology episode occurs with the hiring of a new leader. Current employees are faced with a new individual who they believe has significant power over their careers, and yet they have little knowledge of how the new leader will make decisions, value their role and contributions, and represent them in organizational discussions. Employees have no templates to define what the new leader will do, only uncertainty as to what will happen next. Each new leader brings new values, a new style, and new expectations. While this may not be as dramatic as Weick's hantavirus exemplar of a cosmology episode, such events are occurring more regularly as information technology changes the way work is accomplished (Coutu, 2003). There are fewer and fewer déjà vu events and more and more cosmology episodes.

A cosmology episode is impossible to predict. However, some preparation for when it does occur is helpful. Being alert to minor details, avoiding making assumptions until some discussion occurs, reflecting, and working to make sense of what is happening are appropriate behaviors. Weick advises those in cosmology episodes to work hard to transform the raw experience into intelligible worldviews (Coutu, 2003). Making sense of the cosmology episode lends itself to multiple, conflicting interpretations, all of which may be possible. If an individual or the organization finds itself unsure of where it is going or what it has accomplished, it is essential to be open to many different interpretations. Each action and its consequences assist the leader in editing the list of interpretations down to a manageable set of options. These actions, tempered by reflection, are the critical processes in learning to thrive in a cosmology episode.

STRETCHING

Strategy: Stretching

Taking risks is not the end of the road; it is only the beginning of expanding the capacity of the organization to achieve better results. Stretching one's present skills and abilities to be able to address increasingly difficult situations begins with a strong desire and willingness to move from ordinary solutions to better solutions that improve resource use and clinical outcomes. Quantum leaders provide the vision, which often looks impossible, and continually coach and mentor others to

---

Cosmology Episode

. . . an event or situation in which everything seems strange; a person feels like he has never been here before, has no idea of where he is or who can help him.

Karl Weick, 2003

Cosmology Episodes in Your Organization

Just as the switchboard operators and key punch technicians have gone the way of the history books, current healthcare procedures are changing quickly and dramatically. Less invasive procedures, ear temperatures, and computerized documentation all require the elimination of some work in favor of new work.

1. Identify one procedure/service in your organization that was eliminated last year. What replaced it? How was the new work integrated into the system? Who is now doing new work?

2. Identify one procedure that you believe will be (or should be) eliminated in the next year. What will replace it? How will the new work be integrated into the system? Who will do the new work?

move from novice risk takers to individuals who are not only comfortable with risk taking but also are able to thrive as risk takers while achieving better outcomes.

Consider the situation in which the leader would like to change the patient care delivery system for several of the patient care units. Stretching would involve not only gaining feedback and support for the new model but also extending the ideas to include more clinical departments, roles, and outcomes. The proposed model can be reviewed with the involved caregivers, as well as former patients, community members, and colleagues in other healthcare organizations. Initial feedback can be gained using existing information-gathering networks within the organization and community.

Strategy: Increasing Capacity through Diversity

The complexity of diversity is not always readily apparent. The obvious diversity found in ethnic backgrounds, gender, and age is but the tip of the iceberg. Thinking styles, problem-solving styles, communication styles, decision-making styles, economic status, educational level, and religious affiliation all significantly contribute to organizational complexity and differences within the world of health care. These characteristics are in addition to the plethora of individual values and behaviors.

The fable of the giraffe and the elephant provides an excellent illustration of the multiple realities of the workforce (Thomas & Woodruff, 1999). In this fable, the giraffe builds a house based on the specifications of the giraffe family, which includes high ceilings, narrow doorways, and high windows; the house even wins the National Giraffe Home of the Year Award. In this wonderful house the giraffe has a woodworking shop in the basement. Knowing that his friend from church, the elephant, is also interested in woodworking, he invites the elephant to see his shop and hopes to do work with him in the future. The elephant is delighted and accepts the invitation.

As the elephant attempts to enter the house, he becomes stuck at the front door. The giraffe is not worried because they have installed expandable doors to accommodate wood-shop equipment. Once inside the house, the elephant damages the steps to the basement because of his weight and cannot get through the doorway into the shop. The giraffe responds in amazement; he then quickly recovers and advises the elephant to join the local gym to slim down and to join a ballet class to become lighter on his feet in order to come into his home.

In this story, the giraffe represents the *main* group; it is his house, his design, his rules, and he is in charge. The elephant represents the *other* group. While he is warmly welcomed, in the giraffe's house he will always be an outsider since the house was not built with elephants in mind. The story provides a powerful metaphor of traditional attempts to manage diversity and becomes instructive to us in terms of how we really address diversity.

Diversity is a total collective mixture. It is not a function of race or gender or any other us-versus-them dyad, but a complex and ever-changing blend of attributes, behaviors, and talents. A diversity mixture is a combination of individuals who are different in some ways and similar in others.

The process of building a house for diversity is about finding common ground for all and protecting sacred differences. It is not about building a house for one group and making adjustments to accommodate others. Diversity can be seen as a vehicle toward wholeness, a vehicle in which multiple perspectives are held without judgment. Even with the inherent competition of multiple perspectives, the quantum leader understands the value of each perspective and strives to work to

---

Gem

Even if it is the harder path, even if it is harder to be true to the self, it is far less painful than being out of step with one's values.

Mary O'Connor, 2003

Diversity

Differences	**Similarities**
• Skill types	• Healthcare workers
• Cultural background	• Share common goals
• Gender	• Work in teams
• Age	• Value relationships
• Values	
• Education level	
• Economic status	

Diversity Maturity Behaviors

- Accept personal responsibility for enhancing personal and organizational effectiveness
- Demonstrate knowledge of self and the organization
- Be clear about requirements and decisions about differences and how they impact the ability to meet these requirements
- Understand that diversity is accompanied by complexity and tension and be prepared to cope with these in pursuit of greater diversity effectiveness
- Be willing to challenge conventional wisdom
- Engage in continuous learning

R.R. Thomas, 1999

acknowledge each contribution, accept the differing perspectives, and integrate them in order to succeed as a team able to recognize and thrive in the collective wisdom produced by the integration of many.

Improving one's approach to diversity begins with the recognition of the shortcomings of the traditional approaches of affirmative action, understanding differences, and diversity management.

Affirmative action, which focuses on inclusion and calls for special action to correct the imbalances, does not address the underlying issue of dominant and subordinate factions. For genuine diversity to thrive in organizations, the right climate in which the beliefs and behaviors of all workforce participants are integrated must be created.

Understanding differences is an approach that focuses on relationships and how people get along but does not address structures and organizational policy. There is a reluctance to fully address diversity. The structure or policies represent the needs and values of the main group. The main group identifies differing groups and openly works to acknowledge and accommodate the others. Meeting times, food preferences, and bathroom availability are a few of the typical accommodations made for those with different sleep schedules, cultural food needs, and gender needs.

Finally, the diversity management approach proposes to manage or modify the dominant faction to accommodate the subordinate faction. Diversity tension is inevitable. Regardless of how the giraffe's house is modified, it will never be a mutual house. It will remain the house of the giraffe, modified to meet the needs of the elephant. There are no simple solutions with such a complex phenomenon except to begin with one's internal self and accept personal responsibility for diversity.

Diversity Effectiveness

Creating a climate that integrates and honors differences includes three basic skills and a level of diversity maturity. First, it is necessary to identify the differing components that create the diversity and the related tensions that occur. If young and old patients are attending an education program, an understanding of what the differences are is essential. Examples include reading skills, knowledge levels, concentration span, and writing ability, to name a few. Resulting tensions could include length of time for comprehension of content or differing abilities to understand certain terminology.

The second skill is the ability to analyze the mixtures and related tensions. The analysis is performed to identify which differences could interfere with achieving goals. Not all differences need to be addressed if goal attainment is not compromised. If reading time required by one group is twice as long, when does it interfere with goal attainment? If there is only 5 minutes total, no changes need to be made; if there are 30 minutes, changes should be considered to avoid boredom.

The third skill is to select an appropriate response. What should be done regarding the time for comprehension and use of terminology? If the differences are significant, should there be two distinct classes?

These three skills are developed with practice and become internalized as core diversity skills in order to meet leadership challenges.

Assessing Current Environment Diversity

1. Identify current processes or services that represent a diversity mixture rather than a *main* and an *other* service.
2. How did these processes or services occur? Why are they sustainable?
3. Identify processes or services that are based on a main group of entity.
4. Who are the main groups? Who are the others?
5. What actions could you take to create a diversity mixture?
6. What resistance would be encountered?

Diversity Effectiveness: Challenges for the Leader

Think about a recent conflict in your work environment and answer the following questions.

1. What diversity components were present? List as many as you can.
2. Which component(s) interfered with goal attainment?

Consider also:

3. Did others understand the differences?
4. Was a lack of trust part of the situation?
5. Did others have personal agendas?
6. What will you do differently next time a similar situation occurs?

SUMMARY

Vulnerability continues to be the most significant challenge for leaders in contemporary healthcare organizations. Developing not only competence but also expertise in vulnerability behaviors serves the leader in understanding organizational dynamics, appreciating the complexity of relationships and interactions in an organization, and allowing employees to be all that they can be. The strategies to assist leaders in becoming more vulnerable through controlled risk taking will further support the development of expertise. Finally, the incredible power of the five characteristics of a high-reliability organization can be seen as focusing goals for the organization destined to greatness and excellence.

Gem

There is no time of life past learning something.

St. Ambrose, 340–397, Bishop of Milan

Exercise 1 Vulnerability and Risk Taking

The current patient care delivery model includes only registered nurses and nursing assistants. The availability of registered nurses and nursing assistants is less than adequate to meet the needs. Your team has examined the situation and is proposing a new patient care delivery model. The model includes roles for master's prepared nurses, baccalaureate nurses, licensed practical nurses, patient care technicians, and certified nursing assistants.

- What risks will you be taking with this proposal?
- What are the goals of this approach? The advantages? The disadvantages?
- How will you mediate the risks?
- What measures will you use to determine the value of the new model?

Exercise 2 High-Reliability Organizations

The five characteristics of high-reliability organizations have assisted leaders in providing safer, more appropriate patient care services.

In a recent situation, a team made the decision to replace existing blood glucose monitoring equipment in the outpatient, inpatient, surgical, and emergency departments with new equipment that was less costly and believed to be of higher quality in data management. Within two weeks, problems with accuracy and equipment failure were identified in the inpatient and surgical areas. Over 50 patients were identified to have received inappropriate insulin management.

Consider the five principles of a high-reliability organization. Analyze the results in terms of the principles.

Which principles were followed? What changes should be made to improve operations?

REFERENCES

Coutu, D. L. (2003). Sense and reliability: A conversation with celebrated psychologist Karl E. Weick. *Harvard Business Review, 81* (4), 84–90.

George, B. (2004, Winter). The journey to authenticity. *Leader to Leader, 31,* 29–35.

George, W. W. (2002). Imbalance of power. *Harvard Business Review, 80* (7), 22–23.

Jones, C. B., & Gates, M. (2007). The costs and benefits of nurse turnover: A business case for nurse retention. *The Online Journal of Issues in Nursing; 12*(3). Retrieved February 28, 2008, from *http://www.medscape.com/viewarticle/569393*

Kellerman, B. (2004). Leadership: Warts and all. *Harvard Business Review, 82* (1), 40–45.

Lencioni, P. (1998). *The five temptations of a CEO.* San Francisco: Jossey-Bass.

Maruska, D. (2004, Summer). Making great team decisions. *Leader to Leader, 33,* 38–44.

McGee, K. (2004). Give me that real-time information. *Harvard Business Review, 82* (4), 26.

O'Connor, M. (2003). A look at nursing leadership through the lens of a dancer. *Nursing Forum, 38* (1), 23–28.

Olson, L. L. (1998). Hospital nurses' perceptions of the ethical climate of their work setting. *Image: Journal of Nursing Scholarship, 30* (4), 345–349.

Porter-O'Grady, T., & Malloch, K. (2007). Quantum Leadership: A textbook of new leadership. Sudbury, MA: Jones and Bartlett.

Thomas, R. R., & Woodruff, M. I. (1999). *Building a house for diversity.* New York: AMACOM.

Waldman, J. D., Kelly, F., Arora, S., & Smith, H. L. (2004). The shocking cost of turnover in health care. *Health Care Management Review, 29* (1), 2–7.

Weick, K., & Sutcliffe, K. (2001). Managing the unexpected: Assuring high performance in an age of complexity. San Francisco: Jossey-Bass.

Zimmerman, B., Lindberg, C., & Plsek, P. (1998). Irving, TX: VHA, Inc.

SUGGESTED READINGS

Clancy, T. R. (2004). Navigating in a complex nursing world. *Journal of Nursing Administration, 34* (6), 274–282.

DeMarco, R. F., & Roberts, S. J. (2003). Negative behaviors in nursing. *American Journal of Nursing, 103* (3), 113–115.

Kanter, R. M. (2004). The middle manager as innovator. *Harvard Business Review, 82* (7), 150–161.

Woodburn, L. (2004, June). Stop leading? *Hospitals & Health Networks,* 94.

CHAPTER 6

Innovation Leadership: A New Way of Being

CHAPTER OBJECTIVES:

Upon completion of this chapter, the reader will:

1. Understand the basic concepts of innovation and their relationship to innovation leadership.
2. Describe common innovation resources available to the innovation leader.
3. Examine leader strategies to advance the integration of innovation into the healthcare culture.

INTRODUCTION

In today's healthcare environment, leaders and managers need a wide and varied range of competencies to manage not only the operations of the organization, but also the work of continually adapting to new evidence, new technology, and new processes. The work of adapting to new approaches requires knowledge specific to creativity and innovation. In this chapter, a sampling of key concepts including an overview of innovation, innovation leadership, resources for innovation, strategies to support innovative processes, tools and methods of innovation, the obstacles to innovation, and approaches to the evaluation and measurement of innovation are presented. There is much written about innovation and innovation processes that serious readers should investigate further.

> **Imbalance Challenge**
>
> In general, people are more affected by their fear of creating the wrong idea than they are motivated by the excitement and passion of creating a truly innovative idea.
>
> John Sweeney, 2004

SOURCE OF INNOVATION IDEAS

There is no lack of need for new ideas and processes; nor is there a lack of ideas. The impetus for innovations emanates from multiple sources. Examples of innovation idea sources include the following:

- New science or knowledge such as computer processing or fiber optics
- Needs from service providers (caregivers) such as voice recognition for documentation
- Customer needs for more efficient and effective processes such as drive-through banking

The problems encountered by both providers and users can also become opportunities for innovation. In health care, the motivations for new work have most recently emanated from the patient safety movement. The call for safer patient care, fewer errors, and more predictable outcomes has never been greater.

One caution from Ulwick (2008) when using customers for ideas is the importance of focusing on outcomes or what the customer wants the new product or service to do for them and not the processes to achieve the outcomes. Customers do not have the conceptual tools or knowledge to create new products or services. Those skilled in the tools of innovation should be the creators of new solutions or products that meet the desired outcomes of end users. Similarly, with patient feedback, the emphasis should be on determining the desired outcome and not the processes to achieve the outcomes. For example, patients prefer services in one location rather than visiting many locations; it is up to the innovation team to determine the processes to make this occur.

> ### Point to Ponder
>
> Many established companies fail to make the leap to the new technology because powerful customers persuade them to continue doing what they are doing.
>
> Ralph Katz

Innovation, noun, A change that creates a new dimension of performance (Drucker, 2001)

Innovate, verb, to introduce something new

Innovative, adjective,

Invention, noun, a new process, machine, or improvement that is recognized as the product of some unique intuition or genius.

Innovation leadership, adjective and noun, a leadership competence reflected by the ability to create the context and resources for innovation to occur

Diffusion, noun, widespread scatter or dispersed; a "pull" concept

Dissemination, noun, to spread widely; a "push" or top–down concept

Source: Random House *Webster's College Dictionary*, 1992

INNOVATION IS . . .

There are numerous definitions and descriptions of innovation. These definitions include creating something *new*, something *groundbreaking*, and something that is *better than what it was before*. From the very simplistic description to the more theoretical definition, innovation is about *introducing something new*. Innovation descriptions range from incremental to complete; from improving upon something that already exists to something new to the world that is a departure from current processes. A list of selected definitions and descriptions of innovation and related concepts is presented in **Table 6-1**.

INNOVATION LEADERSHIP IS . . .

Innovation leadership is quite different from the work and processes of being an inventor. Innovation leadership is about creating the context for innovation to occur—creating and implementing the roles, decision-making structures, physical space, partnerships, networks, and equipment that support innovative thinking and testing. This role requires an ability to envision the future, courage to challenge the status quo, comfort with routine risk taking, agility, and significant ego strength. The innovation leader has an understanding of the significance of the collective wisdom that is generated by many individuals and the continual adaptation process that is so powerful that one's ego becomes transparent. Innovation leadership is not about being the best developer of new ideas or being the most creative thinker; it is about facilitating and empowering others to be as creative as they can be.

INNOVATION LEADERSHIP IS NOT . . .

Oftentimes when an individual assumes the responsibility to manage the implementation of a technology product, the perception is that this work is innovation leadership. Innovation leadership is not project management. Innovation leadership is about who the leader is and how the world of work is approached. Project management is about the dissemination of processes using a top-down approach. Traditionally, the work of project management is done by a manager who is following and guiding the implementation of a clearly defined plan. However, as the healthcare industry works to better integrate innovation and operations, an innovation leader can also be a project manager for selected projects. This approach increases cross-fertilization of innovation and operations, and at the same time, it provides real-time opportunities for the innovation leader to correct course or modify the project plan to assure optimal results.

ADVANCING THE HEALTHCARE CULTURE

	Innovative Leadership	Innovation Project Management
Scope	Broad Context specific	Narrow Project specific
Leader Role	Facilitator	Owner
Focus	Change process	New project implementation
	Creativity	Idea testing
Behaviors	Risk taking	Control

Table 6-2 Comparison: Innovation Leadership and Innovation Project Management

Advancing innovation into the healthcare culture presents challenges to even the most skilled leaders. The challenge to assure patient safety, maintain employee satisfaction, and at the same time test and implement new treatments and products is never ending. However, integrating innovation into the healthcare culture so that it is a part of the fabric of the organization rather than an occasional project or study requires a high level of understanding of organizational survival, leadership, courage, and passion to be the best that one can be. While the motivations for innovation range from wanting to retain one's lead position to organizational and personal survival, the reality is that innovation is inescapable. The sooner a leader can engage in an integrated culture for healthcare services, the greater the potential to achieve patient care excellence. The innovation leader necessarily manages the paradox of stability and creativity using more sophisticated skills of critical reasoning and synthesis of complexities of the organization.

The organizational culture supportive of innovation can be a catch-22 situation for healthcare leaders in that a culture supportive of safe practices relies on stability, consistency, and standardization. This is diametrically opposed to the cultural norms and behaviors supportive of innovation. Innovation and health care have an interesting relationship. There is a dual expectation for safety and quality, and at the same time there is an expectation that patients have access to the most advanced state-of-the-art procedures, equipment, and technology. What is not expected nor tolerated very well is the work to consider, test, and implement new and improved solutions. While this is not a new phenomenon for healthcare leaders, the intensity and complexity at which innovations are being introduced and the concerns about the lack of patient safety is different and much more intense. No leader can escape the perceived schizophrenic expectation for tolerance of change and the provision of an infrastructure that supports stable operations *and* the development of new and improved ways to provide patient care services. Health care and innovation are uncommon but essential partners in the patient safety movement. Attaining the critical balance between the two requires new behaviors and expectations for the healthcare team.

In light of this complex and ever-changing environment, healthcare leaders have at least three options when new ideas or technology are available: (1) abandon current processes and move to the new process, (2) work to improve and expand current processes, or (3) hold current process additions and begin to use the new process simultaneously (Katz, 2003). For each new idea or technology, innovation leaders use numerous resources to evaluate which option is most appropriate for the context in which they work.

INNOVATION RESOURCES

Innovation resources are many and varied and include techniques, technologies, and laboratory spaces dedicated to the processes of innovation and that support innovation leadership. Each tool provides a unique approach in the innovation process from idea generation to dissemination and evaluation of new ideas. These resources are useful for the leader to examine and better understand the situation and then to be able to determine if or when to adopt, ignore, or combine new ideas.

Techniques and Tools of Innovation

The techniques and tools of innovation include innovation laboratories or physical space in which innovation dialogue or construction of prototypes can occur, specific activities for idea generation, and Internet sites. All three resources should be considered in the work of innovation leadership. Examples of each are presented to assist innovation leaders in gaining an appreciation of available resources.

Innovation laboratories or spaces are designed for individuals to work together in the generation of ideas, design of prototypes, testing of ideas, evaluation of outcomes, and reworking of projects. For innovation leaders, the physical space includes tables for small-group discussion, electrical outlets for laptops, projection capability, large writing areas for idea documentation, and creative toys or items such as modeling clay, pipe cleaners, building blocks, and construction paper. *Skunk works* is an example of an innovation space designed to provide an environment for project teams with a singular mission and their own quarters. Originally created by Lockheed Martin aerospace manufacturer, skunk works first described a group within an organization given autonomy and freedom to work on special or secret projects.

Innovation Tools

Catchball is a technique in which an idea is tossed from one group to another for the purpose of review, reflection, and modification. This technique is helpful in maximizing input and illustrates the interactive nature of creating optimal solutions. The process continues until optimal improvement is achieved.

Catchball Exercise

An opportunity presents itself for the updating of a patient education resource area. Using the Catchball technique, select two or three teams from different areas to participate in this work.

1. Identify the goal
2. Team 1 develops the idea and includes processes, descriptions of value to stakeholders, metrics for evaluation and timelines.
3. Pass the project on to Team 2 for improvements.
4. Pass the project on to Team 3 for improvements.
5. Pass the project back to Team 1 for comments and so on.

The *deep dive* is a technique for brainstorming that results in highly communicative and innovative ideas in a very short period of time. The deep dive was created by the IDEO Corporation, in Palo Alto, California, a leading product design company that bases its design process on an anthropologic approach. With this technique, several phases are involved. The first phase focuses on understanding the context in which an activity occurs, the market, customers, available technology, and limitations. The second phase involves observation of real people in real situations followed by synthesizing of observations. In the third phase, designers brainstorm new approaches and then create prototypes. The ideas are then refined and streamlined and finally selected and evaluated.

For healthcare workers, non–healthcare sites for the deep dive experience are especially helpful. For example, a group of healthcare students visited a local coffee shop to observe the physical setting, the flow of activities by workers and customers, and their experiences. The students observed, synthesized, brainstormed, prototyped, and selected an improved model. Quite quickly, the students recognized the similarities to patient care throughput issues and were able to translate and transfer ideas to improve patient throughput as a result of the experience.

Directed creativity is a technique developed by Plsek (2003) that emphasizes perceiving things in new ways, breaking free of current patterns, making novel associations, and using judgment in different ways. According to Plsek, the creative process involves connecting and rearranging knowledge in one's mind. With this technique, there is a purposeful production of creative ideas for a specific topic, implementation of ideas, and then enhancing as needed. An important assumption with directed creativity is that the ability to generate innovative ideas for change is a common trait that we all possess. What is important is to recognize that each individual embraces new ideas at different rates and for different reasons.

Empathic design is an idea-generating technique whereby innovators observe how people use existing products and services in their own environments. The purpose of this approach is to learn as much as possible about how a product or service is used and under what conditions. This information is then used in the design process so that the outcome is optimally usable and meets customer needs.

Innovation mapping is a technique that is used to understand work flows. Numerous commercial mapping products are available to document thought and work-flow patterns. The analysis can begin with the caregiver–provider, the patient receiving the care, a specific technology, or a product. Each model produces different information including product, technology, and customer perspectives. This model provides information that extends other techniques in the determination of process efficiency, comparison of processes, and the nature of required resources.

Scenario planning is a technique used to inform the future using a group process. The group shares information to gain greater understanding of issues and then creates several different potential scenarios based on driving forces. These stories then serve to increase the knowledge of the environment and potential interrelated events that could occur.

> Exercise: Innovation Maps:
>
> **Compare and Contrast for Optimal Impact**
>
> Identify an opportunity for innovation for your specific department. Using a mapping approach, create a customer-centered innovation map that identifies what the customer expects and in what order the events are expected. Using the same model, create a provider-based innovation map based on the job responsibilities of the provider. How are they similar, how are they different? Given the knowledge you have gained from examining both maps, what changes could/ should be made to optimize the process?

Internet Resources

Given the varied skill sets and comfort with innovation, Internet innovation resources can be very helpful in not only guiding innovation projects, but also in advancing individuals along the innovation continuum. Resource web sites, blogs, wikis and .ning sites are available to assist innovation leaders with the latest state-of-the-art ideas and information about innovation. **Table 6-3** lists several useful sites to assist aspiring innovation leaders.

While these tools may be attractive and enticing to the novice innovation leader, the importance of personal innovation competence cannot be overestimated. Individuals must be open to new ideas, comfortable with uncertainty and loss of control, and resilient to recover from unsuccessful attempts. Using these tools will not decrease anxiety or increase comfort with the unknown; that must come from within the person for the full benefit of the tools to be realized. Embarking on a deep dive without intention and commitment to explore new ways of being is self-defeating.

www.ted.com	Ideas worth spreading
www.ideo.com	IDEO Corporation, Palo Alto, California
www.ihi.org	Institute for Healthcare Improvement
www.CHCF.org	California Health Care Foundation; Innovations for the underserved
www.innovativecaremodels.com	Health Workforce Solutions and RWJ site
www.simulearn.net/video/virtualleaderorientation2.wmv	
http://www.innovations.ahrq.gov	The Agency for Healthcare Research and Quality innovations resource

Table 6-3 Innovation Web sites

ADVANCING INNOVATION LEADERSHIP STRATEGIES

Developing the competencies and tools that support innovation leadership is the beginning of the journey. The application of tools and techniques can be further enhanced with the specific strategies. The overall purpose of these strategies is to enhance innovation leadership competence.

Strategy No. 1: Learn the Language of Innovation

Similar to other disciplines that have unique languages, so, too, does the field of innovation. The language of innovation includes concepts specific to change, performance, creativity, idea generation, tools for innovation, stages of innovation, and evaluation. The following examples are not exhaustive, but rather representative of the language. The benefits of developing skill in using the language can be far reaching. Individuals learn quickly that innovation is not limited to high-level scientists or the ultracreative. Rather, innovation is common to everyone, just in differing degrees. For example, the language of Rogers (2003), Plsek (2003), and Fraser (2007) (**Table 6-4**) reflects different conceptualizations or approaches to the evolving innovation levels of knowledge or acceptance of new ideas.

Rogers	Plsek (2003)	Fraser
Laggard	Usual thinking	Skeptic
Late majority	Potential better practice thinking	Conservative
Early majority	Clever thinking	Pragmatist
Early adopter	Creative connection thinking	Visionary
Innovator	Paradigm busting thinking	Enthusiast
	Original thinking	

Table 6-4 Comparison of Innovation Spread Concepts: Rogers, Plsek, and Fraser

---

Exercise: Ten Faces of Innovation

Examine a current leader in your organization who is known for innovation using Kelly's Ten Faces of Innovation. Are all faces present? Which faces are the most prominent? Which faces are the least common? How can your team use this information to advance innovation in your organization?

T. Kelly, (2005)

Never give up!

I am constantly and happily surprised by how impossible it is to extinguish the human spirit. People who had been given up for dead in their organizations, once conditions change and they feel welcomed back in, find new energy and become great innovators.

Margaret J. Wheatley (1999)

Strategy No. 2: Understand Your Ego

To be an effective innovation leader, one must first understand oneself from the perspective of the work of innovation. A clear understanding of strengths, range of experiences, abilities to overcome obstacles, areas for development, resources for honest feedback, and personal courage are essential for those leaders dedicated to creating the context for others to thrive and innovate. Empowering others is a selfless process in which the leader of innovation is peripheral to high-profile innovations. The innovation leader is continually focused on personal growth and development as the means to empower others. Most importantly, the innovation leader is comfortable with personal limitations and the reality that one cannot possibly know everything there is to know about any one topic.

Kelly's (2005) Ten Faces of Innovation provides an excellent resource for the ways in which individuals approach innovation. In addition, a list of negative behaviors is listed for the leader to consider both types of behaviors (**Table 6-5**).

Strategy No. 3: Bank on Teamwork

Innovation work requires a team. No one individual can conceive, develop, and deliver an innovation. Numerous individuals with diverse skills are needed to bring an idea from conception to reality. The team makes individuals successful as a result from the emergence of their collaborative efforts and collective wisdom.

Harry S. Truman is known for his comment, "It is amazing what you can accomplish when you don't care who gets the credit." The essence of this comment is not only about minimizing the need for an individual to be recognized for great work, but also about the importance of unrestrained and enthusiastic collaboration among individuals. It is about continually encouraging the human spirit and expectation that the universal human capacity to invent and create can be realized. So, too, is the work of innovation leadership that requires involvement of those key stakeholders in the formulation, design, implementation, and evaluation stages to be successful.

According to von Hippel (2005) the importance of *democratizing innovation* cannot be overstated. Moving the work of innovation from isolated local teams to maximize collaboration and involvement of designers, end users, providers, informaticists, marketers, and the like increases the likelihood of useful, sustainable solutions.

Wheatley (2001), a noted leadership expert, has also recognized the essential nature of teamwork and participation. Including all individuals who are going to be impacted by a change is critical. When we fail to invite these individuals into the creation process, they become resistors and saboteurs. It is not only the management of resistance that the leader needs to consider, but also the recognition and integration of the incredible contributions that others can make.

Strategy No. 4: Recognize and Reward Innovation Work

Traditionally, recognition and rewards in health care are based on the achievement of established goals and targets. Negative feedback and loss of rewards results when targets and goals are not met. Providing negative feedback is inconsistent with the need for creative and innovative thinking and requires significant modification if healthcare organizations are to be successful in both creating new approaches to care and stable patient care services. According to Sweeney (2004), there is a need to reinforce and reward risk taking and creative behavior at a 10 to 1 ratio in order to

10 Faces of Innovation*	Positive description	Negative behaviors
1. Anthropologist	Observing human behavior to understand	Avoids getting involved in new enterprises
2. Experimenter	Takes calculated risks	Requires assurance/guarantee before embarking on new product or activity.
3. Cross-pollinator	Explores other industries and cultures and translates those findings into one's own	Focuses on internal area of expertise only to build a better future
4. Hurdler	Develops skill in overcoming or out-smarting roadblocks	Views roadblocks as endpoints
5. Collaborator	Leads from the middle of the pack to create new combinations and multidisciplinary solutions	Autocratic leadership style that does not seek or desire input from others
6. Director	Gathers together a talented cast and crew and works to spark their creative talents	Works as a director in position of superiority; requires allegiance and obedience
7. Experience architect	Designs compelling experiences that go beyond mere functionality to connect at a deeper level with customers latent or expressed needs.	Stays focused on what is currently being done within the industry/organization and works to make it better on the basis of personal beliefs and values.
8. Set designer	Creates a stage on which innovation team members can do their best work	Relies on research, publications and experts to create new models.
9. Caregiver	Delivers customer care in a manner that goes beyond mere service; anticipates needs and is ready to meet needs.	Focuses on standardized products and services; avoids customization.
10. Storyteller	Builds morale and awareness through compelling narratives that communicate a fundamental value or cultural trait.	Focuses on the facts and outcomes; avoids personal discussions or feelings.

Table 6-5 Kelly's Ten Faces of Innovation with positive and negative behaviors
*Source: Kelly, T. (2005). *The ten faces of innovation*. New York: Doubleday.

counteract an individual's fear of failure. For every success, nine other attempts were not successful, and positive feedback about these nine attempts is needed. Further, this level of positive feedback needs to be in place for a long time before a positive impact occurs. This approach is much like the funnel approach when considering new ideas. Numerous ideas are needed before one workable process or product results (**Figure 6-1**). Little empirical evidence exists for the successful proportion of affirmations to actual successes; however, what is known is that there must be significantly more positive affirmations to produce a single result.

Strategy No. 5: Avoid Reliance on Technology

Innovation leadership is not about introducing new technologies. It is much more about the individual and change; it is about *person* change rather than *technology* change. It is about assisting individuals to look at work differently, reexamining processes for value, eliminating work that no longer produces value, and learning new skills to manage technologies. In health care, the four technologies of the electronic medical record, telehealth, clinical monitoring technology, and distance technology have been adopted by healthcare organizations to improve the quality of health care and are

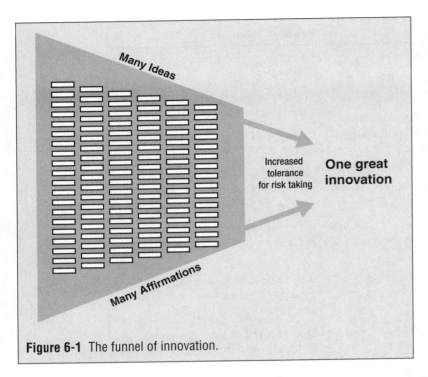

Figure 6-1 The funnel of innovation.

considered tools of innovation—not the essence of health care. From the electronic record, leaders anticipate improved speed in data management, productivity, accuracy, and completeness of records. Decreases in medical errors are also expected. Reliance on the electronic medical record to eliminate medication errors without consideration of human factors involved is unrealistic. There may, in fact, be more new medication errors from the use of the electronic record.

Another consideration in assuring that technology is considered a tool rather than a driving entity is the difference in generations and their experiences with technology. For those born before the technology explosion, most notably the baby boomers, the use of technology is more likely to be perceived as an add-on feature. The challenge to see technology as a helpful tool rather than the primary essence is much greater for this generation than it is for generations X and Y. These generations have grown up with computers, video games, cell phones, and video cameras and fundamentally think and process information differently; they are digital natives. The baby boomers are considered digital immigrants—individuals who began to use digital equipment at a later point in life (Prensky, 2001). Digital immigrants learn to adapt to their environment while retaining the imprinted ways of the nondigital world. For innovation leaders, consideration and sensitivity to these two widely different mind-sets and skill sets is necessary to effect an environment supportive of innovation. What may be required for digital immigrants to innovate may not be needed by digital natives. Necessarily, the innovation leader must become comfortable with the technology evolution regardless of one's status as immigrant or native.

Strategy No. 6: Creating the Business Case for Innovation

Linking the value of innovation with financial data is an expectation for innovation leaders. However, identifying the value metrics and qualitative indicators for innovation is perhaps one of the most challenging processes for the healthcare leader (Burns, 2005). The need to identify value for new work that is yet to be done is important and often requires intuitive estimations and the selection of historical trend markers. What is also important is that evidence and evaluation markers are selected, evaluated, and revised throughout the innovation process.

> ### Point to Ponder
>
> Leaders in one generation of technology are seldom leaders in the next.
>
> Ralph Katz

The evaluation of innovation processes requires a more robust model of evaluation. Specific variables for each of these categories must be considered and monitored in any innovation work. The gold standard for evidence has been the randomized clinical trial (RCT), a rigorous, costly method to determine what actually works and to what degree it works. More recently, clinicians have been challenged to move beyond the RCT to *realistic evaluation* (Pawson & Tilley, 2007). This model requires the consideration and integration of the context which includes the influences of the environment, geographic region, cultural values, economic resources and political components.

Providing the funding for innovation challenges even the most sophisticated organizations. The need for a positive net income margin drives financial assumptions, types of analyses and monitoring tools, and allocation of resources. It is always a challenge to fund innovation in that such ideas are too undeveloped to examine using traditional financial models. The questions of product price, expected units to be sold, developmental costs, training, and desired profit margin are nearly impossible to determine and would be merely guesswork if attempted. Christensen, Kaufman, and Shih (2008) validated the lack of good financial tools for innovation and asserted that using traditional tools distorts the value, importance, and likelihood of success of investments in innovation.

Healthcare organization leaders must courageously challenge existing financial models and create funding resources for idea generation, testing, implementation, and evaluation that support innovative thinking and processes. The designation of funds to support personnel and innovation tools in every department must become the norm rather than an optional expense if long-term sustainability of the organization is the expectation. No process or technology can be considered immune from improvement; thus the support for innovative thinking and design needs to be pervasive.

MANAGING INNOVATION DISPLACEMENT

With the addition of new processes and technologies, old work often becomes obsolete. As part of any innovation implementation planning, attention should be given to what should be given up or eliminated. This causes angst among many workers. Innovation tools, particularly pre- and postinnovation process mapping, can be helpful. A comparison of the two process maps can highlight eliminated work and steps that can also be modified in the job expectations. This objective data can be helpful in guiding teams to make the most appropriate decisions in work redesign.

MANAGING OBSTACLES TO INNOVATION

Some believe that the lack of funding is the greatest obstacle to innovation; however, the importance of relationship and communication skills should never be minimized or overlooked. Indeed, the ability and courage to be an innovation leader may be more significant than the funding. Without strong personal commitment, no amount of funding can advance innovation in any organization.

Kanter (2006) identified the classic traps of innovation that have occurred repeatedly over time. Four categories were identified: strategy, process, structure, and skills traps. In each of these areas, lessons are identified with strategies to manage. Innovation strategy should include small and incremental innovations as well as larger, more significant improvements. Using the innovation pyramid or funnel (Figure 6-1) approach to continually identify, filter, and focus on potential solutions is helpful in avoiding the emphasis on only large projects. The decision-making structure for innovation requires fewer tight, formal controls and greater reliance on interpersonal communication. Also, systems for recognition and reward should be available in addition to traditional performance rewards. Finally, the skill set for innovation requires wide dissemination of knowledge, tools, and resources rather than limitation of these resources to selected individuals or departments.

MOVING FORWARD

Innovation leadership is the norm for contemporary leaders rather than the exception and requires a mind-set for both stability and growth. Significant and regular demonstrations of courage are required to not only balance these two organizational imperatives but also to achieve large-scale spread of new practices. Passion and commitment are equally required in what are sometimes believed to be impossible levels. Yet, the innovation leader ventures on, knowing that the best is yet to come.

REFERENCES

Burns, L. R. (2005). *The business of healthcare innovation.* Cambridge, United Kingdom: Cambridge University Press.

Christensen, C. M., Kaufman, S. P., & Shih, W. C. (2008). Innovation killers: How financial tools destroy your capacity to do new things. *Harvard Business Review, 86* (1), 98–105.

Fraser, S. W. (2007). *Undressing the elephant: Why good practice doesn't spread in healthcare.* Available at *www.lulu.com*

Kanter, R. M. (2006). Innovation: The classic traps. *Harvard Business Review, 86* (11), 73–83.

Katz, R. (2003). *Harvard business essentials: Managing creativity and innovation.* Boston, MA: Harvard Business School Publishing.

Kelly, T. (2005). *The ten faces of innovation.* New York: Doubleday.

Pawson, R., & Tilley, N. (1997). *Realistic Evaluation.* San Francisco: Sage.

Plsek, P. (2003, January). Complexity and the adoption of innovation in healthcare. NIHCM/National Committee for Quality Health Care conference, Washington, DC.

Prensky, M. (2001). Digital natives, digital immigrants. *On the Horizon, 9* (5), 1–6.

Rogers, E. M. (2003). (5th ed). *Diffusion of Innovations.* New York: Simon and Schuster.

Sweeney, J. (2004). *Innovation at the speed of laughter.* Minneapolis, MN: Aerialist Press.

Ulwick, A. W. (2008). *Turning customer input into innovation.* Boston, MA: Harvard Business School Press.

von Hippel, E. (2005). *Democratizing innovation.* Cambridge, MA: MIT Press.

Wheatley, M. J. (2001, Spring). Innovation means relying on everyone's creativity. *Leader to Leader, 20,* 14–20.

SUGGESTED READINGS

Anthony, S. D., Eyring, M., & Gibson, L. (2006). Mapping your innovation strategy. *Harvard Business Review, 86* (5), 104–113.

Berwick, D. M. (2003). Disseminating innovations in healthcare. *JAMA, 289* (15), 1969–1975.

Christensen, C. M., Anthony, S. D., & Roth, E. A. (2004). *Seeing what's next: Using the theories of innovation to predict industry change.* Boston, MA: Harvard Business School Press.

Christensen, C. M., Baumann, H., Ruggles, R., & Sadtler, T. M. (2006). Disruptive innovation for social change. *Harvard Business Review, 86* (12), 94–101.

George, B., Sims, P., McLean, A. N., & Mayer, D. (2007, February). Discovering your authentic leadership. *Harvard Business Review, 87* (2), 129–138.

Getz, I., & Robinson, A. G. (2003). Innovate or die: Is that a fact? *Creativity and Innovation Management, 12* (3), 130–136.

Kirby, E. G., Keeffe, M. J., & Nicols, K. M. (2007). A study of the effects of innovative and efficient practices on the performance of hospice care organizations. *Health Care Management Review, 32* (4), 352–359.

Porter-O'Grady, T. (2007, February). The CNE as entrepreneur: Innovation leadership for a new age. *Nurse Leader,* 44–47.

Rostenberg, B. (2007, February). The cost of innovation. *Healthcare Design,* 18–26.

Verganti, R. (2006). Innovating through design. *Harvard Business Review, 86* (12), 114–121.

CHAPTER 7

Creating a Culture of Safety

CHAPTER OBJECTIVES:

Upon completion of this chapter, the reader will:

1. Identify the challenges of transforming the organizational healthcare culture from one of error avoidance to one in which error is an essential element for improvement.

2. Critique three theories of error and their application to healthcare organizations.

3. Translate lessons from the management of clinical errors to the management of errors in leadership.

4. Identify five principles to guide leaders in facilitating the transformation to a culture of safety.

INTRODUCTION

Traditional society values success and provides winners with recognition, trophies, financial rewards, and promotions. The achievement of goals and best practices receives high recognition while leadership failure is more likely recognized as a scarlet letter, or worse, is not discussed at all. Yet, along the journey to success, leaders do indeed experience failures or less-positive-than-anticipated results. Failure is bound to occur in every organization and in every career.

A new perspective is needed in order to recognize and value the information gained in less-than-successful attempts. Leaders need to reverse many assumptions and learn to embrace situations in which the desired outcomes were not realized. Failures must be viewed as acts of courage and recognized as essential behaviors that do indeed support a culture of excellence for the incredible insight and dialogue that results. A positive and realistic interpretation of the failure experience and the resulting lessons provides all leaders with necessary experiences for a better future. This chapter presents an overview of theories of error, the characteristics of the current healthcare culture of error avoidance, and strategies to transform the healthcare culture to one that values errors as opportunities. Five principles to guide the transformation are presented to assist leaders in this important journey.

Failures and Mistakes Are . . .

- Lack of success, a deficiency, or falling short
- Not achieving something desired
- Portals of discovery (James Joyce)
- The highway to success, as each discovery of what is false leads us to seek earnestly after what is true (John Keats).

A perspective grounded in valuing the experience of error begins with the transition from discipline as the initial reaction to remediation, in which the human factors are identified and an effort to learn from error events is an expectation rather than an option.

THEORIES OF ERROR

Errors are defined in numerous ways, most of which reflect failures or unwanted outcomes. Failures, according to Leape (1999), have been described in two categories: active or system errors that stem from characteristics of communication systems, job design, or equipment; and latent or organizational failures that arise from decisions made by people with indirect responsibilities. Both accidents and recurrent errors result from a series of human decisions associated with both active and latent failures, with active failures having the more immediate and obvious consequences and latent failures undermining organizational efforts to create a safe environment.

Gem

Failure *is* an option . . . when you are dealing with human reality!

Error as Foolishness

Given the reality of human nature and its normal state of imperfection, some scholars have attempted to explain error from an interesting perspective of errors as the result of human foolishness (Kaye, 2000). Humanity begins in a state of perfection, and the journey of life is filled with temptation and distractions. Understandably, humanity partakes from the tree of information and experience that includes both good and evil.

As people mature and stray from the initial state of perfection, errors or mistakes are made. People become distracted and tempted by many things—often the desire for more worldly goods. Not surprising, people follow their desires, losing the awareness of perfection, ignoring the inner voice of wisdom, and giving in to the temptation. Sometimes, individuals risk everything for one more personal thing—another automobile, boat, computer, or vacation—negating the sense of personal wholeness. Error results.

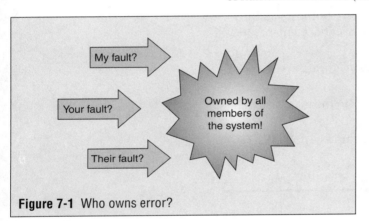

Figure 7-1 Who owns error?

While not all leaders may be comfortable with the theory of errors as foolishness, this mental model provides a framework from which to examine the phenomenon of errors in a more positive way, one that humanizes the error factor. Recognizing that mistakes are expressions of inescapable foolishness rather than the result of malice enables individuals to let the errors go and to avoid taking them personally so that they do not cast a shadow over a lifetime's career. Accepting ourselves and our own mistakes in this way can serve as the basis for responding to the mistakes of others with understanding, rather than responding with anger and resentment (Porter-O'Grady & Malloch, 2003).

Further, the errors-as-foolishness perspective allows individuals to overcome the human tendency to hold a grudge when an error that is believed unnecessary and avoidable is made. Quantum leaders learn to forgive others when a mistake is made and begin to coach others to learn from the event. Moving beyond the resentment of grudges encourages others to expect to be treated as others treat them, with understanding and kindness. Now the leader can move from the need for punishment as the remedy to error to a new mental model in which error is an opportunity for growth. Learning to believe and trust that mistakes may in fact bring great fortune and new opportunities is the only way to move from the toxicity of a blameful culture to one of accountability.

Sagan (1993) identified two theories of error: normal accident theory and high reliability theory. Each theory reflects differing assumptions specific to the basic nature of how organizations operate and analyze complex situations.

Normal Accident Theory

The basic assumption of normal accident theory is that accidents are inevitable in complex systems. In many ways, there is a contradiction to decision-making philosophy: Decentralization is needed to manage the complexity of the system, and centralization is expected to assure tight controls and standardization. System redundancy is believed to be the cause of accidents and further increases interactive complexity and encourages inappropriate risk taking. The theory is similar to a military model that includes strong discipline and control, which is much different than a model of shared leadership and collaborative decision making. There is no way that organizations can train for unanticipated, dangerous, or politically unacceptable situations within this theoretical framework. Finally, the most problematic notions of this theory include the denial of personal responsibility, faulty reporting, and the negative value of reviewing error incidents.

High Reliability Theory

In contrast, high reliability theory assumes that intelligent organizational design and management can avert serious errors when four factors are integrated in the system: safety as a priority; high redundancy in both technical and personnel systems; decentralized operations; and well-developed trial-and-error organizational learning processes. The core belief of this theory is that accidents or errors can be prevented through good organizational design and management. Redundancy enhances safety, as duplication and overlap can render a system reliable rather than unreliable. Continuous evaluation, training, and simulations further support and maintain high-reliability operations. And most importantly, trial-and-error learning from accidents is believed effective and necessary.

THE CULTURE OF ERROR AVOIDANCE

Each of these perspectives offers insight into the existing healthcare culture of organizational error avoidance. The healthcare culture is embedded with complex communication processes and conflicting values. Within most healthcare organizations, unique social hierarchies are dominated by the medical profession. This long-standing social stratification has a profound impact upon the relationships, communication practices, conflict management, expectations for collaboration, displays of emotion, and patient care practices. Dominance of one group over another has contributed significantly to the prevailing practices that support error avoidance and further darken the landscape of error management and the resulting disciplinary processes.

Efforts to address the dark side of discipline require a strong organizational culture that encourages and values safety, accountability, and empowerment of employees to perform responsibly rather than robotically. Standards are necessary for order and consistency but are seldom appropriate for all situations, as the reason for ongoing human evaluation and modification of standards is to assure that the evolving goals of safety and quality are indeed met.

Within the current culture of error avoidance, four common themes have been identified as contributing to the situation: first, long-standing problems that have not been addressed; second, the potential harm was significant; third, the management systems were inadequate; and fourth, little was learned by leaders from repeated errors. Another confounding issue is that time for learning and remediation of systems has been limited or nonexistent in financially strapped organizations. Additionally, the failure to learn from errors is often not caused by the lack of interest in learning to

---

Discussion

Three theories of error, error as foolishness, normal accidents, and high reliability, provide the foundational philosophy for much error management.

- Which theory does your organization or department subscribe to?
- How was this choice made?
- Is there a need for a theoretical shift in thinking?
- How would this shift be accomplished?
- Who would be involved?
- Who are the supporters?
- What are the barriers?

High-Reliability Organizations' Defining Characteristics

1. Preoccupation with failure
2. Reluctance to simplify work
3. Sensitivity to operations
4. Commitment to resilience
5. Deference to expertise

Weick & Sutcliffe, 2001

Culture

The integrated pattern of human knowledge, belief, and behavior that depends upon man's capacity for learning and transmitting knowledge to succeeding generations.

Merriam-Webster's Dictionary

Common Expressions of Culture

- *Observed regularities:* how people interact, their language, customs, and traditions
- *Group norms:* implicit standards and values, such as meetings always starting on time
- *Espoused values:* the publicly announced principles that the group claims to be trying to achieve
- *Formal philosophy:* the broad policies and ideological principles that guide a group's actions toward employees, customers, and stakeholders
- *Climate:* the feeling that is conveyed in a group by the physical layout and the way in which members of the organization interact with each other, with customers, and with outsiders
- *Embedded skills:* the special competencies group members display in accomplishing certain tasks
- *Rules of the game:* the implicit rules for getting along in the organization that a newcomer must learn to become an accepted member
- *Habits of thinking, mental models:* the shared cognitive frames that guide the perceptions, thought, and language used by the members of the group
- *Shared meanings:* the emergent understandings that are created by group members as they interact with each other
- *Integrating symbols:* the ideas, feelings, and images groups develop to characterize themselves, which may or may not be appreciated consciously but become embodied in buildings, office layout, and other material artifacts of the group

Root Cause Analysis: Facilitator or Barrier?

If an unwanted situation tends to occur repeatedly, then it might be beneficial to figure out what is really causing this situation to occur and remove it so the situation does not occur again. This process, root cause analysis, involves finding the real cause of the problem and dealing with it rather than simply continuing to deal with the symptoms. It has become commonplace in health care.

But is root cause analysis really an appropriate phrase and approach when our world is endlessly interconnected and everything seems to influence so many other things? Seeking the root cause may be a reinforcement of a culture focused on finding blame rather than one supporting error as opportunity. Do you agree? Disagree?

improve processes, but rather is the result of the strong disincentives against exposing serious failures. Two sets of records (external and internal documents) further constrain learning opportunities. Interestingly, efforts to internally examine what really occurred and to fully discuss the situation often result in transforming the experiences of failure into successes as a means to mediate liability! (No changes in unsafe systems or behaviors occur to decrease liability exposure.)

Finally, while the attempt to analyze errors through sentinel events and root cause analysis (RCA) has increased awareness and focus on significant errors, the limitations of the RCA are problematic. Few problems can be traced to a single or root cause; most problems or errors are the result of multiple factors in the environment and multiple interactions between multiple providers (Scott, 2004). The RCA is only the beginning step of error analysis, not the end point.

TRANSFORMING THE HEALTHCARE CULTURE

Leaders are called to create better systems for investigating failures, for reporting errors, and for implementing the lessons learned. Eliminating practices that support secrecy, defensiveness, and deference to authority is essential in transforming the current healthcare culture. The next step is to create strong incentives for reporting errors and to support the identification of failures as means to work more effectively.

A culture supportive of safety requires a compelling vision related to patient safety, structures to oversee patient safety and the cultural evolution, systematic approaches to examining and addressing errors, practice and support for team learning, and reinforcement of new behaviors. To begin the journey, much can be learned from clinical error research.

LESSONS FROM CLINICAL ERROR MANAGEMENT

Clinical errors have been analyzed extensively in the recent past and offer information not only about the errors but also about the systems in which the errors occur. The clinical errors that have been studied include unnecessary procedures, treatment complications, and near-miss situations. Fortunately, recommendations from the Institute of Medicine (2001) and Page (2004) have identified many of the specific actions that can improve patient safety. However, overall the analyses provide information that is both alarming and challenging. According to Walshe and Shortell (2004), in most cases of major failure, the systems of quality management in healthcare organizations have been unable to cope with the identified problems. Current systems intended to manage clinical errors are easily bypassed or sidetracked and fail to raise the alarm that something is wrong.

The recommendations from clinical error experiences require changes in not only the culture of the organization but also in leader behaviors for initiating and sustaining practices supportive of patient safety. Error events occur in the processes of leadership as well as in the provision of patient care. For the most part, it is only the leader or the team of individuals responsible for the context of care that can change conditions to minimize both leadership and clinical error as the vehicle to improving patient safety. Given the many perspectives and complex dynamics within the error event, this task is no small challenge.

Leaders need to translate the processes and lessons learned from the analysis of clinical errors and facilitate the needed cultural changes to create the desired culture of safety. They must also examine their own failed practices to provide more reliable systems. Gaining an understanding of fundamental error research, assessing one's organization, creating principles of leadership safety, and facilitating the necessary changes to transform the cultures are all necessary steps in the journey to excellence.

LEADERSHIP ERROR

Unlike clinical error, leadership error is largely uncharted territory in healthcare literature (Chaffee & Arthur, 2002). Many interpretations of leadership error exist and traditionally focus on the failure to deliver healthcare services, the mismatch between an individual and the work to be done, or inadequate educational preparation. Regardless of the perspective of leadership error, a new lens that expects leaders to focus on learning from the experience of the error rather than attempting to eliminate errors is essential in the journey to excellence.

Many lessons can be learned from the recent studies on clinical patient safety. The solutions to problems that address the interwoven contributions of both the individual and the established collective culture of an organization have not been readily apparent. While it often seems straightforward to affix blame to either the individual or the system, solutions that exclusively focus either on the individual or on the organization have been less than acceptable to the healthcare industry. A shift from an error mentality that requires punishment to a mindset that values error as opportunity and includes the realities of human factors such as the amount and type of experience, level of skill, level of fatigue, and motivation affecting a person's ability to perform well is essential in order for progress to be made.

The National Council of State Boards of Nursing's seminal work in the study of registered nurse discipline is the Taxonomy of Error Root Cause Analysis Protocol (TERCAP). Several categories are relevant in the study of leadership error and include initial human factors consideration. The TERCAP categories of lack of attentiveness, lack of professional accountability, inappropriate judgment, poor judgment in the supervision of others, and documentation errors will be presented as vehicles in the creation of leadership safety principles.

ONE IMPORTANT CAVEAT: CULT OR CULTURE FOR TRANSFORMATION

First and foremost, the need for transformation from a punitive culture to an error-supportive culture is not an option. The healthcare industry cannot afford to shield and avoid the reality of errors. Further, it is not a choice about changing policies and report formats to external agencies; it is an expectation from consumers and requires an understanding of the organizational culture and how to effectively begin the long and arduous journey in changing fundamental behaviors, beliefs, and values. Such a journey will not occur quickly or without significant struggle, even though most leaders know in their heart that it should be done quickly and with the support of all of the industry.

The journey to a culture of safety requires more changes in behavior than most can envision initially. The transformation must be focused on sustainable cultural change rather than superficial behavior changes that

Essential Elements for Cultural Transformation

- A vision that identifies safety as a priority
- Commitment to replacing systems that don't work
- Support for continuous learning of all employees to strengthen the system
- Resources within the organization to expect, support, and reward critical thinking

Leadership Failure

- Failure to achieve a specific, defined organizational goal as a result of intrinsic (made by the leader in planning or execution) or extrinsic (system factors not within the leader's sphere of influence) factors.
- The inability to exhibit basic leadership skills of enabling others to do their work, role modeling, challenging processes, and inspiring a shared vision.

Human Factors

- Motivation
- Skill level
- Experience
- Fatigue

Human Factors

- The discipline that tries to optimize the relationship between technology and the human (Kantowitz and Sorkin, 1983).
- The central approach of the human factors discipline is the application of relevant information about human characteristics and behavior to the design of objects, facilities, and environments that people use (Grandjean and Vigliani, 1980).
- The goal of the human factors discipline is to apply knowledge in designing systems that work, accommodating the limits of human performance, and exploring the advantages of the human operator in the process (Yeh & Wickens, 1984).
- The application of the human factors discipline discovers and applies information about human behavior, abilities, limitations, and other characteristics to the design of tools, machines, systems, tasks, jobs, and environments for productive, safe, comfortable, and effective human use (Chapanis, 1996).

Taxonomy of Error Root Cause Analysis
Protocol Categories (TERCAP)

- Lack of attentiveness/surveillance
- Lack of or faulty intervention
- Lack of professional accountability
- Inappropriate judgment
- Missed or mistaken order
- Lack of prevention
- Documentation errors
- Medication errors

Benner et al., 2002

are strongly supported by the leader and champion for safety. Leaders are expected to add value to the organization that is sustainable long after they leave.

Creating a culture of leadership requires the leader to plan to become indispensable as the culture permeates the organization. According to Deering, Dilts, and Russell (2003), if an organization falls apart after the leader departs, the subsequent ruin is, in a sense, a validation of the leader's talent and evidence of the value added during his or her tenure. It is also evidence of the leader's failure to endow the organization with the qualities needed to transcend previous achievements and nurture the conditions under which leadership can exist successfully.

Marx (2001) identified the *just culture* framework as a means to guide both leaders and clinicians in reframing the phenomenon of medical error to eliminate the social condemnation and expectation of discipline for all medical errors. In the just culture model, the emphasis, much like the TERCAP model, is on promoting a culture in which individuals and team members learn from mistakes and facilitate rapid course correction. Human error, at-risk behaviors, and reckless behaviors are the three categories of behavior. The follow-up expected for each type of behavior—from counseling for human error, to coaching for at-risk behavior, to punishing for reckless behavior—is also appropriate from a leadership perspective in addition to the clinical application. The leadership errors of managers and leaders are more likely to be inadvertent mistakes rather than deliberate at-risk or conscious disregard actions, and efforts to learn from these events is more productive than meting out punishment.

Some leaders unknowingly fail to create a culture of leadership and instead foster a personal cult—a rudimentary, incomplete, inherently ephemeral phenomenon that fades away when the personality who created it departs. In contrast, a culture is much more durable and robust, because its survival and strength do not require the presence and personality of a single individual. Culture is something that arises from and is shared by all members of an organization or social system. Organizations with leadership cultures will outperform leadership cults in the following three aspects: anticipating what is needed, aligning values and behaviors, and acting on the basis of priorities that will sustain the culture. Given this, the message is clear to leaders as they embark on changing the current healthcare culture. As leaders facilitate the transformation to a culture in which error is valued as an opportunity, the risk of creating a cult is significant. Too often, changes are viewed as fads and attached to specific individuals rather than integrated into the essential core of the culture. Avoiding creation of a cult in favor of a long-standing, sustainable culture will support the organization rather than render it sensitive to each new superficial fad designed to improve safety.

Personal Cult Versus Culture

A cult is a rudimentary, incomplete, inherently ephemeral phenomenon that fades away when the personality that creates it departs. In contrast, a culture is much more durable and robust than a cult, because its survival and strength do not require the presence and personality of a single individual.

Deering et al., 2003

CREATING A CULTURE OF SAFETY:
FIVE PRINCIPLES FOR LEADERS

Transformation of the healthcare culture requires commitment, a clear and compelling vision, and guiding principles to support progress and serve as checkpoints for evaluation. The following five principles are offered to the leader and are based on current research and publications specific to error research, cultural transformation, and contemporary leadership in complex systems. Each principle includes an overview of the principle, nonsupporting behaviors that should be changed, and supportive strategies to strengthen the processes of cultural transformation.

Principle No. 1: Self-Awareness of Leadership Style, Values, and Beliefs

The first principle is self-awareness of one's leadership style, values, and beliefs. Knowing your values and reactions to clinical error or any failure within the organization is the first and most important step in cultural transformation. Indeed, personal awareness requires careful analysis of how errors are acknowledged, discussed, and documented. For most leaders, a new lens from which to understand failure is needed. While most leaders know that failure of some type at some level is a fact of life, the ambivalence about failure has created an unhealthy state of denial that begins with individual values and perceptions of error as failure that cannot be tolerated and must be eliminated. Our hearts know that failure is inevitable, yet our heads too often tell us that punishment is an essential and expected leader behavior.

Learning to view failure as the result of many factors rather than personal inadequacy is much easier said than done. Working with colleagues to change behaviors and attitudes, acting as coaches and mentors for each other, is the first step in the transformation. Informal, ongoing commitment to new behaviors creates more sustainable change than a one-day seminar. Working in small groups to critique and reinforce each other supports timely dialogue and minimizes the fear of intimidation. Further, leader colleagues can address the unrealistic expectations for performance, assure that adequate time is taken to reflect on one's personal impact and progress in changing behavior, and recognize successful encounters with error.

Poor Judgment in the Supervision of Others

A common leadership error involves poor judgment in the supervision of others. The error could be the result of oversupervision, undersupervision, or inadequate supervision. The span of control for leaders may become unmanageable with overwhelming numbers of individuals to facilitate, leaving many gaps in the key processes of healthcare work. Not knowing what is occurring, it cannot be monitored or modified. This is not to imply that micromanagement is necessary to be sure that everything is done correctly, but leaders need to be cognizant of the real-time effectiveness of processes and be able to course correct as quickly as possible when indicated.

Another example of poor judgment in the supervision of others is the inappropriate assignment of duties to colleagues or managers that is beyond their scope of competence, experience, or communication skills. The situation is further compromised when expectations are not clearly communicated, leaving the individual at risk for failure given that the expectations are not identified. Consider the situation in which an executive requests a newly hired director to attend a physician meeting in his or her place without clear expectations. The director, new to the organization, is unaware of the meeting agenda protocols, personalities of the attending members, and the role of an ex officio. While the director will eventually be quite competent to attend meetings in place of the executive, this situation could quickly become a negative experience and require significant efforts to reverse the impressions of both the new employee and members of the committee if the new employee interacts without background information.

Another example of poor judgment in the supervision of others is inadequate or infrequent monitoring of manager performance and outcomes. While the leader may be aware of the long hours put in by a director and assume that goals are being accomplished, failure by the leader to review outcomes regularly may reveal little or no progress when a review is actually held. It may be that the manager has indeed been

---

Self-Awareness Assessment

- Do I view failure as a personal flaw?
- Do I view failure as the outcome of many factors, individuals, and expectations?
- Am I comfortable in addressing failure as a means to increase the organization's ability to move forward?
- Do I overemphasize my strengths at the expense of weaknesses?
- How did I react to:
  - The last error in budget management?
  - Negative patient outcome?
  - Failure to achieve competency?
  - Hiring of an individual who did not have expected competencies?

Gem

There really is no failure . . . only mistakes that provide feedback and tell us where to go next.

Warren Bennis

Leadership Error

Inappropriate Judgment Examples

- Staff abandonment in times of great uncertainty and risk
- Failure to act due to reimbursement
- Inappropriate priorities (tunnel vision)
- Inappropriate withholding of resources
- Inappropriate acceptance of delegation/assignment

physically present in the facility, but not engaged in work expected for the role. Both the leader and the director would be disappointed and frustrated as both assumed progress was being made. It would be poor judgment to make an assumption that work was being accomplished by the mere presence of the director in the facility. In essence, the leader might be delegating appropriately but not effectively supervising the assignment and could be unknowingly directing substandard care processes.

Strategy: Be Accountable

Increasing professional accountability is an important step in addressing poor judgment issues. The lack of fiduciary or professional accountability has been identified (Benner et al., 2002) as a significant factor in error events. Leaders are expected to create and support the infrastructure for a culture of professional and personal accountability that includes behaviors, organizational norms, and management practices. The culture must eliminate or at least minimize those behaviors that reflect avoidance of accountability and reinforce behaviors supportive of accountability. Several behaviors are identified as not supportive leader actions:

> | Leadership Error |
> | :---: |
> | **Lack of Professional Accountability Examples** |
> | • Lack of respect for staff concerns and dignity |
> | • Lack of integrity; attributes responsibility to others |

- Failing to put the organization (mission, values, and beliefs) first
- Ignoring staff concerns or requests due to time, schedule, resources, or existing policy; denying accountability; delayed decision making in hopes of system self-correction
- Misunderstanding or violating the leader–staff–patient relationship; pointing the finger at others; claiming confusion and lack of understanding or information from recent meetings/communication
- Not acting responsibly in protecting staff, patient, family, and community vulnerabilities; supports physician abuse or poor staffing in favor of controlling expenses and maintaining revenues
- Not notifying others of significant events that impact the reputation and operations of the organization; fearful of feedback
- Lack of insight regarding staff needs; lack of sensitivity to differing generational and diversity needs; behaviors steeped in the values of one generation rather than multiple, diverse needs

> | Leadership Error |
> | :---: |
> | **Faulty Intervention Examples** |
> | • Deliberate error cover-up or avoidance of the issue |
> | • Boundary violations, for example, overmodified policies for selected employees based on personal relationships |
> | • Breach of confidentiality |
> | • Failure to detect faulty or missing information (lack of critical analysis) |
> | • Initiation of new programs without adequate orientation or training |

Reversing these ineffective behaviors begins with a personal assessment of leadership style and adopting the following behaviors:

- *Owning your own circumstances and the results achieved.* Solutions come only after someone takes the initiative to explore, search, and ask questions.
- *Staying engaged.* Commit yourself 100% to the work at hand. When difficult challenges persist, it is easy to give up and stop trying or to wait and see if things will get better on their own. Avoid this trap and consider what *can* be done instead of what *cannot* be done.
- *Recognizing the full reality of the situation and the contributions of multiple individuals.* Create new relationships that involve others you may not have previously considered to be a part of the solution.
- *Challenging current assumptions to support the best processes and outcomes.* Be persistent in formulating new and creative solutions that make progress possible.
- *Avoiding wasting time and energy on things one cannot change.* Acknowledge the reality of problems and challenges.
- *Just doing it, even if it is difficult.*
- *Never fearing learning from one's mistakes!*

Principle No. 2: Plan for Errors

Effective planning for error is about error prevention. That requires leaders assume very little, decrease their reliance on memory, and learn to develop cues that increase awareness of potential problems. The leader must increase awareness for minor but critical signals.

While it is impossible to prevent all errors, it is possible to be more prepared for the future. Reducing the risk of failure is a critical leadership behavior, and this includes the ability to define what might happen in the future and choose among available alternatives as a means to mediate risk. Leaders are challenged to create an infrastructure that will support early identification and open discussion of errors, in order to create better processes that will lead to fewer opportunities for errors and better patient outcomes. Learning to control the areas over which one has control and minimizing the areas in which there is little control is a relatively new mind-set for the quantum leader. Equally important is the need for the leader to not become risk intolerant but to be able to recognize and tolerate enough risk to assure quality and progress into the future, an often difficult position to determine. The level of risk tolerance that the leader selects is necessarily related to the significance of the potential undesirable outcomes.

Nonsupporting behaviors are reflected in the leader's lack of attentiveness to the needs of employees, to the results of ineffective systems, and to the lack of appropriate caregiver skills. In essence, the leader does not know which signposts or events within system processes are critical and require monitoring and intervention. This is different from willful neglect of duty; it is a lack of knowledge about what to observe and what to do. How employees are performing, their level of satisfaction and morale, and the level of clinical outcome achievement are essential variables that require monitoring. In essence, this leader is unaware of the system needs and is unable to develop proactive plans to support positive error management systems.

> ### Gem
>
> If you drop a frog into a pan of hot water, the frog will immediately react to the heat by jumping out of the pan. But if you carefully place the same frog in a pan of comfortably cold water, then slowly raise the temperature, the frog will accept the change, and perhaps without noticing it, stay in the water until the heat kills it.
>
> We all run the risk of getting cooked if we fail to notice the small changes that take place around us.

Strategy: Plan for Error Communication

A very important expectation for the leader in planning for errors is to create communication processes and expectations that allow for timely discussion of error-related issues. The agenda for such a discussion should include a review of overall results, reinforcement of good judgment, identification of situations in which near misses or failure to rescue was identified, solutions to identified problems, and review of the appropriate documentation needed. Participation in error discussion must include those responsible for and involved in the outcome to minimize handoff or communication delays. Limiting discussion to leaders and excluding direct caregivers decreases the potential for timely and comprehensive review of situations, development of appropriate solutions, and support from those responsible for implementing the new interventions. Finally, backup or alternate mechanisms for communication need to be created by the leader to assure that caregivers have timely access to discussion and solutions.

Assuring access to information as well as discussion is also significant for an effective process. Individuals need access to both electronic and paper data as a support for timeliness and quality. Communication of information should include multiple communication modalities: electronic, paper, and face-to-face sharing of information, not one modality exclusively. Using e-mail and the Internet are adjuncts to good face-to-face dialogue, not replacements. Finally, backup or downtime systems for electronic processes need to be established for timely resolution of issues.

Strategy: Manage Professional Licensure

Many caregivers hold professional licenses, including physicians, nurses, pharmacists, and therapists. While less than 2% of licensees are brought to a professional board for discipline, the occurrence of board violations is traumatic to both the organization and the individual.

Quantum leaders develop proactive processes to assure safe and legal practice by providers, and they work to decrease the potential for practice act violations. Developing specific plans to inform license holders of the specific state practice acts and the most common discipline categories is an example of a proactive step to assist practitioners to practice within the law. Approaches that support a proactive approach rather than a reactive approach can increase job satisfaction, reinforce the importance of safe staffing, and minimize situations that require reporting to the professional board.

Review of license scopes of practice and violations is best accomplished as part of new employee orientation and during annual updates. This approach serves to position employees for success, reinforces the legitimate role of the practitioner, and minimizes the potential for violations of professional practice acts. Discussion of multiple roles as a matrix of role accountabilities that identifies role boundaries is a valuable exercise in reinforcing expectations for practice. Discussion of the common licensure violations provides specific information and situations for employees to assist them to avoid such behaviors, which is a proactive approach. Sharing both the specific role accountabilities and the common deviations raises employee sensitivity to vulnerable situations and decreases opportunities for licensure violations. Examples of violations of licensure nurse practice acts in which nurses are disciplined include the following:

- Practicing beyond scope
- Medication errors
- Falsification on employment application
- Alcohol abuse
- Drug abuse/drug diversion
- Positive drug screen
- Failure to supervise
- Failure to assess and intervene
- Sexual misconduct
- Leaving duty station
- Theft from employer
- Theft from patient
- Documentation errors

Strategy: Assure Safe Staffing

An element of safe staffing is the number of hours that caregivers are scheduled to work. Research (Rogers, Hwang, Scott, Aiken, & Dinges, 2004) suggests that the use of extended work shifts and overtime has escalated as hospitals try to cope with the shortage of nurses. The evidence in this first national effort to quantify hospital staff nurse work hours and work patterns and the relationship to errors and near errors is significant, according to Rogers and colleagues. The risk of making an error significantly increases when work shifts are longer than 12 hours, when nurses work overtime, or when they work more than 40 hours per week. The real challenge for leaders becomes one of recognizing and evaluating the impact of this research on current staffing patterns, error rates, and staff availability. No simple solutions to this challenge are on the horizon.

Strategy: Rework the Physical Environment

Several key variables in the work environment have been identified as negatively impacting staff stress levels and increasing patient care errors. Leader involvement in design and redesign of the physical environment for patient care has never been more critical. Design of both work processes and work spaces can decrease medication errors and nosocomial infections. The most notable feature in reducing errors in the design of patient physical space is the provision of single-bed patient rooms rather than multiple-bed rooms or wards (Page, 2004).

The availability of reference material for nurses, unit dose dispensing, bar coding of medications, and smart infusion pumps, as well as physical space for medication preparation that is isolated to minimize distractions (no phone in the medication room) and adequate lighting are features that leaders should assure are present in the work setting (Page, 2004; Ulrich, Quan, Zimring, Joseph, & Choudhary, 2004). The review of over 600 rigorous research articles by Ulrich and colleagues is required reading for leaders who are focused on the physical environment as an important consideration in creating safer built environments for healthcare services.

Strategy: Reduce Handoffs

The transfer or handoff of patients from nurse to nurse, shift to shift, unit to unit, and organization to organization has been identified by Cook, Render, and Woods (2000) as a potential source of errors and adverse patient outcomes. Many errors originate from slips in transfers of materials, information, instructions, and different individuals. Armed with this information, leaders are well positioned to contribute to the planning for new or redesigned physical spaces and work processes, given that the gaps created during the handoff processes are known to threaten patient safety and to waste resources.

Strategy: Conduct Better Project Management

Many organizations have become quite competent in the management of projects and integration of sophisticated project management methodologies. Yet not all projects are successful; some lead to unanticipated and undesired results. When good projects fail, chances are the idea was good but the process of implementation was flawed. Project plans, timelines, and budgets are established to reduce the execution risk, which is the risk that the necessary activities will not be carried out properly. Plans are monitored carefully and systematically. Project teams execute their tasks on time and under budget, and yet the overall project still may fail to deliver the intended results. According to Matta and Ashkenas (2003), two critical risks are often neglected—the white space risk that some required activities won't be identified in advance, leaving gaps in the project plan; and the integration risk that the disparate activities won't come together at the end.

Several strategies can be used to avoid project failures. They include:

- Focus on results first, processes of project management second.
- Challenge the assumptions to be sure the white space or the unknowns are identified as quickly as possible throughout the project. Ask questions such as "Who else cares about this work?" and "Is there someone who can enhance or who will challenge this work?"
- Recognize that it is not possible to identify, plan for, and influence all of the variables in advance; what can be done is the creation of processes to continually challenge the assumptions and having the willingness to modify processes to achieve goals.

Principle No. 3: Create Balance Between Standardization and Customization

The catch-22 of health care must certainly be the need for standardization of processes to achieve reliability and personalization of care to support patient involvement and satisfaction! How does the leader assure consistent processes and still support patient care that considers the diverse values, beliefs, age, education, and culture of each individual? Mandates from regulatory agencies, accrediting organizations,

---

The Cost of Patient Handoffs

1. Potential delays in treatment. The average time from transfer order to arrival in a new room is 5.1 hours.
2. Average cost of labor per transport: $35.17 per hour.
3. Indirect costs of lost productivity, transport equipment, duplication, and rework of patient care documentation, additional linen, and housekeeping expenses.
4. An increase of 0.5 days in hospital stay due to disruptions in the care processes.

Cook et al., 2000

White Space

Examples of White Space:

- Hidden financial costs
- Unknown competing projects
- New legislative mandates
- Unknown project resistors

The Ultimate Dilemma: Standardize or Personalize?

Consider the situation of medication administration. The clinical staff has determined that all medications will be passed at standardized times to assure completion of the task and decrease errors of omission. Recently, patients have requested to take medications at different times more like their own medication times at home.

- How will you address this situation?
- What are the advantages and disadvantages of each approach?
- What changes should or should not be made?
- What is the rationale for your changes and how will you monitor the results?

and professional licensing boards require leaders to create policies supportive of safe practices, clinical standards, and fiscal viability. Coupled with these mandates is the expectation that leaders also create the organizational context that supports personalization of health care. Necessarily, given the complex and multiple accountabilities of the leader, work should be designed to minimize the need for human tasks that are known to be especially fallible. Checklists, protocols, and computerized decision tools should be incorporated whenever possible.

Strategy: Use Evidence-Based Practice

Standardization based on personal agendas and opinions rather than evidence and rationale has resulted in significant redundancies in health care. While there has never been an excess of resources for health care, practice has not been focused on evidence until recently. Efforts to become more judicious in the use of limited resources have elevated the need for evidence-based practices. Thus, it is through the use of evidence that the leader can find solutions to the dilemma of standardization versus personalization. Those practices that are known to support safety must be supported, while those practices that are believed to be effective but not supported by evidence can be negotiated.

Evidence indicates that patients who receive care based on the best and latest evidence from well-designed studies experience 28% better outcomes (Heater, Becker, & Olson, 1998). More recent information suggests that in spite of the numerous studies, few healthcare providers are incorporating research findings into patient care decisions (Melnyk & Fineout-Overholt, 2005).

Leaders can meet the challenge through an intensified focus on first creating the infrastructure and policies that support evidence, then standardization and personalization to assure quality. Evidence-based practice can either integrate the use of published research studies or become the rationale for further study and validation. Integration of a disciplined decision-making process will necessarily support positive outcomes and reduce errors caused from wide variations and personal choice decision making.

Principle No. 4: Continually Ensure Staff Competence

Effective leadership systems provide the context for the right caregiver doing the right task at the right time, resulting in the right outcome. Leaders serve the system well through creating shared leadership structures in which individuals are accountable for their competence and can identify for the organization when new systems as well as new practices are needed to support technology and research. Quantum leaders serve best by role modeling behaviors of maintaining personal competence and an approach to errors that reflects the philosophy of errors as opportunities. Coupled with the structure, the expectation is that individuals are empowered to risk, to fail, and to be able to optimize personal effectiveness. Lifelong learning in the healthcare setting becomes a dynamic process between the leader and accountable professionals.

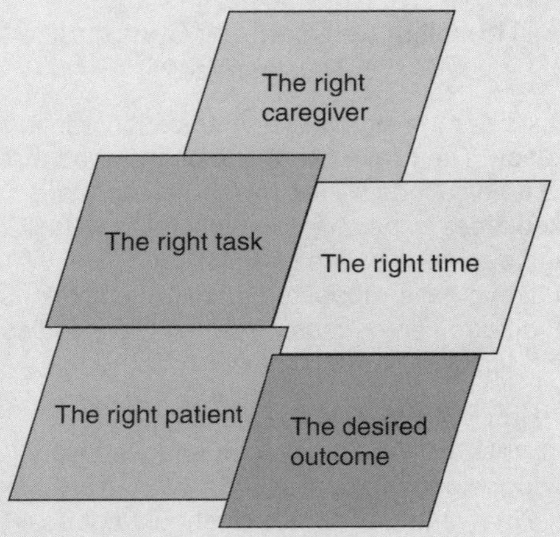

Strategy: Take New Approaches for Old Problems

Competence is about more than having knowledge and technical skills; it is also about the physical and mental capacity of the caregiver. Many times, nurses with knowledge and technical skills are exhausted from long hours but continue to work for a variety of reasons, which include both organizational requests and personal needs. Reluctant to let patients down as well as not meet family commitments, nurses continue to work

---

Research Utilization

The use of knowledge typically based on a single study.

Barnsteiner and Prevost, 2002

Evidence-Based Practice

Evidence-based practice is the conscientious use of current best evidence in making decisions about patient care. It integrates:

- A systematic search for and critical appraisal of the most relevant evidence specific to a clinical question
- One's own clinical experience
- Patient preferences and values

Sackett et al., 2000

Figure 7-2 Safe practice rights.

in highly fatigued states. Given the resounding feedback from nurses and their frustration with excessive patient care assignments and their commitment to the patient, a claim-of-conscience approach may help temper the current adversarial environment.

Nursing is in desperate need of more contemporary vehicles for nurses to objectively express their concerns, discontent, and disillusionments with the work of nursing. The claim of conscience is one strategy that offers a new approach for nurses to address these concerns.

Traditionally, creating claims-of-conscience clauses has been a strategy to respect practitioner moral and/or religious views. While most conscience clauses require that claims are grounded in religious or moral view, in some jurisdictions, claims may be based upon personal judgment or philosophical views.

Claims-of-conscience components include who is eligible to use the conscience clause, procedures covered by the clause, and principles to be cited when using the clause. In some conscience clauses, the issues are limited to reproductive health or end-of-life issues. The responsibility for evaluating claims of conscience is typically shared across several levels of leadership: the immediate supervisor (attending physician/nurse manager), department chairman/chairwoman or director, and administrative executive. Another level includes a review board with members from various ethnic, religious, and academic areas. The review board is intended to represent the diversified demographics within the organization so that all staff might find an advocate.

Creating a new vehicle to address age-old, difficult-to-resolve dilemmas can have a profound application for nursing. The basic principles in evaluating a claim of conscience include:

1. The objection fits within a coherent system of moral, religious, cultural, and philosophical beliefs.
2. This belief reflects a consistently and diligently held core value of the petitioner.
3. The belief is such a key component of the petitioner's internal framework that violation of that belief would cause significant harm to him or her.
4. It would be inconsistent with the petitioner's core values to participate in the procedure or treatment.

Nursing Claims of Conscience

The following is an example of a nursing claim of conscience and serves as a starting point for nurses to discuss complex issues in a framework designed to protect the essence of the discipline of nursing and avoid errors.

1. The objection fits with the nursing code of ethics and is based on a commitment to provide safe, effective, and therapeutic patient care.
2. These beliefs are core beliefs of the nurse. Previous employment records reflect a history of exceptional performance and contributions to the organization and the discipline of nursing.
3. Continued expectations to care for an unreasonable volume and critical level of patients will cause significant stress, probable errors in care, and professional burnout.
4. The nurse is unable to practice under conditions that compromise the core values and beliefs of the profession unless modifications in workload are made.

Attempting to manage the nursing shortage from this perspective creates a new lens from which to examine the work. The outcome must involve negotiation of the workload, prioritization of the specific work to which the nurse is assigned, and elimination of nonvalue-added, nonurgent work. Mediating the demand for services becomes the approach, rather than continually expecting nurses to assume assignments in which errors are inevitable.

Leader Documentation Examples
• Strategic plan • Job descriptions • Performance evaluations • Staffing/scheduling plans and monthly schedules • Progress summaries • Service contracts • Committee records

Principle No. 5: Document Appropriately

The records of the healthcare organization provide evidence of services provided, employee history, and the outcomes of those services. Errors in documentation or lack of appropriate documentation can compromise the work of the organization by failing to recognize its essential work, which necessarily includes the documentation of errors.

The leader is accountable for creating systems that identify appropriate documentation and also bears accountability for deliberate falsification or cover-up of information or failure to document care that was given. Finally, assuring timely processes to review the quality of documentation is essential in the creation of a culture of safety. Those doing the documentation must be involved in the review; reviews performed only by external reviewers or quality management specialists decrease the potential for sustainable solutions.

Creating Sustainable Solutions: Engaging Leaders in a Culture of Safety

Gem
There are not incompetent organizations. Rather, the errors in health care reflect the inherent limits of organizational safety. Recognition of that simple truth is the first and the most important step toward a safer future. Dr. Kathy A. Scott, 2004

It is not easy to avoid being too critical, too insensitive, or too demanding in complex cultures when things do go wrong and the past has rendered us victims of the outcomes. One can only hope that tolerance for mistakes will foster innovations and unleash creative solution finding. When leaders are confident that they will not be held to an impossibly high standard, the process of trial and error will enhance the learning process and encourage all individuals to act with the boldness that should be the hallmark of committed healers. Mistakes are not always indicative of future performance. The lessons of the past provide support and guidance to increasing maturity. Resilient leaders absorb the experiences of failure and incorporate them into their ability to evaluate anticipated actions for the future. In essence, it is the thirst and passion for lifelong learning that drives the leader to reflect honestly on both successes and failures. Further, failures that are not covered up, ignored, or addressed defensively can become the first moment from which lessons can be learned. Much work needs to be done to truly transform the current environment to one that recognizes error as opportunity and expects dialogue among individuals to create a better, more reliable future.

In summary, the following affirmations are offered for the leader aspiring to be effective in managing errors as opportunities:

- I am courageous and consistent in my actions to overcome barriers in achieving the organization's mission.
- My actions and words are consistent even when it would be easier to avoid the issue.
- I expect and encourage discussion of the difficult issues of leadership.
- I do not use my position to fulfill self-interests or further the interests of family, friends, or associates.
- I ensure equitable treatment of patients regardless of socioeconomic group or payor category.
- I demonstrate through organizational policies and discussion with colleagues that overtreatment and undertreatment of patients are unacceptable.
- I protect patients' rights to make their own decisions about care and to have full information about their illnesses, treatment options, and related costs.

Exercise 1 Scheduling and Safe Staffing

Creating a culture of safety is complex and far-reaching, given the research by Rogers and colleagues (2004). That identifies risk for error after 12 hours of work, identify how your organization will use this evidence.

Examine current schedules for numbers of 12-hour shifts that are associated with overtime.

- How many nurses work more than 40 hours per week?
- What are the error rate/near-miss incidents for this unit?
- Are the majority of errors discussed/reported?
- Request that staff nurses identify what changes need to be made in scheduling practices to control and minimize errors.
- What are the supporting factors and barriers to making changes in scheduling practices and policies?

Exercise 2 Remediate Rather than Discipline

This chapter has identified five principles to assist the leader in transforming from a culture of error avoidance to a culture that values error as an opportunity to create a better future that includes improving processes.

In a small group, discuss each principle and do the following:

- Identify the level of performance/competence for each principle as an individual and as a team.

- Develop a plan to celebrate and share the competency achievements with others in the organization.

- Identify actions that would improve leader behaviors.

- Prioritize the actions and develop a plan to achieve greater error management competency as individuals and as a team.

REFERENCES

Barnsteiner, J., & Prevost, S. (2002). How to implement evidence-based practice: Some tried and true pointers. *Reflections on Nursing Leadership, 28* (2), 18–21.

Benner, P., Sheets, V., Uris, P., Malloch, K., Schwed, K., & Jamison, D. (2002). Individual, practice and system causes of error in nursing. *Journal of Nursing Administration, 32* (10), 509–523.

Chaffee, M.W., & Arthur, D.C. (2002). Failure: Lessons for health care leaders. *Nursing Economic$, 20* (5), 225–228, 231.

Chapanis, A. (1996). *Human Factors in Systems Engineering.* New York: Wiley & Sons.

Cook, R., Render, M., & Woods, D. (2000). Gaps in the continuity of care and progress on patient safety. *British Medical Journal, 320* (7237), 791–794.

Deering, A., Dilts, R., & Russell, J. (2003). Leadership cults and cultures. *Leader to Leader, 28,* 36–43.

Grandjean, E., & Vigliani, E. (1980). *Ergonomic aspects of visual display terminals.* London: Taylor and Francis.

Heater, B., Becker, A., & Olson, R. (1998). Nursing interventions and patient outcomes: A meta-analysis of studies. *Nursing Research, 37,* 303–307.

Institute of Medicine. (2001). *Crossing the quality chasm: A new health system for the 21st century.* Washington, DC: National Academy Press.

Kantowitz, B.H., & Sorkin, R.D. (1983). *Human factors: Understanding people-system relationships.* New York: Wiley.

Kaye, L. (2000). The spiritual roots of mistakes. *The Inner Edge, 3* (2), 5–7.

Leape, L. (1999). The causes and prevention of errors and adverse events in health care. *Image: Journal of Nursing Scholarship, 31* (3), 281–286.

Marx, D. (2001). *Patient safety and the just culture: A primer for health care executives* [National Institutes of Health grant]. New York: Columbia University.

Matta, N.F., & Ashkenas, R.N. (2003). Why good projects fail anyway. *Harvard Business Review, 81* (9), 109–114.

Melnyk, B.M., & Fineout-Overholt, E. (2005). *Evidence-based practice in nursing and healthcare: A guide to best practice.* Philadelphia, PA: Lippincott, Williams & Wilkins.

Merrimam-Webster's Dictionary. Retrieved: September 11, 2008. http://www.merriam-webster.com/dictionary/culture

Page, A. (Ed.). (2004). *Keeping patients safe: Transforming the work environment of nurses.* Institute of Medicine, Committee on Quality of Health Care in America. Washington, DC: National Academy Press.

Porter-O'Grady, T., & Malloch, K. (2003). *Quantum leadership: A textbook of new leadership.* Sudbury, MA: Jones and Bartlett.

Rogers, A.E., Hwang, W., Scott, L.D., Aiken, L.H., & Dinges, D.F. (2004). The working hours of hospital staff nurses and patient safety. *Health Affairs, 23* (4), 202–212.

Sackett, D.L., Straus, S.E., Richardson, W.S., Rosenberg, W., & Haynes, R.B. (2000). (2nd Ed.). *Evidence-based medicine: How to practice and teach EBM.* Churchill Livingstone: Edinburgh.

Sagan, S. (1993). *The limits of safety: Organizations, accidents, and nuclear weapons.* Princeton, NJ: Princeton University Press.

Scott, K.A. (2004). *Errors and failures in complex health care systems: Individual, team, system and cultural contributors.* Unpublished doctoral dissertation, Union Institute & University, Cincinnati, OH.

Ulrich, R., Quan, X., Zimring, C., Joseph, A., & Choudhary, R. (2004, June). *The role of the physical environment in the hospital of the 21st century: A once-in-a-lifetime opportunity.* Preliminary report presented at Designing the 21st Century Hospital Symposium, Washington, DC.

Walshe, K., & Shortell, S.M. (2004). When things go wrong: How health care organizations deal with major failures. *Health Affairs, 23* (3), 103–111.

Weick, K., & Sutcliffe, K. (2001). *Managing the unexpected: Assuring high performance in an age of complexity.* San Francisco: Jossey-Bass.

Yeh, Y.Y., & Wickens, C.D. (1984), An investigation of the dissociation between subjective measures of mental workload and performance. *University of Illinois Aviation Research Lab Technical Report Epl-84–01/Nasa-84–1*

SUGGESTED READINGS

Hughes, R.G. (2004). First, do no harm: Avoiding near misses. *American Journal of Nursing, 104* (5), 81–83.

Scott, K.A. (2004). Creating highly reliable hospitals through strengthening nursing. *Journal of Nursing Administration, 34* (4), 170–172.

Transforming Leader Behaviors	Errors to Avoid
1. Know yourself	• Lack of self-awareness of skills and impact on the environment/colleagues
	• Lack of engagement and presence with the healthcare system
	• Interpreting the present in terms of past successes
	• Failure to inspire and create a powerful guiding coalition
	• Undercommunicating the vision
2. Plan for error	• Lack of attentiveness
	• Failing to develop new ways of filtering and managing information; processing information through old perspectives
	• Supporting/tolerating complacency
	• Overreliance on memory
	• Retaining unnecessary procedures
	• Failure to assure safe work schedules
	• Failure to assure safe physical environment
3. Balance standardization personalization	• Lack of or faulty intervention due to lack of skill
	• Continuation of overly complex and confusing processes
	• Overcontrolling information access
	• Egotistical invincibility—my way is best!
4. Continually assure staff	• Lack of advocacy/professional competence responsibility
	• Failing to create short-term wins
	• Lack of passion for the work of nursing
	• Assigning unprepared staff to perform complex tasks
5. Documentation	• Inaccurate documentation
	• Failure to document essential activities of patients, caregivers, and the system

A P P E N D I X

Victim Statements

The following statements are common victim statements. As you read each statement, ask yourself "Does this apply to me?" or "Have I ever felt this way?" Validate your assessments with a colleague. Develop strategies to minimize victimness as a means to creating a culture that views error as opportunity rather than one looking to pinpoint blame.

1. I have been surprised by negative feedback from someone when I thought all along I was doing my very best to solve a problem.
2. I have spent time blaming others and pointing fingers when things did not go the way I wanted them to go.
3. I have spent time "covering my tail" (sending cc: or bcc: e-mail messages) just in case things went wrong.
4. In the last month, I have said, "It's not my job" and expected someone else to solve a problem.
5. At least once a week, I have felt totally powerless, with no control over my circumstances or situation.
6. At times, I have found myself "waiting to see if" a situation would miraculously resolve itself.
7. At times, I am so frustrated that I have said, "Just tell me what you want me to do and I'll do it."

C H A P T E R 8

The Fully Engaged Leader

CHAPTER OBJECTIVES:

Upon completion of this chapter, the reader will:

1. Understand the attributes of the fully engaged leader and the relationship of engagement to organizational outcomes.
2. Review the theoretical underpinnings of the emotional aspects of leadership and the challenges of integrating these concepts into leadership development.
3. Discuss the significance of the leadership calling as an integral component of engagement.
4. Compare and contrast three processes of leadership engagement skill building: self-assessment, valuing others, and sustaining engagement.

INTRODUCTION

An estimated 40% of all managers fail in the first 18 months on the job (Carnes, Cottrell & Layton, 2004). The costs to the organization and to individuals are significant and beg for approaches that will improve the success rate. Unfortunately, the attributes separating successful managers from those who fail are often elusive. No cookie-cutter recipe for leader success has been identified despite numerous studies by leadership experts.

Leader success depends on a wide range of variables that are related to the work to be done, the skills and abilities of the leader and the team, the needs of the team members, the resources available, and the motivation of all those involved. This list is not inclusive, and it continually evolves. The right stuff of leadership may indeed have common characteristics and behaviors, but the reality is that each leader has a unique combination of multiple characteristics, values, behaviors, and ability to get the work done. Most leaders develop their personal essence on the basis of education, experience, mental intelligence, emotional intelligence, and the ability to form meaningful relationships.

Key Concepts

Consciousness
Awareness of one's own existence, sensations, thoughts, surroundings; the thoughts and feelings, collectively, of an individual or of an aggregate of people.

Competence
The quality of having suitable or sufficient skill, knowledge, and experience for some purpose; properly qualified.

Intelligence
Capacity for learning, reasoning, and understanding; aptitude in grasping truths, relationships, facts, meanings; mental alertness or quickness of understanding.

Engagement
The act of being involved or committed to something; a pledge, an obligation or an agreement.

This chapter presents the emerging profile of the engaged leader to gain a greater appreciation of the complexity of leadership and the significance of engagement as a leader characteristic, and to stimulate discussion of the potential impact of engaged behaviors on organizational performance. A brief review of the emotional intelligence literature, processes of the development of engagement, and a new employee interview template that integrates the notions of engagement within a culture of transformation are also presented.

The engaged leader in a healthcare organization has highly developed technical and emotional competence and is fully focused on the work to be done, the necessary relationships to get the work done, and the ever-changing mood of the organization. The environment created by the emotionally competent leader supports employees to experience their own emotions, set limits on expressions when appropriate, and encourages others to be similarly empowered.

First and foremost, emotionally competent leaders acknowledge and respect their own feelings and have the awareness and discipline to not be distracted by the anxieties and stresses of the moment; they actively direct their emotional energy into doing the right thing in the right way at the right time. Emotionally competent leaders not only make self-awareness a priority and are unafraid of their feelings, but they also work to understand the impact they have on others. This high level of consciousness about personal impact is foundational for leaders who are fully engaged in the work of health care, with colleagues and the organization, and, finally, to continuing personal growth. It is no small feat to become a fully engaged leader.

Necessarily, the leader with a high level of emotional competence is not at an end point. Rather, the leader is positioned to continually transcend to higher levels of consciousness, using the skills of emotional competence to relate with others in ways that were previously not possible.

COMPLEXITY LIVE!

Emotionally competent leaders do not dispute or debate the interrelatedness of the processes of leadership, which includes the technical skills of leadership, intentionality, and emotional competence. Perhaps there is no better portrayal of the notion of complexity than what is found in fully engaged leaders and the relationships they form as the means to transform work and the workplace, help others own their own change, undertake the right change processes, and integrate the rules of engagement for the postindustrial age. Engaged leaders are able to both act and reflect upon the events and processes of leading that emphasize the short term but integrate the long-term needs of the community. The complex nature of all healthcare relationships reflects the inescapable interrelationships of all things in the world and the 10 principles of complexity (Porter-O'Grady & Malloch, 2003).

Rather than being overwhelmed by the complex nature of work to be done, the pace of change, the limitations of time, and the endless advances in technology, the fully engaged leader thrives within the following realities of complexity theory:

- Change is endless.
- Information is more readily available than ever.
- Knowledge is no longer a possession but rather an access or utility for good leadership.
- Technology changes the character and content of the healthcare service relationship.

Quantum Gem

You can work with people more successfully by enlisting their feelings than by convincing their reason.

Paul P. Parker

---

10 Principles of Complexity

1. Wholes are made up of parts.
2. All health care is local.
3. Adding value to a part adds value to the whole.
4. Simple systems make up complex systems.
5. Diversity is a necessity of life.
6. Error is essential to creation.
7. Systems thrive when all of their functions intersect and interact.
8. Equilibrium and disequilibrium are in constant tension.
9. Change is generated from the center outward.
10. Revolution results from the aggregation of local changes.

Porter-O'Grady & Malloch, 2003

Self-Reflection: Observe Yourself

Body Language
- Eye contact, arms folded/unfolded

Timing of responses
- Quick, slow, not at all

Inclusion/exclusion of others in discussions

Ask your colleagues to share feedback about your body language, timeliness, and inclusion practices. Is it consistent with your assessment? Which behaviors should be retained? Changed?

Becoming competent in the technical skills of leadership and creating clear organizational goals is much less challenging than developing expertise in building and maintaining relationships, which reflects a high level of emotional competence. Mastery of these people skills is a basic expectation for all leaders, yet the attainment of expertise in relationship-building skills continues to challenge even the most experienced healthcare leaders. As leaders gain an appreciation of the principles of complexity theory and integrate the ideas into the work of leadership, the challenges of new relationships, new technology, and new regulations become much more manageable. Thus, the engaged leader with expertise in technical leadership and relationship building has identified her or his personal and professional purposes and vision for the future and is able to actively facilitate the transformational processes for others. The realities of complexity for the engaged leader include:

> **Emotionally Competent Behaviors**
> - Soliciting opinions of team members in meetings
> - Listening until the other person is finished talking
> - Able to deal with disappointment

- The undeniable interrelationships between all individuals in the organization and the community.
- An emphasis on local health care, namely, the work that occurs at the point of care between the patient and the caregiver.
- Multiple perspectives as essential for survival.
- Failure as an opportunity for improvement.
- *Change* just *is!*

In spite of the undeniable reality of these challenges, commitment to the journey that requires leaders to be emotionally competent and fully engaged is not always valued. Significant pressures emphasize the technical work of strategic planning, budgeting, and controlling. Time and energy to develop relationships or the soft side of leadership are viewed as luxuries, given that they are not believed to be necessarily related to the net income margin.

Developing the people skills of leadership—regardless of what label or attribute is attached to them—provides the most effective vehicle for sustained learning to occur through the recognized power of the collective emotions of the team. It is through people's full engagement with their work that the measurable, sustainable results of satisfaction, quality outcomes, and strong net income margins are achieved. Organizations continue to struggle not only to recognize the quantifiable value of emotional competence but also to inexorably link these attributes to technical leadership processes. Continual reinforcement and demonstration of these relationships is a never-ending process for engaged and enlightened leaders.

> **Emotionally Incompetent Behaviors**
> - Yelling at another person
> - Rejecting or dismissing the opinions and ideas of others
> - Gossip
> - Whirlwinds of hyperactivity
> - Distraught over disappointments

UNDERSTANDING THE PAST: FOUNDATIONS FOR ENGAGEMENT

The evolving body of knowledge dedicated to understanding and guiding people in developing an engaged leadership competence that integrates technical and relational skills continues to offer new and differing perspectives for the leader. Much has been written about the ways in which individuals deal with their emotions, which are an integral part of every leader's personal essence. It is through the understanding of the nature and dynamics of emotions that leaders are able to advance in their journey to a state of full engagement.

Recent variations in the descriptions of emotional intelligence (EI) have raised concerns for some scholars. Some also believe that the significance of EI has been overstated due to the lack of evidence supporting the relationship between emotional intelligence and

> **The Teddy Bear Factor**
>
> Emotional Intelligence involves more than being introspective. It also involves what I call the Teddy Bear Factor—do people feel comfortable with you? Do they want to be close to you?
>
> Manfred F. R. Kets de Vries

workplace success (Vitello-Cicciu, 2002). In spite of the criticisms of the lack of conceptual clarity and overriding behaviors, the basic notions of this work continue to enlighten many leaders about the complexities of emotions and their impact on the workplace.

By its nature, emotional intelligence is a complex phenomenon subsuming theories of emotion, motivation, behavior, intelligence, organizational behavior, and neuroscience. The intersections and overlapping of one's feelings, sense of purpose, knowledge, and attitude vary widely and often unpredictably. New perspectives and new approaches to further engagement and expertise in relationship building can still be learned from the study of the emotional intelligence literature.

The concept of emotional intelligence is significant to understanding emotions. The early definers of EI, Salovey and Mayer (Vitello-Cicciu, 2002), identified three processes as its essence: appraisal and expression of emotion, regulation of emotion, and utilization of emotion. Further studies extended this understanding of EI from one of personal assessment to one that includes the understanding of the emotions of others. New theories identified the ability to perceive emotions, to access and/or generate feeling to assist one's thoughts, and to understand emotional knowledge. Given that the predominant assumption regarding EI is that emotions and intelligence are connected, not all theorists interpreted EI as consistent with the notion of intelligence. Some have misinterpreted the notion of intelligence beyond the definition of mental performance to personality traits, thus creating conceptual confusion (Vitello-Cicciu, 2002).

Goleman (1995) followed the work of Salovey and Mayer and defined emotional intelligence as "the ability to motivate oneself and persist in the face of frustration; to control impulses and delay gratification; to regulate one's moods and keep distress from swamping the ability to think; to emphasize and to hope" (p. 34). The five broad categories of EI defined by Goleman (1995) are: self-awareness, self-regulation, motivation, empathy, and social skills. These are more aligned with motivational intelligence than with EI (Vitello-Cicciu, 2002). Twenty-five competencies have been further identified by Goleman (1998).

These complex phenomena within emotional intelligence are difficult to discretely compartmentalize, and thus they further challenge leadership development experts. While some believe it is difficult for leaders to develop specific standardized approaches to facilitating high levels of emotional competence, the many supporting theories do indeed offer differing areas of focus for leadership development.

Given the recent emphasis on emotional intelligence or the soft side of leadership, leaders have struggled to avoid artificial labels and artificial goals that are based solely on the emotional intelligence aspect and thereby fragment the essence of the integrated leadership perspective. Some leaders have identified values, preferred behaviors, and decision-making styles through the Myers-Briggs inventory, the DISC-Performax assessment, and numerous other assessment tools in addition to the EI survey, gaining an understanding of not only emotional skills but also interpersonal decision-making skills.

At times leaders become overfocused on the style and behaviors of leadership to the extent where one's style (Myers-Briggs or DISC) is identified on the employee badge. Both leaders and employees become focused on the style of decision making at the expense of the desired outcomes. While it is certainly relevant to know that some individuals are ENTJs and make decisions more quickly than others, this information is one piece of the data and does not take into consideration the current context of events and interactions. When there is a need to respond quickly to assure patient safety, the end goal of patient safety must be primary, while individual styles are

---

Goleman's 25 EI Competencies (1998)

1. Emotional awareness
2. Accurate self-assessment
3. Self-confidence
4. Self-control
5. Trustworthiness
6. Conscientiousness
7. Adaptability
8. Innovation
9. Achievement drive
10. Commitment
11. Initiative
12. Optimism
13. Understanding others
14. Developing others
15. Service orientation
16. Leveraging diversity
17. Political awareness
18. Influence
19. Communication
20. Conflict management
21. Leadership
22. Change agency
23. Bonds building
24. Collaboration
25. Team capabilities

Gem

The way a question is asked limits and disposes the ways in which any answer to it—right or wrong—may be given.

Susanne K. Langer

secondary or in some situations irrelevant. The fact that one's primary behavior or decision-making style reflects the need for time to process is secondary to the contextual realities of the situation. The fully engaged leader assures focus on the desired, value-based outcomes that support quality patient care service while information specific to style is supportive but not the driver of processes.

Many scholars continue to offer guidelines for leadership, but there is no widely accepted standardized template of behaviors for effective leadership. Outcomes of good leadership have been identified more consistently than behaviors such as the achievement of clinical outcomes, employee satisfaction, and fiscal stability, which integrate and reflect the unique values, beliefs, and skills of the organization. Regardless of the approach or theoretical underpinning selected by the leader to guide the development of interpersonal or soft skills, the process of development must always be directed to the outcomes; processes must never overtake the significance of the desired outcomes. As previously noted, working to identify one's decision-making style and focusing on the need for expression of that style in deference to achieving organizational goals is inappropriate. The goal is to understand one's style and integrate it into the group decision-making process and achieve the desired goal.

Three developmental processes are identified to assist leaders along the pathway of engagement. The first is discovering the authentic you, the second is valuing others, and the third is sustaining the essence of engagement. Each of these processes is presented with strategies and values that are designed to assist you along your journey.

> **Gem**
>
> Soulful leaders are containers for the *ands* and work diligently to eliminate the *eithers* and *ors*.

> **Gem**
>
> Information voids will be filled by rumors and speculation unless they are preempted by open, credible and trustworthy communication. Pull no punches. When you know an answer, give it. When you don't, say so. When you're guessing, admit it. But don't stop communication.
>
> Jean B. Keffeler

THE AUTHENTIC SELF: A CALLING OF LEADERSHIP

Some days the work of leadership seems like more than a person can handle, yet dedicated leaders continue on through seemingly insurmountable challenges. Most likely, the work of leadership has become an internal calling. The calling to leadership or the inner urge to give away one's gifts and make distinct contributions to the world not only uncovers the joy that everyone seeks but also affirms one's life work and contributions to a better world. It is the calling to leadership that energizes, affirms, and sustains leaders in times of great challenge.

According to Leider (2004), engaged leaders not only know who they are and what they stand for but also are able to assist others to heed their own life callings. They are able to guide others to uncover their embedded destiny and to see beyond today to what they can become tomorrow. This is the ultimate coaching and mentoring process! Thus, the engaged leader with emotional competence is able both to identify personal destiny and to assist others in the journey of discovery and commitment to their calling as a part of the larger design of the world. Not surprising, engaged leaders recognize their calling not as a destiny or goal, but as a wellness issue; leading is doing what needs to be done, and not doing the work of leadership would be frustrating and stress producing.

> **The Calling of Leadership**
>
> Humans search for meaning. Life has some meaning because there is some good in it. The most meaningful lives are the ones in which we directly serve others. Calling joins self and service. When our talents and the needs of the world cross, there lies our vocation.
>
> Richard Leider, 2004

The calling of leadership guides the leader in integrating the internal personal self with the outer world—a struggle that is continuously present in many leaders. Knowing from the internal self what needs to be done and living those beliefs and values in the real world marks the leader's journey. The leader must role model the integration of the personal, authentic self with the real, external world. The journey starts with the self and moves toward others and the needs of the world. The fully engaged leader emulates a high level of consciousness or spiritual connection with those in the world. The leader is fully present in each situation, listens carefully with an open mind, and, on the basis of core values, interacts assertively and honestly.

Gem

The leader's first job is to define reality.

The last is to say thank you.

In between the leader must become a servant and a debtor.

Max DePree, Former Chairman
Herman Miller

Quantum Gem

How can we communicate love? I think three things are involved:

We must reach out to a person, make contact.

We must listen with the heart, be sensitive to the other's needs.

We must respond in a language that the person can understand. Many of us do all the talking. We must learn to listen and to keep on listening.

Princess Pale Moon

Gem

Dimensions of Authentic Leaders

1. Understanding their purpose
2. Practicing solid values
3. Leading with heart
4. Demonstrating self-discipline

Bill George, 2004

THE AUTHENTIC SELF: INTEGRITY

As noted previously, an essential quality that the engaged leader must have is to be his or her own person, to be authentic in every way. Any prospective leader who buys into the necessity of copying the characteristics of other leaders is doomed to fail. Those who are too responsive to others, too quick to deviate from the plan, or unwilling to make difficult decisions for fear of offending others are likely to be overridden by competitors, either internal or external. The authentic leader works to know and be himself or herself.

Within every leader are the questions: What is my professional identity? What do I stand for? Examples of areas of self-awareness that the engaged leader examines include the very basic, such as:

- What is important to me? Balance, family, work, and success?
- Do I value stability, innovation, wealth, happiness, and humor?
- What makes me happy, sad, laugh, cry, stressed, and calm?
- Are behaviors that are gregarious, energetic, impulsive, quiet, and shy tolerable to me?
- How do I treat others? With respect, with indifference, or selectively?
- What impact do I want to have on others? To be liked, loved, and respected?
- How do I react to failure? To myself, and to others who fail?
- How do I describe myself? How do others describe me?

Engaged leaders focus on the deepest dimension of that which defines their uniqueness and potential: the authentic self. Leaders with high degrees of awareness of themselves and those in their environment are described as not just engaged or sensitive to the activities between two people, but sensitive to the larger environment, to the location, other individuals, and the ramifications of the endless interrelationships of the world at large. Consciousness of not only their own self but also the impact of the presence of others and the interactions in which they are involved is a way of being for soulful, engaged leaders. They are known for their continual work in increasing self-understanding of their strengths, weaknesses, values, beliefs, and passions and are able to demonstrate ownership of their behaviors, both the behaviors that contribute positively to harmony and behaviors that are less than perfect. Self-knowledge is achieved in many ways through a lifelong commitment to examination of values, behaviors, accomplishments, and most importantly, the impact on others.

THE AUTHENTIC SELF: NARCISSISTIC

Although it may be difficult for some leaders to acknowledge, narcissism is an essential leadership trait. According to Kets de Vries (Coutu, 2004), all people need a healthy dose of narcissism in order to survive, especially leaders. Narcissism is the engine that drives leadership; assertiveness, self-confidence, tenacity, and creativity are essential to lead. The challenge is to not go over the edge and adopt autocratic behaviors, thus destroying shared decision-making processes. Indeed, leaders can be quite successful in facilitating team processes as assertive, confident, tenacious, and creative individuals. The challenge for leaders is to not overwhelm team members so they become a mirror image of the leader, idealizing and uncritically accepting whatever the leader proposes.

THE AUTHENTIC SELF: TRUTH TELLER—THE WHOLE TRUTH, HALF OF THE TRUTH, OR MY LIPS ARE SEALED?

Authentic leaders behave consistently with identified values and beliefs that have been developed through reflection, study, and dialogue with others. These values form the leader's moral compass. There is a deep sense of what is right and what is wrong. Further, authentic leaders value integrity, which is not just the absence of lying but is telling the whole truth, no matter how painful it might be. Sharing of partial information may be less painful, but sharing of all information is expected by the authentic leader. Telling the whole truth is natural to the authentic leader, just as is admitting mistakes when one falls short and does not succeed. This demonstrates courage to be authentic and honest in all situations.

Engaged leaders speak the truth in a caring, compassionate way, even when the news is not pleasant. Authenticity requires courage to respond when it is easier to be silent and noncommittal and requires courage to avoid partial truths. The lack of response implies agreement to most observers, an impression engaged leaders do not want to give.

Authenticity also often involves telling the stories that no one else will tell, stories that reflect the essence of the human spirit and feelings that range from despair to anger to disappointment. One example involves the termination of a favored employee by a new leader. After finding significant performance issues, the new leader documented the behaviors and began termination procedures. When the new leader informed her supervisor, who previously had been the employee's supervisor, of her decision to terminate, the response from the supervisor was less than typical, but very authentic. The previous supervisor first provided her support to the new leader and then noted that the problem behavior had indeed been present for some time and that she had failed to address it. She thanked the new leader for her integrity and willingness to address a significant issue, something she had been unable to do for a variety of reasons such as a long history with the employee, other priorities, and concern that she would not be able to follow through completely.

The sharing of these stories serves many purposes: building relationships, understanding human frailty, and demonstrating the willingness to recognize that at times others can do a more effective job than you are able to do. Some may perceive this as a failure of leadership rather than the reality of life steeped in complexity, uncertainty, and trial and error. Certain events result from particular combinations of context, timing, and personal energy, rather than behaviors that reflect poor leadership.

Finally, the authentic, engaged leader avoids the tendency to depersonalize a situation or to blame it on an objective entity such as the system. The authentic, fully engaged leader recognizes that individuals create the organization and its culture and are thus the only ones able to change or improve it. Rarely does the leader hide behind the shield of system policies; rather, the leader owns the system policies and is accountable to examine and modify policies if the outcomes can be improved.

Discussion

Authenticity is recognized through both obvious truthfulness and subtle messages. Consider the following questions:

1. Is there such a thing as a truthful budget? Why do some organizations expect an absolute budget that is only negotiated once a year? Why do some believe that the budgeting process is used as a shield to discourage some expenditures and at other times to provide flexibility for an uncertain future? Why do some leaders believe the budget is a guideline rather than an absolute and specific allocation of resources?
2. Is the performance appraisal ever totally honest? Or is the process a reflection of partial, nonspecific information that minimizes the opportunity for healthy dialogue and ultimately employee growth?
3. Which principle(s) of complexity guide each perspective?

Gem

When wealth is lost, nothing is lost;

When health is lost, something is lost;

When character is lost, all is lost.

German proverb

VALUING OTHERS: LISTENING FROM THE HEART

There can never be enough emphasis on listening to others with a stilled mind. Soulful leaders use a communication style that begins with personal focus and clearing of the mind, questions for greater understanding, and then response. Receptive, open communication is about the willingness to embrace many perspectives and creative ideas.

The engaged leader not only recognizes that there are many perspectives within a team or organization but also seeks out the differing viewpoints in order to recognize and give value to all dimensions. Efforts are not focused on eliminating the differing ideas but rather on working to sustain healthy tensions in which diverse polarities are present: peace and war, conservative and liberal, nursing and nonnursing, traditional medicine and alternative therapies. There is no rubber stamping of like-minded ideas or like-minded individuals.

Receptive communicators also understand the importance of *suffering presence*, which is the willingness to tolerate (while perhaps suffering on the inside) others' viewpoints, values, beliefs, thinking styles, and even the same story for the second time. Receptive communicators are truly present; they are engaged in the dialogue and are not merely marking time until they can interrupt and speak their mind. Finally, receptive communicators do not intimidate others in order to make a point or gain support for their position.

> ### Quantum Gem
>
> The real art of conversation is not to say the right thing in the right place but to leave unsaid the wrong thing at the tempting moment.
>
> Lady Dorothy Nevill

VALUING OTHERS: AVOIDING THE RUBBER STAMP

The established, successful leader can be unintentionally intimidating to others, particularly new members of the team. Engaged leaders do not want members of the team to merely echo their ideas and proposals, even when they are new to the team. Engaged leaders create the context for open, healthy dialogue to elicit new ideas, discard suboptimal processes, and create new strategies from the collective wisdom of the team.

Resisting the power of flattery is an important skill that is seldom taught in management programs. The quantum leader is well served to periodically examine the dynamics of the team and affirm that he or she is not in a hall of mirrors, being continually flattered and reinforced, hearing only ideas that echo those of the leader, and seldom receiving challenging feedback. The leader does not need mirror images of himself or herself; it is healthy debate and dialogue that is needed by the leader to achieve great results.

Engaged leaders are sensitive to the tendency to quash creativity, and they work to avoid responses such as, "We've always done it this way," and "We tried that last year, and it didn't work." Continuing emphasis is placed on eliminating these reactions from both the leader's and other members' vocabularies.

> ### Avoiding a Hall of Mirrors
>
> 1. Focus on vision and values.
> 2. Make sure people disagree.
> 3. Cultivate truth tellers.
> 4. Do as you would have done to you.
> 5. Honor your intuition.
> 6. Delegate, don't desert.
>
> L.R. Offerman, 2004

VALUING OTHERS: FINDING COMMON GROUND

Finding common ground when it seems nonexistent is also a characteristic behavior of the engaged leader. Rather than allow conflicts to persist, leaders brainstorm with those who may have differing ideas and work to identify areas of common interest that can be used to reinstate healthy dialogue and minimize conflict. Too often, the emphasis is on differences rather than on finding areas of common ground that could serve to begin healthy dialogue. Negative issues may be highlighted rather than mediated. For each conflicting situation, there is always common ground to be identified. It may begin with the commonality of being a healthcare worker, the need for a job, or the current shift worked. Other commonalities that can serve as openings for less stressful conversations include gender, age group, ethnic background, birthplace, college attended, and sports interests. Once dialogue has begun in a less stressful manner, individuals can move on to discussing and resolving areas of conflict.

> ### Finding Common Ground
>
> Adversaries are often believed to be archenemies; yet, there can be common ground that, once identified, can be used to mediate the conflict-ridden situation. Consider the following four relationships that are often adversarial:
>
> - Physician–nurse
> - Labor union–professional practice advocates
> - Day shift–night shift
> - Finance–nursing
>
> 1. Identify three specific areas of common ground for each of the dyads of conflict.
> 2. Identify three specific areas of conflict for each of the dyads of conflict.
> 3. Can you identify new ways to create new and better relationships within the dyads?

VALUING OTHERS: ENDURING RELATIONSHIPS

The capacity to develop close and enduring relationships is one mark of a leader. The detached style of leadership in which leaders remain aloof from those they supervise does not work in today's workplace. Employees demand more personal relationships with their leaders before they will give themselves fully to their job (George, 2004). They expect access to leaders and know that openness and the depth of relationships with the leader are the foundations for trust and commitment to the organization. These enduring relationships—the soft skill outcome—are built on connectedness and shared purposes and serve as an important element in achieving far-reaching and once believed impossible goals.

> **Self-Awareness: My Legacy**
>
> As a leader, the legacy you leave can range from a very positive difference, no perceived change, or a very negative impact.
>
> Consider your legacy on a daily basis:
>
> 1. What difference did you make today?
> 2. Who did you affect?
> 3. What opportunities did you miss?
> 4. What do you need to change?

VALUING OTHERS: COMPETING FAIRLY

Leaders are highly competitive individuals driven to succeed in whatever they take on. Authentic leaders know that competing requires self-discipline in order to be successful. There are two views of competition: the positive or win-win side and a negative or win-lose side. When individuals compete with each other to establish superior and subordinate positions, someone wins and someone loses, and competition is considered negative. When individuals compete against their own performance to achieve higher levels, the competition takes on a more positive aspect. There are only winners in this approach; the past is improved upon, and new outcomes increase the value of the results. For example, when patient care units compete against each other for the highest patient satisfaction scores, one unit always wins and the others lose. It is seldom possible for an oncology unit to exceed the satisfaction scores of a postpartum unit due to the nature of the clinical situation. It is possible for each unit to compete with last month's score and work to achieve higher ratings within the unit. All units can potentially be winners.

Being competitive does not have to be negative; it is an essential quality of successful leaders, but it needs to be channeled through purpose and discipline. It is not uncommon to mistake competitive individuals, those who generate results by improving organizational effectiveness, for genuine leaders. Achieving operational effectiveness is an essential result for any leader, but it alone does not ensure authenticity or long-term success.

SUSTAINING ENGAGEMENT: SELF-DEVELOPMENT

The lifetime learning process requires discipline as well as the internal passion to want to learn more about new ideas, historical perspectives, and the successes or failures of initiatives. Both are necessary for sustainable learning. Yet, sometimes having passion for learning is not enough in the complex and ever-changing healthcare environment. The imbalance of excessive operational demands often displaces the preferred balance that integrates operations, continuing development, and time and energy management, further challenging the engaged leader to determine effective strategies to regain the balance.

According to Edgar Schein (Coutu, 2002), in reality, few companies ever succeed in genuinely reinventing themselves; they rarely get to the point of challenging deeply held assumptions about strategies and processes and thinking and acting in fundamentally altered ways. Rather, most end up doing the same thing in superficially tweaked ways—practices that fall short of what is needed to compete in the 21st century. Further, Schein (Coutu) notes that in spite of the optimistic

> **Discussion**
>
> **Coercive Persuasion and the Electronic Medical Record**
>
> Edgar Schein, noted organizational theorist, described coercive persuasion as a situation in which people cannot physically escape and are pressured into adopting new beliefs.
>
> Consider the emergence of the electronic medical record (EMR) and its impact on caregiver behavior and the use of paper. Giving up or at least minimizing the printing of reports and using notebooks in favor of the electronic devices is a significant challenge for all caregivers.
>
> Removing printers and the supply of paper is an example of coercive persuasion. What other examples have occurred in your organization?
>
> Do you agree that change or learning occurs best through coercive persuasion? Why? Why not?

rhetoric that learning is fun, learning is often more about guilt and anxiety. Indeed, some may enjoy and revel in the learning process, but more change is believed to be accomplished through indoctrination and coercive persuasion!

Engaged leaders are indeed accountable for their own lifelong learning. They are sensitive to the radical ideas of coercive persuasion and realize that there is an inherent paradox surrounding learning; anxiety inhibits learning, but anxiety is also necessary if learning is going to occur. For many, the presence of anxiety stimulates and reinforces the need for change, given that real change begins after the organization or the individual experiences some threat that thwarts progress or desired outcomes. The leader works with the anxiety of learning and channels activities into situations in which people learn together, minimizing the anxiety of looking foolish in the process.

Consider the recent organizational changes to support patient safety initiatives. Patient safety has always been important to healthcare workers, in spite of the documented high numbers of errors and tweaking of the systems that resulted in errors. Not until major reports from the Institute of Medicine were presented did significant change in practices specific to patient safety begin—an example of coercive persuasion. Organizations were mandated by regulatory and accrediting agencies to make specific changes within defined time frames. Such learning and change is indeed reality, and the engaged leader works to use both the anxiety of the situation and the dedication of healthcare workers to create sustainable solutions that improve patient safety outcomes.

SUSTAINING ENGAGEMENT: MEASURING SUCCESS

The measuring stick of the highly engaged leader is more than the accumulation of wealth, jewelry, homes, and automobiles. The engaged leader perceives success as much more than material goods. Enduring success is the result of multiple forces and multiple skills: success gets leaders where they want to be, with rewards that are sustainable for them and those they care about. It is about success that is emotionally renewing, not anxiety provoking.

Further, each engaged leader perceives and values success in unique ways that may indeed change over time. There is no standardized format for success; rather, there are commonalities that serve to nourish the mind, body, and spirit. Nash and Stevenson (2004) identified four components of enduring success:

1. *Happiness:* feelings of pleasure or contentment about one's life
2. *Achievement:* accomplishments that compare favorably against similar goals others have strived for
3. *Significance:* the sense that one has made a positive impact on people one cares about
4. *Legacy:* the way to establish one's values or accomplishments so as to help others find future success

Each of these components is important in creating feelings of success. For example, achieving significant wealth from a corporate position without the ability to experience pleasure does not lend to a feeling of success. Or, if one had a significant power base of thousands of employees but did not allow for the creation of positive impacts on others, success would also not be felt. Success is never satisfied by just one category; it encompasses one's personal life, achievement at work, significance to family, and legacy to the community.

Engaged healthcare leaders recognize the need for balance and focus in all four categories; focusing on one factor leads to knowing that you are doing what is right but still feeling unsuccessful. The achievements and pleasure of one category fade

---

Discussion

Enduring Success

Nash and Stevenson (2004) have identified four components for enduring success: happiness, achievement, significance, and legacy. In a group, consider each of the four components and identify as many possible examples of each component that are unique to nurses as you can.

1. Which area of success is the easiest to attain?
2. Which one(s) are the most challenging?
3. How can you develop a more balanced approach to achieving enduring success?
4. Who can assist you along the way?

as soon as they occur. Working diligently to create a legacy without sensitivity to operational responsibilities, failing to spend time with family, and unhealthy diet and exercise habits become short-lived and frustrating.

In contrast, enduring success that recognizes all four categories is enriching and sustainable. Synergy is created in single events and the combination of activities. As the leader takes time for family and coworkers while creating a new healthcare center, giving to the community, and attending continuing education workshops, the balance of activities is focused and sustainable. The integration of activities at this level does not occur without thought and reflection and regular adjustments.

SUSTAINING ENGAGEMENT: SOULFUL OPTIMISM

Engaged leaders are filled with optimism, resilience, and the belief that the future is brighter and that one can, indeed, make a difference. They understand that disharmony or stress is caused by forces external to them in the world and that the way to reduce stress is to gain internal control, not more control of the world. For example, when the engaged leader is caught in a traffic jam, the stress level does not automatically increase due to the annoyance of being late; rather, the slowdown is managed as an opportunity to relax. The challenge is to change the view of the world from the inside to sustain calm and harmony!

HIRING FOR ENGAGEMENT AND PRESENCE: THE BANNER ESTRELLA MODEL

Interviewing for and retaining employees who are committed to full engagement in the organizational culture begins with an interviewing process that is aligned with organizational values among all employees, not just those in leadership positions. As a new facility, Banner Estrella Medical Center (BEMC) recognized the incredible opportunity to create the ultimate organizational culture and physical environment supportive of healing and at the same time to remedy behaviors that had been barriers to quality patient outcomes, a safe environment, and employee satisfaction. BEMC leaders worked with the community to identify the desired values, services, and outcomes that would support the best health care possible. The collective effort not only identified the characteristics of the physical facility that would architecturally support healing, but also the culture that would transform the healthcare experience.

Early in the process, the newly hired leadership team created an interviewing template that integrated core values and behaviors of the parent organization, Banner Health, and the expectations for all employees seeking to be a part of the transformational culture. The team clearly appreciated this opportunity to correct previous undesirable behaviors and practices and thus created an interview template to guide all interviewers in preparing for the interviews and to inform those being interviewed of potential questions. The interviewing template follows at the end of the chapter in Appendix 1.

SUMMARY

Achieving full engagement is not a destination; it is a lifetime journey that is filled with varying degrees of engagement. Leaders may be focused and fully engaged in the work at hand. Or leaders may be overchallenged by the intensity and quantity of work, personal health status, and family needs, and are thus unable to be engaged at the desired level. Recognizing the difference and accepting the reality is healthy and stress reducing for the engaged, emotionally competent leader. Achieving full engagement in a world based on complexity theory is at best a highly sought-after state that exists only intermittently, based on the degree of change present in the modern world, available time, and technological advances. Continuing activity limits the opportunity for minor engagement with others and the system, much less full engagement. This is not to dissuade leaders from striving for engagement as means to improve relationship effectiveness and outcomes, but it is a reminder of the reality of a world steeped in complexity.

It is much like reaching for the stars; the destination is ever present and inspirational. The lack of success in reaching a star does not deter one from continuing to envision the process and continually aspire to greater achievements.

Exercise 1 Discovering Full Engagement

The profile of the fully engaged leader includes the following characteristics:

- A high level of self-awareness with specific criteria that have emerged over time
- Valuing others
- Commitment to continuing development
- Application of values and beliefs to daily operations

For each of the four characteristics, list the behaviors and specific actions that should be taken to assure a high level of engagement. Also, identify behaviors that should be eliminated to improve engagement.

Exercise 2 The Hall of Mirrors

Healthy dialogue requires sharing opinions, challenging assumptions, and encouraging new ideas. Leaders may find themselves in a hall of mirrors, with everyone agreeing and praising the leader for his or her views, proposals, and progress. No one challenges the leader. Often the result is organizational dysfunction, a disrespectful culture, and little or no progress.

Are you in a hall of mirrors?

Consider proposing an unrealistic idea and assess the response. If the response is the mirror of yourself, begin to assess the behaviors and rationale, for member reluctance to engage in healthy dialogue.

Identify at least one strategy to support open dialogue and decrease the rubber stamping of ideas.

Identify the potential improvements as a result of this change.

REFERENCES

Carnes, K., Cottrell, D., & Layton, M.C. (2004). *Management insights: Discovering the truths to management success.* Dallas, TX: CornerStone Leadership Institute.

Coutu, D.L. (2002). The anxiety of learning. *Harvard Business Review, 80* (3), 100–106.

Coutu, D.L. (2004). Putting leaders on the couch: A conversation with Manfred F. R. Kets de Vries. *Harvard Business Review, 82* (1), 65–71.

Goleman, D. (1998). *Working with emotional intelligence.* New York: Bantam.

Goleman, D. (1995). *Emotional intelligence: Why it can matter more than IQ.* New York: Bantam.

George, B. (2004). The journey to authenticity. *Leader to Leader, 31,* 29–35.

Leider, R. (2004). Is leading your calling? *Leader to Leader, 31,* 36–40.

Nash, L., & Stevenson, H. (2004). Success that lasts. *Harvard Business Review, 82* (2), 102–109.

Offerman, L.R. (2004). When followers become toxic. *Harvard Business Review, 82* (1), 54–60.

Porter-O'Grady, T., & Malloch, K. (2003). *Quantum leadership: A textbook of new leadership.* Sudbury, MA: Jones and Bartlett.

Vitello-Cicciu, J.M. (2002). Exploring emotional intelligence: Implications for nurse leaders. *Journal of Nursing Administration, 32* (4), 203–209.

Banner Estrella Medical Center Technical and Cultural Interview Guidelines

INTRODUCTION

The hiring process is extremely significant in creating and supporting a culture of health care that will transform the healthcare experience. To identify the most qualified applicants, multiple encounters by multiple individuals are believed essential in determining the knowledge, values, and cultural fit of the applicant. The following guidelines are recommended to assist leaders and managers in the selection of Banner Estrella Medical Center (BEMC) employees.

BASIC INTERVIEW STEPS

1. Human resources staff:
   a. Screens candidates for basic qualifications.
   b. Notifies hiring manager of qualified candidates.
   c. Coordinates interview schedule with candidates—recommended scheduling:

   NOTE: Human resources individual interview scheduled same day as manager interview (45 minutes). The individual interview with hiring manager (30 minutes–1 hour) is scheduled for the same day as human resources interview to prevent applicant having to come in twice.

   NOTE: Final two applicants will complete steps d and e.

   d. Panel interview of the applicant with 2–3 of the hiring manager's peers (1 hour)
   e. 3–6 BEMC employees attend an audition by the applicant; 15-minute presentation by the applicant and 15 minutes for debriefing

2. Hiring manager coordinates with other interviewers on team to determine which behavioral and skills-based questions each person will ask. Balance skills-based and behavioral-based questions during each interview.
3. Hiring manager will prepare applicant for step 1d by providing an overview of BEMC's culture and vision of "Transforming Health Care for the Future" (fact sheet available by e-mail or hard copy given to candidates to help them prepare).

4. During interviews, each interviewer notes the highlights of each candidate's responses to questions and completes a score sheet.

5. After interviews, the hiring manager schedules discussion with the interview team to review candidates and make hiring recommendations.

NOTE: Try to keep the same interview team for all candidates interviewed for a single position for consistency.

BANNER ESTRELLA MEDICAL CENTER SELECTION TOOL

There are nine competency categories that will be assessed for the BEMC applicant. Each section includes required questions (in **bold**) and optional questions. Items can be considered for leaders, clinicians, and staff positions on the basis of the recommendations of the interview design team and are noted in their respective columns.

Behavioral Based Competency No. 1	Leadership
Indicator:	• Provides an environment for people to experience caring, healing, and learning. Treats people with dignity, respect, honesty, and fairness. Recognizes the value of individual differences and the collaboration of people with different strengths and expertise. • Engages people in integrating the values, code of conduct, and service standards in daily activities by modeling expected behaviors and reinforcing behaviors demonstrated by others. • Is diligent in efforts to recognize and reward contributions. Provides timely feedback in a constructive manner. Partners with employees to develop meaningful action plans for development.

Questions	Leader	Clinician	Staff
1. Interviewer: Describe the environment of care for BEMC. Ask: How/why are the values, skills of employees, relationships, and financial accountability included in the leadership role? What experience have you had that connects to this environment?	Yes	No	No
2. What are the core values of your current or former organization? What did you do to ensure your team integrated them into their daily activities? What methods did you use to reinforce desired behaviors? Give me some examples of deliberate attempts on your part to model the values.	Yes	Yes	Yes
3. Delegation is a challenge to many leaders. Describe your process for delegating. How do you know when delegation is not working? How would you improve it and why? Give an example.	Yes	Yes	No
4. Share a time when you provided an employee a unique opportunity to use his/her strengths. What were the circumstances? How did you know this employee could perform the job? How did the system or department improve because of this effort?	Yes	No	No
5. Tell me at least one nontraditional way you provide learning and development to your team. How did this impact your team?	Yes	No	No
6. Describe your most challenging performance assessment. What were the challenges? How did you overcome them? What do you do differently today because of this experience?	Yes	No	No
7. Describe your system for recognizing and rewarding the people on your team. What have you found people most want as rewards and recognition? How did you develop your recognition system?	Yes	No	No

Behavioral Based Competency No. 2	**Achieve Results**
Indicator:	• Business awareness/focus: Focuses on quality, cost effectiveness, and services to improve processes and outcomes. Results include streamlined systems and increased patient, customer, and employee satisfaction. • Manages resources: Manages resources efficiently to achieve the best outcomes including people, finances, equipment, materials, and supplies. • Makes values-based and evidence-based business decisions. • Demonstrates commitment to quality and safety.

Questions	Leader	Clinician	Staff
1. What indicators have been necessary to measure results in your area? Describe your utilization of those indicators in your department's/team's daily operations.	Yes	Yes	No
2. What responsibility have you had with managing the costs of a department or organization? What were the resources in that experience? What did you do to ensure they were used efficiently? How did you know whether or not you were successful?	Yes	No	No
3. Describe a time when you needed to cut costs and you knew your staffing ratio was already very lean. What did you do to realize savings without cutting needed staff? How did the decision impact the business? How did your supervisor respond to your decision?	Yes	No	No
4. What are the areas that you believe are the most important to assuring a safe environment for employees? Patients? Colleagues? Describe a situation in which you improved the safety for one of these groups.	Yes	Yes	Yes
5. Tell me about a process improvement effort you initiated that resulted in improved patient outcomes that was cost effective. What stimulated your effort? What were the steps you took? What were the results or changes in practice/performance that occurred? How did you measure the results? What was the impact on employee satisfaction?	Yes	Yes	Yes
6. How do you evaluate turnover? Is all turnover negative? Why/why not?	Yes	No	No

Behavioral Based Competency No. 3	**Effective Communicator**		
Indicator:	• Active listener • Clear, concise verbal and written communication • Effectively manages conflict • Accessible • Follows through		

	Leader	Clinician	Staff
Questions			
1. Describe the most significant written document, report, or presentation you have had to complete. How did you pull the information together? What was the response from your target audience?	Yes	Yes	No
2. Having difficult conversations is an essential skill for open and positive environments. How have you learned to: • Express your own strong feelings? • Deal with abusive people? • Deliver difficult decisions to an individual or group? • Deal with conflict? • Say no to someone you like? Please give a specific example from your past experience.	Yes	Yes	Yes
3. Describe a time when you realized you needed to make an improvement in your communication skills. How did you manage it?	Yes	Yes	Yes
4. As BEMC is dedicated to advanced computer technology, electronic charting, and wireless communication, employees will need to be competent to work in this environment. Describe your computer/technology skills and how quickly you believe you will adapt to this environment. Also, describe the training that you believe you will need to become competent within 1 month.	Yes	Yes	Yes
5. In a recent work experience, how have you differentiated appropriate information from inappropriate information to share with patients and customers? Describe the situation. What was the outcome?	Yes	Yes	Yes

Behavioral Based Competency No. 4	Customer Service
Indicator:	Service Excellence Skills: 1. Treats people he/she serves as guests. Is courteous, makes eye contact, smiles, introduces self, addresses people by name when possible. 2. Presents a professional image. Name badge highly visible. 3. Answers telephone with a smile. Identifies self and asks how he/she can help. 4. Listens to the people we serve and coworkers. Responds promptly and reliably. 5. Anticipates the wants and needs of the people we serve. Asks, "How can I help?" 6. Practices open and honest communication with those with whom he/she serves and works. 7. Keeps the people we serve informed. 8. Maintains a clean and safe environment. 9. Acts to reverse negative service situations using the anticipate, acknowledge, apologize, and amend service recovery process. 10. Respects the privacy and confidentiality of the people we serve. 11. Strives to master skills needed to do the best for the people we serve. 12. Positively represents BH and BEMC in the workplace and the community.

Questions	Leader	Clinician	Staff
1. **Describe an environment that promotes caring, healing, and learning. Give me an example of an action you've taken to create this type of environment in the workplace.**	Yes	Yes	Yes
2. **Give me an example of a time you provided outstanding customer service.**	Yes	Yes	Yes
3. **Describe a time when you found it difficult to treat a patient or customer as a guest. What was the situation? What made it difficult for you? What did you end up doing?**	Yes	Yes	Yes
4. Think of a recent situation in which you were able to identify a customer's or patient's needs before he/she asked for help. What did you do? What was the patient's response?	Yes	Yes	Yes
5. How have you handled negative customer situations? How have you calmed an angry or upset patient/visitor/coworker? Cite a specific example.	Yes	Yes	Yes
6. What would make you proud of the way we treat our patients?	Yes	Yes	Yes

Behavioral Based Competency No. 5	Teamwork		
Indicator:	• Understands and incorporates relational wholeness into actions (avoids silo behavior) • Collaborative: Takes opportunities to work with others to find solutions to problems • Accountable: Follows through on commitments • Becomes a resource for other team members • Plays to own strengths and stretches out of comfort zone in team interactions • Shares information so others may be successful • Supports groups' solutions to problems		

Questions	Leader	Clinician	Staff
1. Tell me about the last time you collaborated on a project with others. What were the circumstances? Who was involved? What did you do to contribute?	Yes	Yes	Yes
2. Under what circumstances is it difficult to be cooperative on a team? Describe a time when you've faced these challenges. How did you handle the challenges? How did it turn out?	Yes	Yes	Yes
3. Tell me about a team decision in your current or past position that you were not in agreement with. What was the decision? What was your idea that wasn't used? How did you respond to the decision? What did you do to demonstrate support of the decision even though you did not agree with it?	Yes	Yes	Yes
4. How would members of your most recent team describe you?	Yes	Yes	Yes
5. What prevents people from sharing information or skills with others? What have you done to overcome these barriers?	Yes	Yes	Yes
6. Coaching is about providing feedback for growth, improvement, and/or correction. Describe your skills with each situation. Tell me about a time you've used these skills well.	Yes	Yes	Yes

Behavioral Based Competency No. 6	**Personal Attributes: Job Fit**		
Indicator:	• Energized • Confident • Respectful • Open • Fun-loving • Creative • Honest		
	Leader	**Clinician**	**Staff**
Questions			
1. Describe how you have gone about developing an environment that promotes caring, healing, and learning. Please be specific. What were the circumstances? What did you do? What were the results?	Yes	Yes	Yes
2. How can you help BEMC transform the healthcare experience? Give specific examples.	Yes	Yes	Yes
3. How do you treat others with dignity, respect, honesty, and fairness? Please provide a specific example.	Yes	Yes	Yes
4. Have you ever had the opportunity to work in an open architecture, cubicle-type environment? If yes, give me an example of how you worked in that environment. What worked well? What didn't work so well? If no, what types of issues might you have working in this type of environment and how would you handle these issues?	Yes	Yes	Yes
5. Tell me about your greatest professional accomplishment. What made it especially challenging? What type of feedback did you receive? What makes you the most proud of this?	Yes	Yes	Yes
6. If you took out an ad in the New York Times and had to describe yourself in only three words, what would those words be and why?	Yes	Yes	Yes
7. Describe your ideal work environment.	Yes	Yes	Yes
8. Tell me about a work situation that irritated you. What did you do?	Yes	Yes	Yes
9. What responsibilities do you want and what kinds of results do you expect to achieve in your next job?	Yes	Yes	Yes

Behavioral Based Competency No. 7	**Problem Solving and Creativity**		
Indicator:	• Seeks a variety of alternatives/approaches • Identifies a variety of sources • Solves problems effectively • Can articulate a problem-solving process • Takes calculated risks • Critical thinking skills—confidence, flexibility, intuition, open-mindedness, perseverance, questioning, and reflection		
		Leader	**Clinician**	**Staff**

Questions	Leader	Clinician	Staff
1. How do you define critical thinking? Give me an example of a nonroutine or more difficult problem you had to solve. How did you work through to a solution?	Yes	Yes	Yes
2. Tell me about a time when you did your best, but were unable to solve a problem. What were the barriers? What did you do to remove them? What did you learn from the experience?	Yes	Yes	Yes
3. Give an example of a situation in which you took a calculated risk in a recent position. What were your considerations? What was the outcome?	Yes	Yes	Yes
4. Please describe the last creative solution you came up with in response to a problem. What was the problem? How did you work through to your solution?	Yes	Yes	Yes

Behavioral Based Competency No. 8	**Manages Change**		
Indicator:	• Manages ambiguity. • Understands behaviors and change management techniques and theory. • Asks questions so he/she can support decisions. Does not resist changes in the organization. • Communicates throughout change process.		
	Leader	**Clinician**	**Staff**
Questions			
1. Tell me about a recent change in your workplace. What did you do to learn more about the rationale for the change? What did you learn? How did it affect your ability to manage the change?	Yes	Yes	Yes
2. When was the last time you initiated a major change in your life? Please provide a specific example. What drove your decision to make the change? What did you do to ensure the change went as you expected it to?	Yes	Yes	Yes
3. Describe a work situation in which a project you worked on and felt was important was delayed or postponed due to other changes in the organization. How did you handle this situation?	Yes	Yes	Yes

Behavioral Based Competency No. 9	**Manages Time/Sets Priorities**		
Indicator:	• Organized • Manages multiple projects effectively • Meets deadlines with quality work		
	Leader	**Clinician**	**Staff**
Questions			
1. Tell me about your work experience in managing multiple job priorities with varied deadlines. When and how do you determine priority and deadline changes?	Yes	Yes	Yes
2. You are on the phone with another department resolving a problem. The intercom pages you for a customer on hold. Your manager returns your monthly report with red pen markings and demands corrections within the hour. What do you do?	Yes	Yes	Yes
3. Think of a typical day when you had plenty of things to do. Describe how you scheduled your time.	Yes	Yes	Yes

BEMC Interview Guide Summary Sheet for Leadership Roles

Date of interview:
Candidate name:
Position:
Interviewer:

Competency categories	(1–5 Score) 1 = unacceptable 2 = below average 3 = meets minimal expectations 4 = above average 5 = outstanding	Question number(s)	Candidate responses
Leadership			
Achieves results			
Effective communicator			
Customer service			
Teamwork			
Personal attributes: job fit			
Creativity and risk taking			
Manages change			
Manages time/sets priorities			
TOTAL SCORE			

Would you recommend this person for hire?
If yes, what are the key reasons for hiring this person?
If no, what are the key reasons for not hiring?

Contact Connie Harmsen, former CEO, at charmsen1@cox.net for additional information on the interview guide.

CHAPTER 9

CHAPTER

Turning Toxic Behaviors into Transformational Actions

CHAPTER OBJECTIVES:

Upon completion of this chapter, the reader will:

1. Differentiate between healthy and toxic leader behaviors.
2. Examine selected behaviors of new employee hazing, destructive confidants, poor communication, and feedback dysfunction as sources of toxicity in the organization.
3. Formulate at least three strategies to decrease toxic behaviors as a developing quantum leader.
4. Critique the value of story telling as a meaningful leader strategy.

INTRODUCTION: HEALING IS OUR BUSINESS

Healing is our business, and yet not all healthcare leadership practices result in outcomes that reflect therapeutic intentions. Many outcomes are in fact quite negative and detrimental to not only individuals and teams but also the organization as a whole. In this chapter, sources of toxicity that are specific to the healthcare marketplace, organizational structure, individual behaviors, and team processes will be examined, along with strategies for eliminating toxic practices and replacing them with therapeutic behaviors more reflective of the healer.

TOXICITY IS...

Healthy behaviors seldom get the attention that toxic behaviors or negative outcomes receive. Consider the question often posed by nurses, "What is most evident when it is missing?" The response is nursing. When nursing is being practiced in healthy and meaningful ways, the attention it receives is minimal compared to when nursing does not occur as expected. When there is shortage of

> **Gem**
>
> A toxin is a substance or poison that has an inherent tendency to impair health and destroy life.

nurses, nursing care cannot be delivered in the same way as when there were more nurses. Shortages lead to lack of care, missed treatments, low morale, high turnover, and ultimately high costs to consumers. Understanding the optimal way health care should be provided, as well as what happens when the outcomes are less than

<table>
<tr><td colspan="2" align="center">Impact of Nurse Staffing
Selected References</td></tr>
</table>

• Patient mortality	Aiken, et al. 1994; Cho, 2003
• Length of stay	ANA, 1997; Flood & Diers, 1988; Pronovost, 1999; Thungjaroenkul, Cummings, & Embleton, 2007; Mark, Harless, & Berman, 2007
• Medication errors	ANA Report Card, 1995; Blegen & Vaughn, 1998
• Nosocomial pneumonia	ANA, 1997; Blegen et al., 1998
• Turnover	Keeler & Cramer, 2007;
• Failure to rescue	Clarke & Aiken, 2003
• Cost to consumer	McCue, 2003; Unruh, 2008

Quantum Discussion

Healing *Not* Behaviors

In your workgroup, identify those behaviors that are believed to be healing, but in reality are *not*. How can you begin to eliminate such behaviors and replace them with more appropriate behaviors for a healthcare organization?

Examples include:

- Withholding feedback/key information
- Smiling sarcasm
- The devil's advocate role

optimal, can help us determine when healthy processes become toxic and negatively impact healthcare service.

SOURCES OF TOXICITY

Toxicity in organizations seldom occurs blatantly or in resoundingly strong practices and behaviors. Organizational toxicity is often subtle and seemingly insignificant as it spreads its highly venomous substance, destroying the essence of health and healing cultures. Toxicity seldom results from one source or a single activity; it is a consequence of several factors and pressures that, once understood, can be reversed by the collective actions of competent leaders.

The Marketplace

Failure to provide service of the highest quality in the eyes of the consumer, regardless of social or economic status, personal attributes, or the nature of health problems has been identified as the most significant ethical issue encountered in healthcare organizations (Cooper, Frank, Gouty, & Hansen, 2002). Marketplace forces seriously challenge the ability of the leader to achieve and sustain financial viability. The chosen strategies to achieve organizational goals may compromise the essential work of the organization, namely, providing effective, value-based healthcare services. Thus, from seemingly good intentions, negative, toxic outcomes result. The organization may be financially solvent, yet patient care outcomes are marginal and healthcare workers are disenfranchised, angry, and often leave the organization searching for less toxic and healthier organizations.

Organizational Structure

The pathways for communication and decision making in organizations can be a subtle but significant source of toxicity. When the organization espouses shared leadership and yet reinforces practices of double-checking others believed entrusted with the power and authority to make decisions, the situation is in conflict. The message of this double standard diminishes the integrity of organizational leadership and trust among employees and creates more toxicity. What a conundrum when professional nurses believe they are members of a shared leadership council with decision-making accountability and authority and yet the decisions they make are changed or overridden without their input. In many organizations, shared leadership councils are created below the traditional executive leadership team chaired by the chief executive officer. The executive team reviews all council decisions and often overrides or redirects councils to shift or reconsider decisions. This approach creates confusion for council participants and discourages future participation. In time, employees are demoralized, and trusting relationships are forever undermined.

TOXIC INDIVIDUAL BEHAVIORS

Not all toxicity can be attributed to the organizational structure. While poorly designed and ineffective systems make it difficult for good individuals to do good things, the need exists for leaders to take action to assure that both the individual and the system are examined for potential shortcomings. System policies and procedures, computer system effectiveness, reward strategies, and individual behaviors require analysis prior to choosing a correcting strategy. Denial and resistance to examining current system attributes will serve only as ineffective rationalization and will avoid addressing the fundamental issue.

Individuals within organizations may fail to embrace established values and cultural norms for several reasons. These reasons or rationalizations are related to system functioning, but the accountability for behavior rests squarely with the individual. Hofmann (2004) identified the following seven reasons why good people behave badly.

1. *Lack of organizational loyalty.* Often short-term employees have not established allegiance to the organization but merely are earning a paycheck. High staff turnover further contributes to such behaviors and lack of commitment to the organization.
2. *Pressure to succeed as defined by the organization.* Some organizations have placed emphasis on net income above clinical outcomes and value conformity over candor, resulting in personnel who act inappropriately and unethically. The recent fraud and abuse violations of several national healthcare systems was most likely motivated by an overemphasis on financial criteria.
3. *Rules are for the others.* Driving 5 miles per hour above the speed limit to get to an important meeting on time, believing that one's business is more important than following rules, is a simple example of this behavior. Certain employees assert that they should not be subject to certain policies and procedures.
4. *Believing their actions are not illegal.* Being ethical is more than being compliant with statutory regulations. Not every action and behavior is governed by statute, nor should they be. Yet, some believe that ethical acts and legal acts are synonymous. To be sure, there are many unethical actions that are not legislated.
5. *Pressure from peers.* The combination of strong-willed colleagues with those who are inexperienced, easily influenced by others, or conflict avoiders sets up conditions for toxic behaviors. Acquiescing to overbearing colleagues diminishes the probability for effective dialogue and high quality decision making.
6. *Lack of resources.* Much like the pressure-to-succeed behavior, when resources are limited, individuals attempt to cut corners as an excuse for unsatisfactory work rather than work to adjust demands to more closely match available resources. Eliminating safety evaluations and safety measures are examples of cutting corners inappropriately.
7. *A sense of entitlement.* An inflated sense of self-importance and an absence of organizational pride contribute to the belief that the organization or the community owes one something. An example of entitlement abuse can be the use of earned sick time. In those organizations that have separate sick hours benefits, employees often use the sick time at will rather than solely for sickness in order to not lose the earned time.

New Employee Hazing: Tolerating Change Avoidance

When leaders do not walk their talk, do not live the values and policies they endorse, yet still speak to these values from the podium, members of the organization recognize the inconsistency and interpret the actions as a serious lack of integrity. Frequently, leaders assume new positions with expectations to take the department to a higher and more productive level. Everyone in the interviewing process agrees that changes are needed and needed quickly. However, something very different occurs.

Discussion

Ineffective System Processes

Consider the following routine interactions in most healthcare settings. Each process has at some point in your career been identified as less than optimal.

- Patient admission
- Acquiring capital equipment

Discuss each process from the perspective of supporting policies and procedures, computer system support adequacy, and individual competencies to perform the processes.

- What is working?
- What changes would make the process more timely and value based?

Discussion

Rules for Others

List the rules or policies that are routinely ignored without consequences.

What actions should be taken to decrease the noncompliance?

- Reinforce the value of the policy and expectations?
- Modify the policy?
- Eliminate the policy?

Examples to consider for discussion:

- Hand washing
- Returning from breaks on time
- Documentation
- Eating in designated areas

Discussion

New Employee Hazing Assessment

Meet with the last five individuals hired in your organization. Discuss their expectations and what really happened. If the expectations are not close to reality, discuss what happened and how to reduce the gap.

Eliminate employee hazing!

As new employees join organizations, a subtle but toxic process may occur: employee hazing. This situation of toxic mentoring follows the selection and hiring of the new employees. Although leaders overtly believe that innovative ideas are the lifeblood of any organization, especially in today's rapidly changing healthcare environment, obstacles are often covertly placed in the way of new employee innovation. After intense rounds of interviews, the candidate with the best believed fit with the vision of the organization is hired and touted as the key to future success.

The new leader joins the organization and is quickly met with messages and guidance that are intended to assist in the orientation and socialization process but provide obstacles to those innovative ideas on the very first day of employment! New leaders are told of the failures of the past, why certain strategies did not work, or current policies and regulations that would make it impossible to consider innovative ideas. Current employees reflect on long-held traditions, the need to ensure peaceful relationships, the importance of not upsetting long-term employees who have given so much to the company, and finally the need to go slowly in introducing and implementing any changes to assure employee support and buy-in. Seldom are new leaders met with passionate optimism and enthusiasm to figure out how to test new ideas in the face of the established organizational culture.

When the organization is not getting individuals with the new and truly innovative ideas necessary to stay ahead of the competition, the organizational culture and norms may be hazing the innovation out of them. Examination of organizational policies and procedures specific to orientation of new employees is essential. Inclusion of expectations to bring innovative ideas rather than expectations of blind acceptance with cultural norms is the first step to the elimination of hazing and support for innovation.

Destructive Confidants

Organizational toxicity may also emanate from destructive confidants. Traditional leaders avoid any hint of dependency on others, yet the need for a close confidant is rooted in childhood, the need to feel close to someone, to feel understood, cared for, and loved. Having a trusted confidant with whom to discuss challenging issues, share fears and experiences, and gain unfiltered advice adds to the leader's competence. Given the isolated position of the leader, selecting a confidant deserves special attention to ensure that the goals and motives of the confidant are congruent. Too often, individuals in the organization shelter the leader from unpleasant or conflicting information. Executive coaching programs can be designed to assist leaders is recognizing the values and pitfalls of confidants.

According to Sulkowicz (2004), many confidants end up hurting, undermining, or otherwise exploiting CEOs when they are at their most vulnerable. Although intentions may be honorable on the surface, confidants become close friends who affirm the leader, rather than serving to challenge and sharpen the leader's effectiveness and keeping the leader's best interest at the forefront. When a confidant becomes dangerous, the leader is often the last one to know when and how the relationship became toxic. Admitting that the relationship is toxic further demoralizes the already isolated and vulnerable leader.

Consider the situation in which a confidant preys on the leader's anxieties about certain competitors, relationships with others in the community, and personal characteristics. Rather than challenge the reality of the anxiety, the toxic confidant reinforces the hopelessness of the negative relationship or the potential for further negative actions. Another situation is in the selection of key members of the leadership team. Destructive confidants reinforce selection of less competent members to assure they are not exposed. Selecting those with less experience, less education, and less

---

Quantum Tip

Eliminating New Employee Hazing

- Avoid the tendency to "correct" new employees into the current culture.
- Encourage new ideas. At the end of each day, ask new employees what observations they have made and potential changes that could benefit the organization.
- Evaluate your own behaviors:
  - How long does it take new employees to look and act like everyone else?
  - In what subtle ways have you doused new employee ideas?

Quantum Point

Three Destructive Confidants

Reflectors—Confidants who mirror the leader
Insulators—Confidants who prevent critical information from getting out or getting in
Usurpers—Confidant who ingratiates him- or herself with leader in a desperate bid for power

K.J. Sulkowicz, 2004

competence under the guise of mentoring severely limits the organization's capacity for innovation and growth.

Avoiding these destructive relationships may seem impossible for many leaders, given the often narcissistic role of the leader. Yet these narcissistic behaviors are also essential in creating, achieving, and sustaining organizational visions. To minimize the destructive confidant syndrome, several strategies are worth examining. Watch for the warning signs of a destructive relationship:

- Employees complain that you are not accessible
- You feel no one but your confidant understands you
- Your confidant discourages you from getting other opinions or counsel

These signs may be reflective of a larger problem as well, such as procrastination, mediocre communication skills, or lack of trust in others by the leader.

Effective leaders have many confidants or colleagues whom they trust, and they value their wisdom rather than a single confidant. Having only one confidant can be stunting and immobilizing for the leader who desires realistic mentoring for dialogue and reflection. When leaders hear only positive feedback, the alarm should sound and the search for confidants to represent complex dimensions of healthcare leadership should begin in earnest.

Communication Gone Awry

Communication among employees, patients, and physicians has long been a challenge for organizations. Delivering the right message to the right person, at the right time, with the right intent does not occur consistently for a variety of reasons. The rationale for delivering partial or poorly timed messages is often due to impulsive or spontaneous actions that simply override good sense! The challenge to continue to work toward effective communication remains with all individuals.

Abuse of Power: Verbal Abuse

Abusive communication is not always expressed loudly and profanely. Often, verbal abuse is in the form of a believed kind and generous sharing of information. Much attention has been given to overt disruptive behavior in organizations.

Abuse of Power: Decision Making

Leaders often abuse power in their eagerness to remedy system imperfections. Efforts become aggressive and nonparticipatory when the issue is believed to be critical and urgent.

Toxic Mentoring

The need to create succession plans for future leadership often serves as a vehicle for toxicity, continuing those practices that are no longer effective and even detrimental to organizational creativity and energy. While not overtly toxic, mentors may emphasize the continuation of previous practices that were controlling and reinforced the hierarchical nature of a command and control decision-making model. These behaviors unintentionally serve to reinforce past practices that were appropriate for the industrial age. Believing that such strategies are also effective for the information age belies the reality of the new age and all of its characteristics. The past is reinforced as appropriate, and the future is denied.

Discussion

Uncommon Verbal Abuse

This statement was made by a smiling supervisor in the presence of patients and coworkers: "It's hard to believe that with your experience and skills, you did not provide the information to this family. I'm sure that you will take care of this quickly." It is disrespectful, confrontational, and demeaning without the typical aura of verbal abuse.

1. Identify three situations in which verbal abuse occurred that did not involve yelling, arrogance, profanity, or physical threats.
2. What strategies can you identify to address these behaviors and to avoid them in the future?

Decision-Making Characteristics

Traditional

- Compartmentalism
- Focus on analysis to determine cause and effect
- Standardization of processes
- Emphasis on structure and process
- Individual leaders dominate
- Control mechanisms to minimize variation

Shared Leadership

- Collaboration
- Synthesis of ideas
- Teamwork
- Collective wisdom: Recognition of individual strengths as contributions to the whole
- Attention to the whole system
- Emphasis on value-based outcomes

Discussion

Hiring for the Future

The CEO hires a CNO with less than the traditional years of experience, but with the appropriate confidence, ability to form effective relationships, desire to perform in the role, and basic skills reflective of collaboration and consensus building.

1. What are the advantages/disadvantages of this decision?
2. What are the facilitators/barriers in your organization to a similar decision?
3. How would you prevent new employee hazing into the old way for this individual?

Consider the situation in which a leader believes that 5 years of experience is required to understand and function in a particular position. A candidate for the position has 2 years of experience, the desire to serve in the role, the confidence, and the technical and relational competence. Current leaders encourage the candidate to gain the experience and then apply for the position. The traditional time for paying one's dues is sustained, and the opportunity to coach and mentor a strong candidate is missed. Mentors from outside the organization may be more appropriate than current leaders from within. When a mentor can be objective about situations without the historical bias of the organization, the leader learns to challenge existing practices and structures in the journey of leadership. New leaders do not need to change everything but rather need to clearly know the rationale for existing practices and become comfortable learning when to sustain practices that are effective.

Managing the Unmanageable Leader

Not all leaders are competent in their positions. Employees who are not getting along with their leader are often challenged to get along or move on. Before moving on in utter frustration or just tolerating the incompetence, they should give serious consideration to other options. The following steps are recommended to assist you in making wise decisions before things really get out of hand, even when the leader is the clone of every disastrous leader you have ever read about, heard about, or had nightmares about:

1. Meet with him or her and clarify what is expected in terms of style of getting the job done. The priorities of your former boss and current boss may be very different in basic work methods.
2. Carefully confront criticism in private. Express your desire to communicate effectively, discuss your negative perceptions of the interaction, and finally ask for guidance in how to communicate effectively with him or her (no matter how difficult it is!).
3. Check the mirror! Your own attitude may be part of the problem. Have you been helpful since this new person joined your organization? Standoffish? Annoyed? Neutral—neither negative nor helpful? Is your body language outrageously loud? Are facial expressions and tone of your voice telling of your dissatisfaction?
4. Reflect on the issues. Is your shadow showing? The style, mannerisms, and communications that annoy us the most are often behaviors of our own that we ourselves struggle to manage.
5. Make your decision. Do not dawdle as the toxicity may only increase.

Feedback Dysfunction

Gaining an understanding of what others are thinking is essential to good communication and teamwork. Often coworkers become caught up in the need to share their feelings openly and honestly, and the result is less than satisfactory. Communications are interpreted as whining or complaining without purpose or accountability. Perceptions of personal attacks, global commentaries on vague issues, opinionating about conditions not under one's control, and failing to address issues to the appropriate person result in toxic communication. These communications serve no useful purpose, waste valuable organizational time, and too often are no more than idle gossip destructive to the culture.

TOXIC TEAM PROCESSES

In the best of all worlds, the processes that emerge in organizations are the result of deliberately designed authority and decision-making structures and are then embraced and practiced by the individuals in the organization. Given the realities of organizational dynamics, which includes the recency of the structure design, the match of individual skill sets to the established vision and values, and the personal motivation of each leader to actively support the defined culture, disconnects between what is stated and what is practiced occur, all too often resulting in toxic conditions.

Consider the organization that has designed shared leadership structures but does not always achieve the processes to support these structures. Shared leadership council structures have been identified and created. The need for member skills of collaboration, negotiation, and facilitation, and the ability to surrender the once-required strong, authoritarian ego are also agreed to and included in performance expectations. In reality, decision making is offered to councils but is often overridden, negated, or ignored. Recommendations by councils are seldom integrated into organizational policy, thus rendering the work of councils insignificant.

SOURCES OF TOXICITY: TEAM PROCESSES

Shared Decision Making: Rhetoric or Reality

Toxic behaviors can be present in decision-making processes. Transitional leaders or those leaders who began their careers in organizations steeped in command and control require significant support in moving to a shared leadership model. Ongoing dialogue and reflection are essential to ensure that all members of the team are in fact living in the new participative model. McMurry (2003) notes that often leaders become overenchanted with participative processes, yet still operate from an autocratic model.

McMurry (2003) describes three types of leadership: group autocracy, blind autocracy, and benevolent autocracy. They can be very subtle but highly toxic to the organization. The phenomenon of group autocracy typically occurs in large, bureaucratic organizations in which strategic decisions are not officially made by the leader, who lacks courage and takes refuge in the principle of unanimity. The leader maintains bureaucratic autocracy without leadership, imagination, or drive while functioning under the guise of shared leadership.

As healthcare leaders transition from autocratic behaviors to leading from a shared perspective, with the expectations to produce optimal results, respond quickly, and assure positive employee satisfaction, there is a tendency to subtly slip into group autocracy behaviors. In essence, leaders are preaching shared decision making yet operating as autocrats.

Both blind autocracy and benevolent autocracy behaviors belie the guiding principles and values of shared leadership. Leaders firmly entrenched in autocratic practices believe that, although the democratic participative philosophy of management is more productive in the long term, stimulates creativity and development, and improves morale, the probability of such behaviors succeeding is minimal. Lower and middle managers have not been given opportunities to demonstrate shared leadership practices, making the prospects for this new model of leadership negligible. Current managers are dependent upon strong autocratic leaders to provide specific direction and appear insecure and

---

Tips for Effective Feedback: Managing Others

1. Establish formal and informal review processes. Monthly discussions should be the minimum frequency for feedback.
2. Address potential fear of feedback issues. Create expectations for open and honest communication.
3. Avoid the tendency of providing superficial feedback. Provide objective feedback specific to established goals.
4. Avoid angry confrontations, defensiveness, ambivalent conversations.

Three Types of Decision-Making Autocracy

Group Autocracy: Decisions discussed by the group, but in reality made by the leader who is hiding in the group process.

Blind Autocracy: Decisions made by the leader who directs others to trust his or her decisions due to the competence of the leader.

Benevolent Autocracy: Decisions made by the leader on the assumption that others cannot make optimal and effective decisions in a team setting.

R. McMurry

Toxic Versus Humanistic Values

Toxic	Humanistic
• Overcontrol	• Trusting
• Reminding of past failures	• Focus on new approaches to improve the past
• Identifying mistakes	
• Double-checking work	• Valuing unsuccessful attempts
• Controlling processes	• Expecting personal accountability

ineffective. Thus, leaders assume that the only way to get the work done is to create a benevolent autocracy model of leadership. The lack of emerging behaviors from lower and middle managers requires the autocrat to continue with the current behaviors.

To shift from this dehumanizing and toxic model, leaders are required to transition to a new and more humanistic approach that values the contributions of each employee as the more appropriate vehicle to higher organizational performance. Not surprising, this transition requires time, energy, and patience, which are not always readily given to the process.

Black, White, or Neither or Both?

Another source of toxicity can be found when the zeal to implement shared leadership overrides common sense. The notion that the only way to work is through teams can be problematic. Embedded in a shared leadership model are the expectations that at certain times group participation in decision making is not possible and members of the team must make autocratic decisions in certain situations. Attempting to live in the absoluteness of one style or the other creates uncertainty and toxicity in the organization. When employees are expecting one process exclusively and then experience several processes, the trust level within the organizations declines dramatically. It is the allegiance to the defined values and mission of the organization that must remain the constant in all decisions, regardless of the decision-making process.

Decision Making

Unilateral
- Following laws
- Facility licensure requirements
- Nurse practice act
- Accreditation requirements

Shared
- Processes to meet laws, licensure requirements, nurse practice act, and accreditation requirements

---

Toxicity emerges when the council structures are mere window dressing and decisions continue to be made autocratically on the basis of inconsistently defined values, not only at the executive level but also at the unit level. Most importantly, toxicity can be reversed by clarifying council charter expectations for work to be managed and outcomes to be achieved.

A recent situation resulting from the failure to distinguish unilateral from shared decision making involved an emergency department. The state department was conducting a survey, following a complaint from a patient who believed she suffered unnecessary pain in the emergency room. Upon investigation, the complaint was not substantiated. However, the state department was duty bound to cite the organization for failing to follow its own policy on pain management. The unilateral decision from the state required each department to have a policy specific to pain management for patients in the emergency department. The department director created a policy and an expectation for nurses to assess 10 factors related to pain for each patient upon admission and upon discharge. During the review of records, zero compliance with the facility policy was noted; thus, the facility was cited. While some may believe that regulatory agencies impose unreasonable and bureaucratic standards, it is often the organization that has overinterpreted the standard. The unilateral state requirement is nonnegotiable. The processes and content developed by the organization to meet this requirement should be developed by the team to reflect the nature of the patient care in each department.

Covert Greed or Competition Gone Bad

Within leadership teams, the enthusiasm for success can often move beyond reasonable success to that for greed. Greed is a trait that we typically attribute to others, as it is a profoundly negative quality. Given that money and things are often considered measures of success, the desperation to acquire things can become toxic not only in one's personal life but also in the workplace. When individuals become aggressive and manipulative in acquiring goods and money, the behaviors become pathological greed (Coutu, 2003).

Recent events in corporate America have exposed the negative outcomes of greed. Chief executive officers have desperately worked to amass more and more fortune for unknown reasons. Fortunately, greed is tempered by social norms and can be harnessed to serve social ends. In less than 50 years, the management of hospitals and health systems has shifted from a passive, custodial, and largely benign administrative tradition to an aggressive, growth-oriented, entrepreneurial management framework (Goldsmith, 1998). Not surprising, the economic position of healthcare systems has also improved significantly with the new technologies and the transition from primarily inpatient services to multisite ambulatory settings.

The desire for success can become toxic or be considered unhealthy greed when the desire for more profits and more buildings overshadows the fundamental need for preservation of the healthcare mission and organizational survival. Traditionally, the profoundly negative essence of greed has not been associated with healthcare services. Yet, increasing numbers of organizations prioritize shareholder gain as the priority. When expectations and reward structures designed to support primarily shareholder gain drive decision making, the chasm between leaders and professionals is enlarged; as leaders discard the core accountabilities of quality healthcare services in favor of personal gain, greed of a very unholy nature exists! In some cases, not-for-profit organizations are also at risk for unholy greed. The desire for more equipment, more technology, more physical locations, and higher net income margins can easily create toxic conditions. In the healthcare marketplace, there will never be enough dollars to provide the highest quality patient care, the most progressive technology, and the newest physical settings. Yet, some leaders work to achieve these goals at the expense of providing value-based healthcare services.

It is no surprise that this success has an undesired outcome—the alienation of professionals who are the lifeblood of health care and who bear most of the moral risk of the healthcare transaction. The cultural disintegration resulting from organizational greed has impacted nurses, physicians, technicians, and social workers, who see themselves transformed into commodities and marginalized by the corporate culture of healthcare services. The chasm between leaders and professionals remains, while financial strength is at its peak and expansion abounds. The tension of this paradox is certainly recognized by leaders and providers, yet the hostility remains as healthcare systems continue to grow to the point of dwarfing both the patient and the caregiver who must work within them. Some organizations have grown beyond human scale and have lost their focus on the daily life-and-death struggles occurring within their walls, thus fueling toxicity.

Greed can be seen not only in healthcare leaders but also in patients who believe they are entitled to every medical treatment known to man, even without evidence of probable success of such treatments or commitment to therapeutic supportive behaviors. In many situations, patient advocacy and informed consent that clearly delineates all of the advantages and disadvantages can assist patients and their families in making more realistic decisions.

Personal greed and selfishness often transfer to the workplace and interfere with group commitment and willingness to take appropriate action. Individuals gauge decisions on the basis of their personal wants, at the expense of effective team collaboration and decision making. Decisions that ought to be good for patient care are not made, in favor of personal expectations of obtaining more time off and more overtime pay than is reasonable.

Healthcare workers can be guilty of greed in the expectations of excessive benefits and hourly wages. Employees may be caught up in the situation or strongly influenced by a labor organization to always ask for more from an employer without a corresponding contribution. Channeling greed to constructive purposes is a necessary leadership skill that is seldom recognized or articulated. Assisting employees to understand the marketplace value that each contributes (or does not contribute) as well as competitive wages and benefits within the industry elevates wage and

---

Quantum Point

Tempering Greed Assessment

1. Assess your motives for new projects—is it for personal recognition, contributions to the industry, or solely to make money?
2. Are the mission and values of the organization congruent with the work of the organization?
3. Is the organization achieving the best possible outcomes, or are more resources needed at the bedside to assure excellence?
4. Is consideration given to Earth's limited resources?
5. Does a spirit of altruism permeate the healthcare organization and its work?

True Success Characteristics

- Values are clear and known to others.
- Service to the public is achieved.
- Resources are used appropriately.
- Services are value based and make a difference in healthcare outcomes.
- Integrity is never challenged.

benefits discussions to a much higher and more appropriate level. Employees must first know what difference they make to the organization's mission before demanding more from the employer. Further, when employees clearly understand their role and importance in the organization, morale is increased and efforts to continually enhance those contributions occur in a much healthier manner.

Valuing Fragmented or Partial Leadership

Organizational toxicity can increase when good and effective leadership is equated with partial leadership skills. Strength in some areas of leadership does not make a quantum leader. It is no secret that some expert technicians do not possess expert relationship skills, or that some leaders have outstanding relationship skills and little ability to envision and lead a team through health care's challenges. It is also not a secret that these individuals hold and sustain significant leadership positions and continue to demonstrate only partial leadership competence.

For example, the nurse executive with exceptional financial management skills may not possess exceptional or even average relationship skills. This nurse executive is continually rewarded for financial performance while employee satisfaction ratings are less than average, resulting in high turnover. Valuing of partial leadership by senior leaders can be acceptable for the short term but disastrous in the long term. Partial leadership erodes trust and negates the values of holism, values that form the essential patient care experience and include physical, social, financial, and technical components.

Arizona Nurse Leadership Model

Recognizing the limitations of current healthcare leadership models, nurse leaders in Arizona developed the Arizona Nurse Leadership (ANL) model to offer a comprehensive approach, which included six essential competencies of the quantum leader for the information age (Malloch, 2003). This model defines skills of nursing as managing relationships; communicating the role and contribution of nursing; creating effective working environments; impacting public policy; defining the value of nursing in marketplace language; and assuring that the work of nursing is in concert with the mission of health care. These skills form the framework of the larger model that encompasses the traditional activities of coaching, mentoring, and facilitating. The lack of these highly developed skills in leadership roles leads to frustration, disenfranchisement from the healthcare organization, partial leadership, and, all too often, resignation from the healthcare system. The six competencies of the ANL model, based on the work of Longest (1998) are described in the next section. These characteristics are requirements for not only leaders, but also staff nurses and nurse educators.

Conceptual competency includes both the knowledge and skill to envision one's place in the organization and within the larger society. The leader must be able to visualize the interrelationships that exist in workplaces and to integrate the cultural and historical development of values, beliefs, and norms of nursing within the workplace. Clear articulation of the role of nursing and its fit within the organization provides for the visible yet integrated role of nursing in the provision of health care.

From the staff nurse to the manager to the leader to the educator, the ability to model the vision for nursing is fundamental. Recognizing its historical development, leaders must continually evaluate, modify, and connect the role of nursing to the realities of the social, economic, and political environment. The understanding of the conceptual fit of

---

Leadership: Examples of Partial Versus Comprehensive

Partial

- Highly competent in clinical and relationship skills; poor governance skills
- Excellent manager of technical aspects; poor financial skills
- Excellent financial and productivity management skills; poor conceptual and interpersonal skills

Comprehensive

- Highly competent in clinical, relational, financial, conceptual, and governance skills
- Able to identify ongoing needs to continually enhance skills
- Able to coach and mentor others to achieve comprehensive leadership skills

---

Arizona Nurse Leadership Competencies

- Conceptual
- Technical
- Interpersonal
- Political
- Commercial
- Governance

Conceptual Competency Checklist

1. Am I able to articulate where nursing services fit within my organization? In my community?
2. Does the vision for nursing reflect the defined fit of nursing?
3. Do principles of systems thinking and systems analysis serve to further explain the complex dynamics of the work of nursing?
4. Am I continually adjusting the role of nursing, i.e., creating and adapting, as an evolutionary process supporting the comprehensive healthcare system?

nursing with society serves to assist the leader in clearly articulating these interactions and accountabilities. Living by the American Nurses Association social policy statement and knowing the contributions of nursing to the health of society and the cost of nursing care are some of the essential conceptual competencies of the nurse leader.

Technical competency of leaders encompasses those skills and knowledge specific to planning, designing, evaluating, and measuring performance. Specifically, technical competence encompasses the skills the nurse leader must have to ensure that nursing care is provided in the environment for which she or he is accountable. These skills are the fundamental work of leaders and are often believed to be the majority of the required skills, rather than only one facet of the role. Too often, the emphasis is placed primarily on technical skills at the expense of the integrated leadership skill set.

The technically competent leader is able to use problem-solving skills at the team level; understands the psychology of work satisfaction that translates into commitment, retention, and high productivity; and is able to measure performance based on established goals and standards. Also within the technical competency realm is the ability to create an environment for employees that is safe, challenges them to think critically, and encourages professional development and innovation.

Interpersonal competency embodies the knowledge and skill of human interactions and relations through which one leads other people in pursuit of common objectives. The ability to form collaborative relationships among caregivers, patients, and community members in the provision of care as well as in socializing others to the profession cannot be overstated. Forming relationships is the cornerstone of healing services, and nurses must be experts in this area. Nurses must relate effectively with patients, other healthcare professionals, members of the community, and the formal organizations of nursing to assure that the role of the nurse is explicitly enacted in the social setting as defined in the social policy of nursing.

Expertise in interpersonal competency for nurse leaders includes the expectation that the current knowledge of the profession is represented and personal development is self-directed to remain contemporary with the profession. The link with not only individuals and teams but also the profession of nursing embodies relationship expertise for nurse leaders. Nurses with expertise in interpersonal relationship building are respected for their integrity, trust, respect, presence, and ability to form meaningful alliances. Further, diversity of thought, culture, and demographics are seen as essential to ensure that each person is able to contribute in unique and different ways for meaningful relationships.

Political competency is the dual capacity to accurately assess the impact of public policies on the performance of one's domains of responsibility and to influence public policy making at state, federal, and international levels. The nurse with political competency knows what the rules or policies are for the profession and the industry, knows who or what organization created them, the rationale for their existence, and how they impact the provision of healthcare services. When an existing policy is identified as no longer appropriate or as negatively impacting health care, the nurse leader is both proactive and reactive in addressing the need for change.

One example is the multistate licensure of nurses. At one time, state-supported nurse licensure was appropriate. In the global world in which nurses are increasingly mobile, this model for licensure no longer protects the public as well as a multistate licensure model would. Thus, the politically competent nurse is knowledgeable of the policy

---

Technical Competency Checklist

1. Are you able to manage complex multidisciplinary meeting processes and achieve desired goals?
2. Are your project management skills adequate?
3. Are employees/team members able to solve problems effectively?
4. Is decision making based on evidence?
5. Are customer needs and expectations managed?
6. Is there a succession plan in place?
7. What skills are you missing?

Interpersonal Competency Guidelines

1. Listen carefully to others.
2. Be fully engaged when others are speaking; do not think ahead or of other things.
3. Ask for feedback about your trustworthiness.
4. Ask for input and guidance, not only about new ideas but also about daily routines.
5. Request feedback regularly from those outside your normal group to determine how your work is impacting others.

Political Competency Guidelines

1. Be aware of the impact of the state board of nursing, Centers for Medicare & Medicaid Services, and the department of health services within your state on the practice of nursing.
2. Participate in organizations that impact the practice of nursing.
3. Expect colleagues to actively participate in nursing and healthcare policy organizations.
4. Meet with your state legislator at least every 3 months.
5. Invite legislators to your organization to share ideas and influence policy.

of the state board of nursing, the rationale for the policy, and recommendations to change current policy to more appropriately support the provision of safe patient care. Nurses must be able to clearly state the impact of fiscal policy on healthcare outcomes. Most importantly, the politically competent nurse is proactive about the issue rather than reticent to comment.

Commercial competency addresses the economic exchanges between buyers and sellers in which value is created. It is the knowledge and skill to establish and operate value-creating situations in which economic exchanges between patients/learners and the healthcare system occur. The nurse with commercial competency is able to identify and provide care that makes a difference in patient outcomes within the boundaries of available resources. This competency is more than understanding basic cost accounting principles and the mechanics of developing a budget. The nurse with commercial competency understands reimbursement models as opportunities for nurses to demonstrate their unique contributions, understands the relationships among reductions in revenue, patient safety, quality outcomes, nurse satisfaction, and professional standards, and is able to use research to demonstrate which nursing interventions are consistent with cost-effective patient care. In essence, the nurse with commercial competency has the financial knowledge necessary to make decisions that integrate the clinical and business aspects of health care and value cost effectiveness.

Governance competency addresses the establishment and enactment of a clear vision for the organization and includes the knowledge and skill to establish and enact the vision. Nurse leaders with expertise in governance competency are able to integrate the values of nursing within the organization and to create a culture that supports realization of the vision while providing care in the organization. Governance competency is about consistency among organizational values and beliefs, the tenets of the discipline of nursing, and the actual work of the organization. Examples of governance competency include ability to role model patient rights and welfare in decision making, formalization of nursing's vision, mission, and objectives, ensuring performance from nursing by establishing standards of care and a work setting that promotes quality care, and creation of a cultural system that allows teams to deliver patient care and hold professionals accountable for practice, work processes, teamwork, and outcomes.

Commercial Competency Guidelines

1. Seek out financial experts for the mechanics of accounting—you can't know it all.
2. Identify the economic value of nursing in the marketplace using evidence-based research.
3. Document cost effectiveness of nurse interventions in your department/service/ organization.
4. Recognize the limitations of the current financing system and its impact on access to care.

Governance Competency Guidelines

1. Articulate one clear nursing vision for the organization—avoid the tendency to create a vision for every department.
2. Translate and review the mission, vision, and values for all employees at least annually.
3. Proactively evaluate the protection of patient rights—establish measures to demonstrate that the rights are protected.

Organizational Transparency Versus Overmanagement of Information

With the proliferation of management information systems, the amount and types of data generated are overwhelming. Leaders are expected to protect proprietary information and preserve the reputation of the organization. Leaders are also expected not to create roadblocks to information access when access to that information is appropriate. Creation of unnecessary roadblocks adds additional work for staff and frustrates those requesting the information. The ability to know the difference is an essential leadership competency. At times, healthcare leaders have worked diligently to conceal information under the guise of protecting one's license, avoiding liability, and minimizing patient and family upsets. According to Kerfoot (2004), this concealment is at the heart of an organization's dysfunctional relationship among staff, patients, and families. Concealing information creates additional work processes that do not achieve the desired outcome and that cause employees to overanalyze information and wonder what is missing, creating a sense of caution and distrust.

Consumer Information

Openness or information transparency in organizations benefits the community, employees, and patients. Secrecy paralyzes learning, and performance cannot be improved without full disclosure (Berwick, 2004). As consumers become the directors of their own health care, openness with patients in healthcare organizations is essential. Patients are indeed the best source of truth about their personal health, and healthcare professionals need to provide information they have gained to enhance the patient's ability to manage his or her own health care.

Caregiver Information

Consumers can easily access information on the Internet specific to appliances and vehicle safety. Similar information and resources must also be available from and accessed by healthcare organizations and providers.

Caregivers should know the outcomes of their patient care process, what is being measured, how they compare to other units and similar units in other organizations, and what improvements are possible to continue the journey to excellence in patient care.

Organizational Information

Records of outcomes, satisfaction, and costs serve to assist consumers in making informed decisions. Access to this information becomes the accountability of the organization in order to assure that consumers not only know services and potential healthcare interventions, but also the level of performance of organizations that provide those services. Both the numbers of cases and outcomes should be readily available to current and potential consumers.

Differentiating confidential information from readily available and often public information requires knowledge of the owner of the information, regulatory requirements, and expected use of the information. Taking time to determine what really should be protected and what information is readily available to the public is important for minimizing the creation of unnecessary bureaucratic processes. Creating a more trusting organization or organizational transparency should be the norm, rather than concealing information. Leaders need to be willing to share information that belongs to patients and to enter into meaningful dialogue to explain issues and decisions that are within their ability to disclose. This reinforces the value of trusting relationships. In contrast, leaders resistant to information sharing, fearful of dialogue in which patients will challenge the information, and belief that others will not understand the issues further reinforces a culture of secrecy and skepticism.

Patient Care Unit Outcomes

1. Average number of patients/day; average length of stay
2. Patient satisfaction level
3. Number/type of medication errors
4. Number of patient falls
5. Number of urinary tract infections
6. Number of nosocomial pneumonia infections
7. Employee satisfaction level
8. Percentage of RNs/LPNs/NAs providing care
9. Cost of registry RNs
10. Average cost of care/day

Rewards Without Evidence

Another source of toxicity is within the reward and recognition systems of an organization. Linking recognition and rewards to the desired competency and performance of caregivers continues to challenge the healthcare industry. Multiple roles, multiple clinical settings, and multiple generational values provide a backdrop that does not support single or standardized reward and recognition programs. Yet, given this complexity, most organizations offer standardized benefits and pay structures in the name of fairness and consistency. The emphasis in this mind-set is on the processes of rewards and recognition rather than the desired outcomes of performance.

One of the most troubling practices is the annual awards banquets. Employees who have been physically present in the organization for numbers of years are recognized and rewarded in one of the most significant and costly events of the organization. This occurs in the face of organizational marketing touting clinical excellence, community involvement, and an environment of patient safety, none of which receives the level

Rationale for the Nebraska Medical Center Clinical Ladder

- Recognition of clinical expertise is essential to retain clinical experts.
- Responsible management of resources in anticipating and providing support for applicants is expected.
- Responsible budget forecasting that begins with clear goals will assist in long-range planning.
- Candidates will be supported to be successful!

Examples of Award Criteria for Excellence

1. Patient satisfaction scores above the norm
2. Development of innovative plans for individualized patient care
3. Resource to new and experienced nurses
4. Accountability for ongoing competency

of reward and recognition of the annual employee attendance banquet. The challenge remains to recognize and reward employees who have contributed to the outcomes of quality patient care.

Nursing clinical ladders offer opportunities to transition from the traditional attendance reward system to one based on clinical competency and outcomes. The Nebraska Medical Center met the challenge of creating an effective management tool to recognize and reward clinical excellence by the creative use of consultants. The medical center identified the need to revise its clinical ladder to increase the credibility of the program and to ensure that rewards were linked to patient care outcomes and system goals. Using a nursing consultant and a human resource consultant as a team, goals were clarified, clinical excellence was redefined, and realistic financial incentives were created.

Key features of the program included:

- A specific annual dollar amount dedicated to the program
- An identified number of positions that would be available each quarter
- A clinical expert/nurse manager sponsor required, to assist the nurses in achieving the designation of clinical expert
- The majority of nurses recognized as proficient
- Level 2 of the program included nurses with national certification and a specific percentage salary increase
- Rewards for the expert status were segmented into 30% of the dollar amount for continuing education and 70% of the dollar amount in a lump sum or other financial options
- Recognition of expert nurses as donors of knowledge along with other hospital donors identified with plaques in the main entrance

Members of the clinical ladder program developed the following list of behaviors and competencies essential to the role of the expert. The unique feature of the program is the requirement for the presence of all competencies as described below. Nurses at the expert nurse level possess the competencies and must be able to provide evidence. Five categories of behaviors include:

1. *Clinical Excellence (Nurse Content).* The expert nurse is able to manage complex patients with multiple diagnoses, requiring multiple interventions. Managing family stress and customized patient education are examples of patient complexity. The nurse demonstrates clinical forethought, anticipation of patient needs and proactive planning, and ability to assist patients and their families to manipulate/navigate the healthcare system using complex critical thinking skills. Documents services accurately, concisely, and legibly.
2. *Patient Advocate.* The expert nurse promotes excellence through patient advocacy. The expert nurses questions inappropriate clinical actions, behaviors, and/or orders and initiates system changes to avoid repeat behaviors. The expert nurse challenges the system appropriately, i.e., in a timely manner and in a respectful manner. The expert nurse takes risks to modify the system rules to assure patient safety.
3. *Expert Resource.* The expert nurse serves as a confident and credible resource to others through the following roles: preceptor, which includes orientation to technical and relational behaviors of the organization; coach, which provides intermittent assistance with technical and relational behaviors and course corrects when appropriate; and mentor, which includes specific commitment to an individual for a designated time period. The expert nurse demonstrates and shares knowledge about the organization and the healthcare environment.

4. *Role Model.* The expert nurse role models therapeutic behaviors, i.e., behaviors that improve the status of the individual following an interaction. The expert nurse is a team player and is viewed as a stress reducer rather than a stress producer. The expert nurse is able to refocus a stressed group of team members or patients/physicians. The expert nurse delegates duties to appropriate individuals and intervenes to ensure there is appropriate delegation.

5. *Accountability.* The expert nurse is able to demonstrate accountability for personal/professional development during the last 3 months. The expert nurse is knowledgeable about the changing practices of nursing and current healthcare system processes.

The Magnet Bandwagon

The desire for recognition within the industry can become toxic when there is a disconnection between the infrastructure, goals, and processes to achieve those goals. The recognition and award should be the result of practice excellence, not the driver of the process just because others are doing it. Leaders may be able to envision the goals needed to achieve quality outcomes but cannot envision and create the appropriate supportive infrastructure with organizational processes and the desired goal. The endpoint of clinical excellence is recognized, while the processes of achieving the recognition are negated or not valued. Merely desiring an organization to be known for excellence is not enough; the infrastructure, processes, values, and commitment to cultures of excellence must be present and in the right relationships. All elements fully integrated are essential components to achieve the goal of organizational excellence.

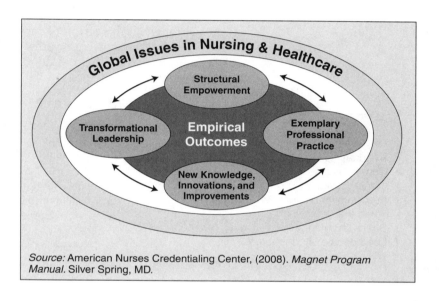

Source: American Nurses Credentialing Center, (2008). *Magnet Program Manual.* Silver Spring, MD.

The Magnet bandwagon is one recent example of a toxic behavior. As many organizations achieve Magnet status, the attractiveness of the recognition and attempt to get on the bandwagon is escalating. Some view Magnet recognition as merely a process to document current practices rather than evidence of organizational systems, processes, and outcomes that reflect the highest level of excellence in patient care and the organizational culture supportive of nursing. Even more problematic are the challenges to change Magnet standards to be more reflective of the current reality! Consider the efforts to modify the credentials of the chief nurse executive and allow nurse executives without a baccalaureate in nursing to be reflective of nursing excellence. While the nurse executive may have a bachelor's and master's degree in a health-related field, the lack of at least a bachelor's in nursing is inconsistent with excellence in nursing. Excellence in nursing leadership is about knowledge, relationships, effective processes, and achievement of exceptional outcomes—a comprehensive model rather than pieces.

Shared leadership is another example. Magnet standards include the expectation of shared leadership rather than autocratic models of decision making. Organizations declare shared leadership in their quest for Magnet status, then establish the traditional councils and continue to make decisions on the basis of individual role and position. The councils are merely window dressing for the survey process. The past is couched in the structure of new policies and language, but it is readily evident to members of the organization that past practices continue to be the norm. The Magnet journey is devalued to the Magnet bandwagon. Changing organizational structure and processes should be made to reflect the vision, mission, and intention of the organization, not the desire for a certain credential or award.

REVERSING TOXICITY: CREATING SUSTAINABLE SOLUTIONS

The work of healers is never finished. Removing negative influences and creating healing conditions is the essence of the healthcare leader. This work necessarily requires understanding the broad landscape of human behaviors and knowing which behaviors fit with one's personal and organizational vision and which behaviors cannot be tolerated if the healing journey is to continue. The challenge will always be to differentiate between the appropriate behaviors and inappropriate behaviors and to sustain and enhance the positive while isolating and minimizing the negative influences.

ONE MORE STRATEGY

Throughout this chapter strategies to reverse toxicity have been presented to assist the leader in creating healthy, healing cultures that will meet the needs of patients, employees, and the community. The additional strategy of storytelling is presented to continue this journey.

Stories as Motivators

Most leaders are comfortable with the analytical process as a way of thinking to discover factual information and minimize myths, gossip, and speculation. The strength of the analytical process lies in its objectivity, its impersonality, and its heartlessness (Denning, 2004). Yet, to motivate individuals to live the vision and values of the organization with enthusiasm and energy, a more personal and heartwarming approach is needed to supplement the traditional PowerPoint presentations.

The age-old practice of storytelling can be one of the most effective tools of the leader. A story that has applicability to current practice and identifies both desired and undesired behaviors provides a method of teaching values that can achieve several goals.

A colleague was once asked to present a keynote address to a healthcare audience. Knowing that the audience had heard it all about healthcare reform, the leader opted to tell a story of two experiences. Her address, "The state of healthcare?" did not have objectives, a beginning, or a well-developed middle, but it did have a thunderous ending. This story touched each person in the room in ways that were never anticipated, thus forever changing the practices of each person in the audience. The story is as follows:

An elderly woman was admitted into the small-town hospital by her son and daughter-in-law for circulatory problems. Most caregivers knew the patient and worked to make her feel comfortable. The patient was evaluated and determined to need surgery. Unfortunately, the surgery could not be performed at the small hospital, so the patient was transferred to a large, urban facility. The first night of the patient's stay in the large facility was quite eventful. The patient was found out of bed in the middle of the night roaming the hall and was determined to be incoherent and subsequently restricted to bed. The patient begged for her son to be called, to no avail. The next day, nurses informed the family that a sitter was needed to assure the safety of the patient. In discussing the situation with the patient, it was learned that the patient needed to go to the bathroom and did not want to bother anyone; thus the confusion and subsequent restrictions. The next night the patient needed to go to the bathroom (at about the same time!) and attempted to get over the rails and blankets that were placed around her. Not surprisingly, the patient fell and fractured her hip. The speaker ended the story with, "So what's wrong with healthcare today—we're disconnected, overautomated, and can't get the basics of human elimination in the elderly managed, and my mother-in-law has a broken hip." The room was silent.

Storytelling Rationales

- Spark action
- Communicate who you are
- Transmit values
- Foster collaboration
- Tame the grapevine
- Share knowledge
- Lead people into the future

Stephen Denning, 2004

Such stories are all too common and provide insight and instruction to more issues than a textbook could. Using stories to make healthcare services better can only help us be better healers.

SUMMARY

Most organizations are diligently working to meet deadlines, address national initiatives, achieve quality outcomes, and of course, make money. Unfortunately, many leaders get caught up in the busyness of their roles, and the intended work of healing does not occur. Some very toxic practices and behaviors can emerge and undermine the hard work of all members of the organization.

This chapter offers new perspectives about the sources of toxicity, not to demoralize the leader but to offer insights that others have shared and strategies to correct negative processes. The realities of new employee hazing, destructive confidants, poor feedback, and working with those who just don't want to change should serve to motivate the quantum leader to assist all employees to be aware of these behaviors, call them to participate in minimizing the negative impact, and continue the quantum journey of leadership in the new age of technology.

Exercise 1 Partial Leadership

The description of the cardiovascular surgeon with exceptional technical skills, good patient outcomes and very poor interpersonal skills is familiar to nurses. All too familiar also is the manager or leader with partial leadership skills—good negotiation skills, ability to develop a reasonable budget, and very poor performance evaluation skills due to the lack of ability to address conflict. Thus the overall reputation of the manager leader is less than stellar.

1. In your leadership group, discuss the differing skill levels of essential leadership behaviors. List the essential skills.
2. What skills are most often present?
3. What skills are often lacking? Develop a plan to address partial leadership.

Exercise 2 Removing the Barriers to Information

Technology now allows Internet access in each patient's room, wireless, real-time computerized documentation, integrated laboratory, medical imaging/diagnostic, and clinical progress. While these advances are relatively new and still being refined, the consumer now wants to be in charge of his or her data.

1. Given the availability of data and capabilities of the system, how would it be possible for patient information to go directly to the patient before or at the same time as the ordering provider receives the results?
2. For the patient to review and edit progress notes made about his or her care?
3. What expectations would need to be defined specific to the ordering of diagnostic tests?
4. What new skills would providers need to support these processes?
5. What security/access requirements would need to be in place to assure compliance with HIPAA?
6. What other issues need to be addressed?

REFERENCES

Aiken, L.H., Smith, H.L., & Lake, E.T. (1994). Lower Medicare mortality among a set of hospitals known for good nursing care. *Medical Care, 32:* 771–787.

American Nurses Association (1995). *Nursing Care Report Card for Acute Care.* Washington, DC: American Nurses' Publishing.

American Nurses Association (1997). *Implementing nursing's report card: a study of RN staffing, length of stay and patient outcomes.* Washington, DC: American Nurses' Publishing.

Berwick, D. (2004). *Escape fire: Designs for the future of health care.* San Francisco: Jossey-Bass.

Blegen, M.A., Goode, C.J., & Reid, L. (1998). Nurse staffing and patient outcomes. *Nursing Research, 47:* 43–50.

Blegen, M., & Vaughn, T. (1998). A multisite study of nurse staffing and patient occurrences. *Nursing Economic$, 16,* 196–203.

Cho, S., Ketefian, S., Barkauska, V.H., & Smith, D.H. (2003). The effects of nurse staffing on adverse events, morbidity, mortality and medical costs. *Nursing Research, 52* (2), 71–79.

Clarke, S.P., & Aiken, L.H. (2003). Failure to rescue: Measuring nurses' contributions to hospital performance. *AJN: American Journal of Nursing, 103,* 42–47.

Coutu, D.L. (2003). I was greedy, too. *Harvard Business Review, 81* (2), 38–44.

Cooper, R.W., Frank, G.L., Gouty, C.A., & Hansen, M.C. (2002). Key ethical issues encountered in healthcare organizations: Perceptions of nurse executives. *Journal of Nursing Administration, 32* (6), 331–337.

Denning, S. (2004). Telling tales. *Harvard Business Review, 82* (5), 122–129.

Flood, S., & Diers, D. (1988). Nurse staffing, patient outcome, and cost. *Nursing Management, 19,* 34–43.

Goldsmith, J. (1998, July 5). Operation restore human values. *Hospitals & Health Networks, 74.*

Hofmann, P.B. (2004, March/April). Why good people behave badly. *Healthcare Executive, 40.*

Keeler, H.J., & Cramer, M.E. (2007). A policy analysis of federal registered nurses safe staffing legislation. *Journal of Nursing Administration, 37* (7/8), 350–335.

Kerfoot, K. (2004). On leadership: The transparent organization: Leadership in an open organization. *Nursing Economic$, 22* (1), 33–34.

Longest, B.B. (1998). Managerial competence at senior levels of integrated delivery systems. *Journal of Healthcare Management, 43* (2), 115–135.

Malloch, K. (2003). Leaders of the pack: Leadership model focuses on RN's authoritative role to boost uniformity, job satisfaction. *NurseWeek, 8* (7), 9–10.

Mark, B.A., Harless, W.F., & Berman, W.F. (2007). Nurse staffing and adverse events in hospitalized children. *Policy, Politics & Nursing Practice, 8* (2), 83–92.

McCue, M. (2003). Nurse staffing, quality and financial performance. *Journal of Health Care Finance, 29*(4), 54–76.

McMurry, R.N. (2003). The tyranny of group-think. *Harvard Business Review, 81* (7), 20.

Pronovost, P.J., Jenckes, M.W., Dorman, T., Garrett, E., Breslow, M.J., Rosenfeld, B.A., et al. (1999). Organizational characteristics of intensive care units related to outcomes of abdominal aortic surgery. *JAMA: Journal of the American Medical Association, 281*(14), 1310–1317.

Sulkowicz, K.J. (2004). Worse than enemies: The CEO's destructive confidant. *Harvard Business Review, 82* (2), 65–71.

Thungjaroenkul, P., Cummings, G.G., & Embleton, A. (2007). The impact of nurse staffing on hospital costs and patient length of stay: A systematic review. *Nursing Economic$, 25* (5), 255–265.

Unruh, L. (2008). Nurse staffing and patient, nurse, and financial outcomes. *American Journal of Nursing, 108* (1), 62–71.

SUGGESTED READING

Lencioni, P.M. (2003). The trouble with teamwork. *Leader to Leader, 29,* 35–40.

10

The Leader as Mentor and Coach

CHAPTER OBJECTIVES:

Upon completion of this chapter, the reader will:

1. Clarify the need for a coach and mentor relationship and articulate its value in advancing leadership skills.
2. Describe the elements of coaching in the new age of leadership with emphasis on 21st-century leadership development.
3. Articulate the components of coaching and mentoring and apply them to the exercise of leadership at every level of the organization.
4. Identify the value of coaching and mentoring as a fundamental part of the management process and making it a part of the exercise of leadership.

INTRODUCTION

We're clearly deep into a new age for leadership. New skills are required in order for success in the exercise of the leader role. The 20th-century models for leadership rested primarily on the role of leader as a controlling agent. This notion of control and an historically defined, gender-driven management incorporates a whole range of skills that were essentially parental in nature and hierarchical in expression. This understanding of leadership as a hierarchical, controlling role drove much of the understanding of competency and content of the leadership role during the whole of the 20th century.

The Role of the Industrial-Age Leader
Planning
Organizing
Leading
Controlling
Evaluating

The problem with a controlling and hierarchical leadership is reflected specifically in its role expectations and performance requirements. In exercising the role of the leader in a hierarchical organization, there is a need on the part of the organization for the leader to represent the best interests of the organization and to see to it that workers' efforts are directed to the organization's goals. As a result, the leader's role historically has been focused on assuring that the organization's goals were met consistently and with the level of expectations the organization had for the work. The role of the leader was primarily expressed in the functions and activities related to supervising and controlling workers' actions and activities. It was assumed that the followers needed constant attention and supervision in order to do their work well. The leader was primarily required to act as a parent, and the organization assumed that in this role the leader would ensure that the workers (the children) of the organization did as they should or, at least, as they were directed. The organization represented the belief that workers would not meet its goals or fulfill its requirements if they did not have appropriate supervision and direction, which was provided by a good leader. This notion of directing the activities of others gave the leader role authority and responsibility for ensuring that work was appropriately done. Certain assumptions regarding the leader's skills and abilities were made under the rubric of supervision. It was assumed that the leader had the same knowledge about the work as the workers did and that the subordinate's level of knowledge and the leader's positional authority ostensibly gave the leader greater skill and deeper understanding of the work than those who had actually performed it. The authority for work outcomes was essentially invested in the exercise of the leadership role rather than in the performance of the work role.

The control function in the organization predominantly defined the managerial role. The expectation of the leader was that the department or service was well run, orderly, controlled, and disciplined, quietly and efficiently achieving predetermined outcomes. Essentially, the workforce was to see to it that the work was done, and the leader's job was to ensure that happened. Disciplining the workforce and keeping workers focused on the work were the requisites of leadership, as was doing so with a minimum level of "noise." Leaders who were successful in running their departments or services kept the staff noise level down, minimized the acting out of problem workers, and reduced the number of worker problems, thus enhancing productivity and assuring that the organization's outcomes were met. The notion of control drove the value of excellence and performance within the context of the role of the leader.

Of course, this contextual framework for the role of the leader was not sustainable. In organizations today, it is recognized that adult-to-adult relationships are essential to organizational effectiveness. They replace notions of parent–child models of leadership and relationship. Current research shows that these new leadership models that reflect partnership, interaction, and adult behaviors actually facilitate work, as opposed to the controlling models, which were more of an impediment to effective work than an assist to it.

The 20th-Century Leader Expectations

- Kept workers focused on the job.
- Made sure workers were not "noisy."
- Ensured work was focused and detailed.
- Kept workers happy.
- Disciplined workers appropriately.
- Resolved inevitable worker conflicts.
- Supervised workers closely.
- Was specifically directive with clear expectations.
- Saw that the work was done well.

Controlling Versus Engaging Leadership

Controlling

- Hierarchical
- Assumes superiority
- Directive style
- Highly positional
- Detailed supervision
- Criticism based

Engaging

- Equitable
- Role based
- Inclusive
- Reflects parity
- Horizontal dialogue
- Exploratory

Managing Professionals

What is unique in the space of the last few decades has been the growing emergence of the professional or knowledge worker. This worker is unique insofar as the requisite for a preexisting level of knowledge necessary to undertake work obligations. Because of this need for preexisting knowledge, the ownership of knowledge has increasingly affected the worker–workplace relationship. Managing knowledge or professional workers requires a unique set of skills different from those in production or process-oriented workplaces. In addition, for licensed professionals, there is a social expectation for individual accountability and performance that represents a unique contract between the individual and the society that licenses them. In this unique set of circumstances the social obligation of the individual circumscribed by the licensed relationship between the individual and the community creates an additional set of factors that influence the character and kind of relationship between the individual and the organization.

For these licensed professionals, their individual accountability is enumerated in the direct relationship between the practitioner and the patient in a way that precludes unilateral organizational control. Furthermore, this organizational control is additionally limited by the obligation of the profession for defining the requisites of membership; performance; and discipline-specific requirements evidenced in codes of ethics, standards of practice, educational requisites for membership, professional performance expectations, and the professional obligations of members' relationship to the profession and to the community. In truth, the professional owes his or her allegiance to the society that licenses the individual professional, not to the institution. For the professional, the view of the institution is either as facilitator and enabler of the professional relationship between the individual and the patient or an impediment to this relationship. The traditional employee-defined relationship between professional and organization simply does not operate in professional workgroups, and managing them in the same way as other organizational constructs for nonprofessional workers simply doesn't work. In fact, attempting to do so creates an internal organizational dynamic that ultimately becomes incongruous and conflict based; ultimately fails to support the work of the professional; and consistently fails to obtain the outcome both the profession and the organization intends. The professional worker needs an entirely different relationship and context within which to adequately and appropriately define and perform the profession's work in a way consistent with its sense of social obligation and professional performance mandate.

Leaders are predominantly context creators. In creating an appropriate context, the leader builds a frame of reference within which the organization can operate. This context either creates opportunities for meaningful work and positive relationships or draws away from the environment necessary to do good work and to achieve meaningful outcomes. The leader understands the relationships necessary to produce positive outcomes and maintain a meaningful work environment. The leader also recognizes that all people are social creatures and thus reflects the understanding of the necessity of good social interaction and positive relationships in order to maintain high levels of productivity. The challenge is that the leader must recognize that workers (most specifically, the professional worker) are essentially partners who must establish collaborative and meaningful relationships in order to sustain productivity and to enhance the work of the organization.

As with all relationships, the leader recognizes that interaction must go through a number of stages, each of which must be thoroughly addressed, in order to ensure the highest levels of integrity and work quality. In this set of circumstances, the leader is primarily a coach working in a framework that fully enables individuals to be successful. The leader knows that encouraging and strengthening the relationships between leader and workers and between workers creates circumstances and a context that assures meaningful, purposeful, and energy-filled activity directed to fulfilling the purposes and goals of the organization and of the profession.

Different Expectations for Communication
Adult-to-Adult
• Respect based
• Acknowledges unique talents
• Inclusive
• Reflects equity
• Eliminates hierarchy
• Open and free-flowing
Parent–Child
• Safety based
• Developmental
• Instructive
• Reflects superiority
• Vertical dialogue
• Directed and clear

COACHING AND EXPECTATIONS

The leader must reflect in his or her coaching role an understanding of performance expectations and others' related behavior. The leader is always aware that performance is an integral part of the fulfillment of the demands of work. Furthermore, relationships demand a clear understanding of what people expect from leaders. The leader does not leave role expectation to accident.

The wise leader establishes a framework for expectations. In fact, this leader contracts for expectations so the roles, functions, and activities performed by individuals either in a team or in relationship to the leader are clear and understandable in advance of establishing the relationship. When coaching is discussed, it is often exemplified in relationship to a one-on-one interaction. In truth, coaching relates to the individual as leader and to the leadership of groups. No leader simply establishes a relationship with one individual and then focuses solely on that person to the exclusion of the relationship with all others. Coaching involves the collective relationship between all those with whom the leader interacts. The leader exemplifies in her or his behavior the expectations for performance and for the relationships that the leader seeks to see in others.

The greatest concern in most organizations is the conflicts that are often generated, problems associated with relationships, and interactions between individuals. This focus on facilitating positive interaction frequently becomes the major focus of the leader's work. These behaviors and interactions are continually influenced by the ebb and flow of the group members' interaction and communication with each other. The leader attempts to build as positive a framework for these interactions as is possible and attempts to identify conflicts or impediments to smooth functioning relationships between and among team members.

The leader is always concerned with the interaction of the team. In the coaching role, the leader attempts to represent in her or his own behavior best practices in terms of expression, communication, interaction, and problem solving. Here, the leader is most interested in ensuring that a model of sound leader behavior is created and exemplifies this model of behavior in her or his own conduct. The challenge here is the consistency and continuity of the behavior in the message of the leader as coach. In this role, the leader clearly presents an example or set of behaviors that potentially can be exemplified in the expectations of the conduct of others. The leader is attempting through this behavior to create a model of expression and interaction that others can replicate in their own behavior.

The leader's context for coaching includes an understanding that the leader's expression represents the truth of who he or she is as a person. While others are listening to the message of the leader, what is more important is that they are watching the behaviors and practices of the leader with determined consonance between who the leader is and how that gets represented in what the leader says and does. Of paramount importance to the leader as coach is how well he or she characterizes the expression of the role of a leader in a way that clearly articulates the best in the leader with personal attributes and a consistent framework of expression.

> ### Gem
>
> Coaching relates to all the relationships of leadership. The coach recognizes that all relationships serve as a potential for ideal behaviors and commitment to growth. The coach is available to all through the representation of the role as an exemplar. The coach models the role so that all people are informed by it and seek to include the ideal behaviors in their own practices and roles.

THE LEADER IS ALWAYS "ON"

The leader is never "off." (**Figure 10-1**) The leader's expectation is that all behaviors will be consistent and will be sustained. In this way, others can incorporate new patterns of leader behavior in their own roles because they witness good leader behavior as consistent and congruent. The leader becomes a living witness to the expectations of interaction, performance, and role behavior that serves as a model for each member of the work team. As a result, there are no times in which the leader can assume that he or she is not being observed or heard in any time in the expression of the role. There are no accidental moments, side conversations, informal interactions, and personal expressions in the role of a leader that do not have some significant implications for persons and the organization in a way that is perceived as important. No matter how seemingly inconsequential, the expressions and behaviors of the leader are constantly observed

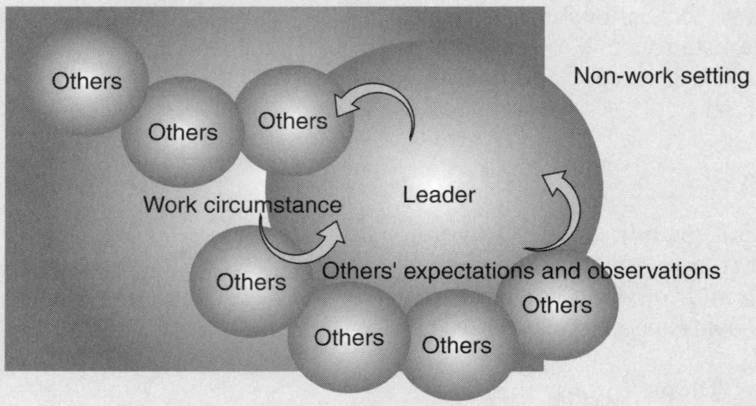

The leader is never "off," always interacting and being observed, creating a context for relationships and work.

Figure 10-1 The leader is always on.

and do, in fact, have meaning and consequences whether intended by the leader or not. Therefore, it is critical for the leader to recognize the need for congruence patterns of behavior and consistency of message.

CONTRACTING FOR EXPECTATIONS

A contract for expectations is simply a delineation of those performance factors that must be most often considered and exemplified in the role of each team member. This contract is entered into as an agreement among all members of the team and with the leader. In this contract, there are specific elements that are critical to the expression of expectations and commitments made by team members to each other:

> **The Coaching Contract Basics**
>
> - The contract is voluntary.
> - The language is specific and clear.
> - The leader lives the elements of the agreement.
> - The contract can be adjusted as reality requires.

1. The leader is clear at the outset that the contract is voluntary, underscores mutual expectations and behavioral determinations, is clearly an agreement to behave in a particular way, and is understood and accepted by all members of the team.
2. The contract is specific and clear. It is not left for team members to guess the expectations and performance factors that they must exemplify in their relationship with each other.
3. The leader agrees to not only abide by the contract and the commitment made by team members, but to exemplify those behaviors in his or her own role. The team leader exemplifies membership and collaboration with team members by virtue of her or his own collaborative and interactional role characteristics.
4. The team commitments are not cast in stone, as behavioral expectations and patterns of relationship will shift. Change in the content of the charter should also reflect a mutual understanding of the commitment of all parties. Each shift in expectations and performance factors should be included in the charter, reflecting it as a living document. As this contract moves and shifts in content, it can be redesigned to reflect the new expectations and different patterns of behavior.

Not all contracts have to be written agreements. The notion of contracting reflects an understanding between the team members and the leader regarding certain sets of behaviors and expectations that they have agreed to between and among themselves. Written documentation of these processes simply acts as a certification or verification that these agreements have been entered into. Whether or not the contract is written down, all parties to the contract assume some responsibility for ensuring that their behaviors will be consistent with their agreement and with the expectations for performance.

Accountability with regard to performance requires that individuals be willing to commit to reviewing and evaluating each other with regard to certain expectations (see **Figure 10-2**). The leader clearly must be aware that these evaluation processes are fraught with general difficulties and much noise. When one is evaluating another individual, there are a number of sensitivities that emerge that must be addressed carefully and thoughtfully if such evaluation is not to degenerate into untenable and unacceptable critique. This requires that some measure of performance expectation and evaluation be discussed and clarified before performance evaluation occurs. Each member of the team, building the expectations for other members of the team, must be clear about how to approach and interact with others during evaluation of an individual's performance or behavioral pattern. The challenge for the leader is to exemplify good communication and conflict management

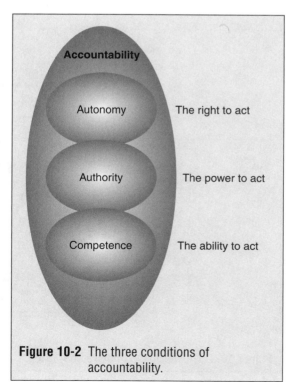

Figure 10-2 The three conditions of accountability.

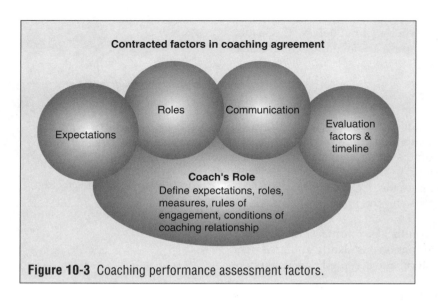

Figure 10-3 Coaching performance assessment factors.

patterns in her or his own behavior so that these patterns can be reflected in the behaviors of those he or she leads. In a coaching situation, team members will be looking critically at the role of the leader as that person undertakes the active evaluation of another, assessing performance or adjusting behavior.

Again, the leader's role is to exemplify desired behaviors in the leader's own behavior. Perhaps this is the central heart of all mentoring and coaching relationships. Staff is continually observing leaders and learning what their consistency is in terms of their own behavior and just what the vagaries of that behavior is (**Figure 10-3**). The leader must know that every moment she or he is being observed within the context of the leadership role.

It is often said that leaders have no friends. This is especially true in a coaching and mentoring situation. Yet it's surprising how many leaders forget that leadership is a particular role, one in which friendship is not, by definition, an element. The mentor and coach leader must always recall the role that he or she plays in relationship to those being mentored or coached. The relationship between leader and those being coached has a particular set of structures and characteristics that is unique to it. The leader recognizes this reality and does not attempt to confuse those he or she is coaching by exemplifying other kinds of relationships not appropriate to the role. The notion of always being in role is a critical part of understanding the role of the leader, especially in the process of mentoring and coaching. Leading implies setting direction and moving others to embrace the journey and to incorporate it into their own experiences and lives. The coach and mentor helps others engage their own reality, identify their own role in relationship to it, and embrace the activities and functions necessary to achieve it. This is done by the leader exemplifying the degree of commitment and by embracing and engaging the dynamics of change and the demands of the role in the life of the leader. Using this living example as the frame of reference for coaching and mentoring becomes the most viable tool the leader has to advance and incorporate appropriate and desirable behaviors in others, especially in regard to interaction, relationship, and embracing the future.

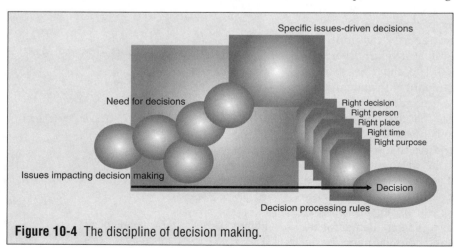

Figure 10-4 The discipline of decision making.

DEMONSTRATING GOOD DECISION MAKING

Besides exemplifying good behaviors, interactions, and collaborative relationships, the leader must exemplify the skills of good decision making. The leader's application of the skills and ability to develop and expand decision-making talent (see **Figure 10-4**) becomes a foundational skill set for those the leader coaches and mentors. There is, perhaps, no other skill more important to the development of leadership than the ability to make effective decisions.

Decision making is not an accidental process. Decisions are not effective simply because people make them (**Figure 10-5**). Good decisions require insight, creativity, and methodology. The good leader recognizes and understands that if good decision making is to be replicated it must involve a process that is organized and systematic and can be replicated. In working with the team, the leader represents in her or his own behavior a specific discipline or set of processes within which decision making unfolds. The leader does not make decisions for others. Instead, the leader positions other individuals to make decisions by ensuring that the appropriate decisions, skills, and patterns of decisional behavior are incorporated into the role of that person that he or she mentors.

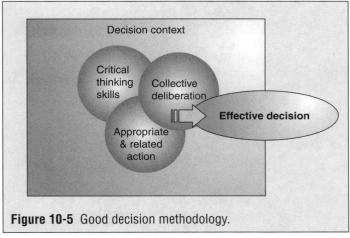

Figure 10-5 Good decision methodology.

There are essential characteristics to effective decision making. Good decision makers always understand that there is a discipline to decision making, as there is to any other organized work activity. Good decision making involves a number of process steps to ensure that the decision will be effective and produce the desired results:

1. *The use of good methodology.* A leader recognizes that decisions have components and elements expressed in stages. When articulated and defined clearly enough, these processes can be followed and replicated in all decision processes. The leader recognizes that critical thinking, deliberation, and responsive action all work together to create a framework for the effective application of decision making. Building a clear methodology is an essential cornerstone for effective decision making, regardless of who is involved.

2. *Gathering information.* All good decisions are made with as much information as possible under the circumstances. What is important to remember is that no one has all the information needed to make effective decisions. The point is not to have every bit of information that is available, but instead, to have sufficient information to make the right decision with the resources available at the time of decision making. The leader recognizes that decision making must be well informed to the extent possible at the needed time and recognizes that a lack of information is a part of the process. Therefore, the leader takes whatever information is available, aggregates it with other sources of information, synthesizes it, and decides the best course of action to take under the circumstances. Recognizing and managing limited information resources is not only good information management, it is good leadership.

3. *Good critical thinking skills.* Nothing replaces the ability to think clearly, logically, and appropriately at the right time and arrive at the right answer. Critical thinking reflects the ability of the individual to organize thoughts and to make decisions based on the integrated relationship of ideas, information management, and good response in a way that most effectively meets the demand of the situation or circumstance. Decision making simply is the result of having carefully considered all the elements related to and affecting a decision and proceeding with action followed by evaluation.

4. *Effective evaluation of decisions.* The leader always assesses the effectiveness of decision making in a meaningful way. A good mentoring and coaching technique is to involve others in evaluating an individual's decision making. The competent and balanced leader is not afraid of an evaluation of his or her own decision making because this helps clarify, refine, and improve that

---

Maximizing Information Sources

- Review what is at hand.
- Determine what can be readily accessible.
- Use Internet sources.
- Access readily available historic data.
- Have conversations with key stakeholders.
- Speak with colleagues who have previous experience.
- Sort the relevant from the merely interesting.
- Focus information within the defined time frame.
- Select information based on priority of impact.

Evaluating Good Decision Making

- Did the decision relate directly to the problem?
- Was the desired outcome achieved?
- What information was helpful in arriving at the decision?
- What was the relationship between the information, the decision, and the outcome?
- What information was most helpful?
- What information was of least value?
- How do others perceive the decision and its outcome?
- What would you do differently next time?
- What information was missing?
- What process barriers did you confront?
- What learning did this decision and its outcome provide for you?
- How will you proceed differently next time?

Gem

Error is not a source of fear or punishment. Error is simply an opportunity for learning. The only errors that are unforgivable are those that are repeated. The continual repetition of the same error is a sign that little has been learned from it and that the participants in the error are doomed to continuously repeat it. Error is to be celebrated, acknowledged for its contribution to learning, and responded to appropriately and in a timely fashion. Doing so gives error its proper place and assures its role as a teacher bearing renewable fruits.

Corrective Action Processing

1. Locating the critical event (error)
2. Enumerating again the characteristics of an error
3. Identifying the learning embedded in the error
4. Naming the impact of the error
5. Discovering the source or foundation of the error
6. Delineating the process elements leading to the error
7. Listing effective corrective steps
8. Defining evaluation of corrective steps
9. Clarifying corrective steps and successful actions
10. Celebrating and sustaining newly defined behaviors

skill, both in the leader as well as in the mentor. In fact, the leader usually develops a formalized evaluation process so that evaluation is not simply a periodic and perhaps optional undertaking; it is, instead, a structured routine that is incorporated into the fundamental activity of decision making and of evaluation.

5. *Good error assessment processes.* The leader is not afraid of error. In fact, error is understood as a fundamental part of the experience of deliberation and decision making. No matter how effective the decision maker is, there will always be an element of error embedded in every decision and action. Ineffective decision making is not the greatest problem with regard to leadership. But the ability to successfully and effectively address errors at the right time and in the right format is essential. Error is not an untenable part of the activities of human life. The good mentor and coach demonstrates the ability to engage his or her own experience of error as part of the evaluation and deliberation process. The leader can mentor staff and coach new behaviors through exemplifying his or her own ability to self-evaluate and make critical judgments about the decision. The leader adjusts or changes patterns of behavior based on what the evidence reveals about the process, methodology, or outcomes of decision making. In this way, the leader demonstrates that error is not a source of fear or punishment; instead, it is an opportunity to learn, engage, and adjust performance and behavior based on what the evidence reveals.

6. *Creating effective corrective action processes.* Recognizing the inevitability of error, the leader incorporates that understanding into the process of responding to error. The leader indicates this through an organized and systematic corrective action process, demonstrating to those he or she is coaching or mentoring the engagement of corrective action as a normative and functional part of critical decision making. All decisions require assessment. Out of this assessment comes the need for a change in practices, behavior, or processes. The leader demonstrates the ease of incorporating the need for new practices and behaviors as a result of evaluating past practices and behaviors. Incorporating this understanding into leadership practices demonstrates for those being mentored and coached the desirability of evaluating of decision activities, the value of applying a critical method to evaluation processes, and the growth and development that results in the individual from undertaking this discipline. Error is thus transformed from a negative aspect of decision making to a positive part of the cycle of decision making. Error can become a fundamental part of the entire decision process and serve a critical role in helping to develop the decisional effectiveness of individuals and the excellent application and ultimate productivity of error management in the course of decision making and in advancing the quality of work.

IDENTIFYING COACHING GOALS

Coaching focuses on the needs of the person being coached. A part of establishing these needs is identifying the goals and specific objectives that the individual seeks to address through the coaching process. The goals initially are negotiated and agreed to by the coach and the person being mentored. Ultimately, however, the goals and specific objectives of the individual being coached must be owned and exercised by that individual. The individual looks to the coach for support and encouragement, as well as indicators and patterns of behavior that can be replicated and developed. Individuals are responsible for their own development and growth. It is the goal of the coach to make those being coached as independent as possible, needing as little coaching as possible. In fact, the primary role of the coach is to ensure that the individual being mentored has no extended need for the mentor and has developed sufficient skills to be able to act independently. In the coaching and mentoring relationship, the ultimate sign of success is when those being coached and mentored themselves become coaches and mentors to others. It is this goal of obtaining independence and being able to operate at the same level of facility or skill as the coach that becomes one of the primary operating criteria for a good coach–mentor relationship. The coach is always aware that the coaching relationship is short term. The coach does everything possible to ensure the growth and development of the individual being coached, to the extent that the individual will no longer need the same developmental processes and activities as at the beginning of the coaching–mentoring relationship.

When the coaching and mentoring goals are clearly defined and the expectations and performance against those goals unfolds, as they should, the coaching and mentoring relationship becomes developmental. As the developmental process unfolds and the individual being coached becomes more successful in his or her own patterns of behavior, two things occur. One key element is that the coaching relationship changes in form and substance as the individual matures and becomes increasingly independent. The second critical factor is that the coaching role transitions into a collaborative partnership role that continues the dynamic of relationship but simply changes the form in which it is expressed. It is in this relationship that the most significant value is obtained from the coaching–mentoring interaction. This relationship is one that can best delineate for those being coached a very specific valuing of purpose, achieving the highest level of outcome from the process.

A NEW AGE FOR LEADERSHIP

Leadership is unfolding in a time of great change. Mentoring and coaching means bringing people into a new era of leadership that requires different skill sets and roles. This evolution in organizational forms matches a significant change in the social culture and the global community. A part of the challenge for leaders is recognizing that the leader is now leading movements to a new age. This notion of leading movement is critical to understanding the role of the leader and the changes in the expectation and performance of leadership.

Movement into the global community means a change in all organizational constructs. Furthermore, it means a change in the kinds of relationships and interactions that must unfold in order for organizations and systems to be successful. The challenge for the leader is having the ability to identify in her or his own behavior the kinds of role changes necessary to lead an organization into a quickly evolving world. Further complicating this challenge is the requisite that the leader be able to change her or his own behavior in a way that represents or characterizes a new set of expectations for expressing the role of leader. Being able to translate the skill sets necessary to lead in a new age and adapt those skill sets to a new model of organization is another critical exemplar for the role of leader as coach and mentor.

The mentor and coach now must incorporate in his or her own leadership behaviors mechanisms for building partnership, constructing

---

The Coaching and Mentoring Relationship

- Short term
- Goal driven
- Owned by the person being coached
- Centered on learning
- Developmentally focused
- Performance based
- Contains elements of evaluation
- Peer based
- Ends when goals are achieved

The Coaching–Mentoring Partnership

- Is equity based
- Represents a set of defined expectations
- Involves negotiated roles
- Includes continuous evaluation of effectiveness
- Incorporates a regularly scheduled dialogue
- Has other collaborators identified by the coach
- Includes team review
- Clarifies time expectations
- Has clearly defined relationship outcomes
- Features regularly reviewed performance expectations

Managing Movement

Leaders do not manage people. People manage themselves. The role of the leader is to create a safe context where people can adjust their patterns of work behavior to fit an ever-shifting context. The leader recognizes the movement of change, translates it in a language the follower can comprehend, and finally enables the follower to fully engage the changes affecting the dynamic of work in a way that can continue to produce positive and meaningful outcomes.

Using Competition Versus Cooperation for Obtaining Goals

Competition

- Creating opposing forces
- Generating energy in opposition
- Beating others toward a target
- Harnessing internal resources
- Focusing action externally
- Identifying a common foe

Cooperation

- Creating converging forces
- Enjoining group energy
- Consolidating around a common goal
- Gathering all relevant resources
- Focusing energy on the group's efforts
- Surpassing the group's own standards

Questions of Ethical and Moral Leadership

- Is our position or initiative consistent with our corporate values?
- Is our position or initiative legal?
- Does our position or initiative reflect defined standards of practice?
- Does our position or initiative violate any cultural norms?
- Are individuals purposely disadvantaged or harmed by our position or initiative?
- Do our efforts reflect sound business practices?
- Would our organization be ashamed if our efforts were made public?
- Do we have a mechanism for auditing and evaluating our work processes?
- Will the outcomes of our efforts have a negative social or environmental impact?
- Do our efforts raise our standard of performance and enhance the organization's image?

Entrepreneurial Leader Characteristics

- Creatively individualistic
- Is a self-starter
- Sees things out of the box
- Has a powerful personal charisma
- Is idea driven
- Explores all avenues
- Engages others in creative work
- Is able to move ideas to goals

---

alliances, defining new directions and constructs for the organization, negotiation and conflict resolution, and the management of complex systems and relationships. Each of these skill sets brings with it a specific set of demands that alters the leader's expectations and performance obligations.

Organization around team-based approaches requires a different kind of facility with regard to leadership. Hierarchical relationships often defined the past, traditional approach to leadership. Now, because systems are membership communities, the leader must exemplify a different set of more horizontally aligned behaviors. The leader must form partnerships and alliances in an effective array of interactions and intersections that help organizations move in concert toward the goals necessary to thrive. The challenge in a complex world is the balance between competition and cooperation. Leaders must exemplify for those they are coaching and mentoring that neither competition nor cooperation are unilaterally effective in undertaking or advancing the organization's work. The leader must exemplify in his or her own behavior those times when cooperation predominates within the system, perhaps even with competitors. On the other hand, the leader also must exemplify those times when competition is necessary in order to advance the viability and success of the organization.

At the same time as the leader is handling concerns regarding competition and cooperation, ethical and relational issues emerge as increasingly important concerns. With communication and technical advances in systems processes affecting the work itself, a new sensitivity to the importance of ethics as incorporated into relationships, business practices, and corporate and organizational intersections emerges as a critical element of new leadership. The leader must exemplify in his or her own behavior those skills necessary to delineate the moral and ethical elements of relational, decisional, or operational issues. This has become increasingly evident in the current business environment. The leader must represent to the person being mentored or coached the moral and value implications in all processes of decision making. The leader must also represent the incorporation of these behaviors into the activities necessary to positively express sound leadership in any circumstance. Decision making and effective decision processes should include the ethical and moral implications as a part of the planned process of effective decision making. Furthermore, mentors and those being coached should themselves exemplify the incorporation and evaluation of these patterns and practices of ethical and moral behavior in all decisions and actions.

DEVELOPING NEW ERA LEADERSHIP COMPETENCIES

In this new era of changing organizational forms and structures, leaders will require a certain level of entrepreneurial freedom as well as a set of self-directed skills that exemplify a new kind of engagement with the organization and its journey into a preferred future. In the industrial age, the leader represented for those learning new leadership skills a stronger orientation to function, effectiveness, and process. Although these elements are certainly important, they are no longer the centerpiece of work or the role of the leader. In the development of leadership in others, the leader must exemplify within the role a deeper understanding of its relationship to an organization's or system's journey and a willingness to perceive the response to that journey within the context of a larger social construct.

In a mentoring and coaching model, the leader must exemplify the notion of managing movement in a way that characterizes the pace and the direction of change for the organization. The leader sees the role within a much longer and larger trajectory. Using approaches that take into account the changing circumstances, conditions, innovations, and social challenges, the innovative leader undertakes appropriate responses configured to position the organization well within the context of its continuing journey. This fluidity and flexibility in approaches and response will be a critical foundational element if the leader is to influence and exemplify learning flexibility when both mentoring and coaching new leaders.

The leader exemplifies the skills of anticipation as a part of the development of sound leadership practices. The leader's talent for reading the signposts is an important transformational characteristic for coaching and mentoring. Reading signposts means taking the various factors that indicate imminent shift or changes at the sociological or organizational level and applying them to the unique work circumstances for which the leader is accountable. In this way, the leader reads the conditions, circumstances, and indicators that tell the story of the organization's journey in a way that anticipates the next steps. Through this leadership strategy of vectoring or signpost reading, the leader represents a willingness to engage the foundations of change and to bring form and substance to the direction of the change (see **Figure 10-6**). It is this notion of bringing congruence between the direction of change and the response to the demand of change that most influences the appropriate development of leadership skills in others around the notion of harnessing talent for the future.

It is important to emphasize that the leadership coach and mentor doesn't underestimate the traditional values and role competencies related to cost effectiveness, organizational congruency, human relationship skills, decision making, and conflict resolution. What happens instead is that the leader also represents additional sets of behaviors that represent the changing context for leadership. The industrial age clearly had a more institutional, structured, and functional frame for the expression of leadership. In the sociotechnical age, contemporary roles of the leader are dramatically shifting to reflect the new characteristics of high technology, global communication, and fluidity and flexibility of work systems and organizational pursuits. This fundamental change in the notion of work and its exercise causes the coach and mentor to change the content and the frame for leading others and modeling that leadership for the future. Coaching and mentoring now become a set of challenges that helps individuals alter their frames of reference for leadership and form a new foundation for understanding and exercising the role as they learn it.

> ### Managing Movement
>
> The contemporary leader understands that managing movement means helping people engage the challenges of their own journey. This leader recognizes that the failure of individuals to embrace the demands of their own personal change and to join that with the inevitable changes in work performance and expectation is most problematic. Leaders recognize that they exemplify willingness in their own behaviors and through personal example model agreement and engagement to continuously embrace every movement in the dance of change.

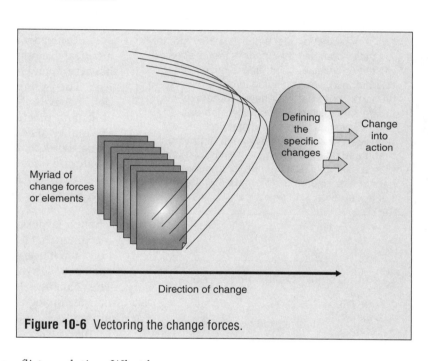

Figure 10-6 Vectoring the change forces.

DEEP CHANGE: NEW WAYS OF BEING AND DOING

Thus far, the focus has been on the elements and constituents of coaching and mentoring the emerging leader into a new set of leader behaviors. Equally important

---

Deep Change

Real and sustainable change cannot occur unless there's a strong personal commitment on the part of the individual to undergo significant personal change. All of the mentoring in the world will not achieve successful outcomes if individual personal commitment is not present. In the mentoring and coaching process, the individual agrees to engage many challenges and vagaries associated with learning and growing and consents to not pull back from the demands of change when they become uncomfortable and raise potential personal difficulties.

Modeling Change

Leaders cannot expect that those they mentor will make changes that leaders themselves will not undertake. Mentoring is essentially role modeling: exemplifying in one's own behavior those same behaviors one expects to see exemplified in those one mentors. Leadership is a lived circumstance that requires leaders to give evidence of having embraced specific changes in their own roles before asking others to change. Leaders cannot ask for change in others that they have not undertaken in themselves.

20th-Century Behaviors for Leaders

- Directing
- Organizing
- Leading
- Controlling
- Informing
- Parenting
- Telling
- Managing
- Evaluating

21st-Century Behaviors for Leaders

- Serving as clearinghouse
- Enrolling
- Investing
- Conflicting
- Challenging
- Moderating
- Inquiring
- Facilitating
- Stretching

---

is the commitment of the individual being coached or mentored to his or her own deep personal change. While leadership is clearly an important area of discussion and certainly a critical pursuit in the changing workplace, what is equally important is the need to understand that new leaders must represent an entirely different foundation for behavior. The coach must exemplify within the role a clear commitment to personal change through her or his own efforts and activities. Subsequent to any real change occurring, the people being mentored and coached must also evidence their own commitment to the "noise" of deep personal change.

This understanding of deep personal change goes further than a simple understanding of the change process. Deep personal change means adaptability and willingness to change. The person being coached or mentored needs to be able to express a willingness to undergo the challenges of change. This individual must greet a new paradigm for practice that incorporates the notion of managing continuous and endless movement and transformation within the context of individual personhood, as well as within the framework of the organization.

For the leader who is coach and mentor, exemplifying this behavior is a critical exemplar for the expression of good leadership. Leaders must always remember that they are constantly being watched by those they lead. The exemplar is the leaders' commitment to never forget their own behavioral patterns and the impact those patterns have on the skills and practices of others. This notion of willingness to embrace the reality of constant change and to engage it in a meaningful way using the skills identified here is the critical subtext for coaching and mentoring others.

COACHING FOR DEEP CHANGE

Change leaders and coaches must help those they are mentoring to recognize that leadership now is different in its expression and application than it was in the past. The move out of the industrial age is calling leaders to see their role differently as the context for leadership shifts. The challenges that emerge in the new age relate to the introduction of new technologies, global communication technologies, digitalization of information, and the application of new work processes to health care. In this shifting context, the coach represents in her or his own behavior a willingness to address what these challenges mean and how they call for a change in leadership behavior.

The coach must articulate for the learning leader a completely new frame of leadership skills. The primary role of the leader in today's world is to help others make the transition in their own practice and behavior to represent a much more fluid and mobile work environment. The coach exemplifies this in willingness to meet the challenge related to unfolding the new framework for work and new work processes. Because of this, the coach begins to challenge the learning leader to see the role in a different light and to begin to articulate those skills that will be necessary to facilitate the changing role and work of others.

The coach seeks in the learning leader an ability to facilitate adaptation and to crystallize within the role positive behaviors that model willingness, availability, vulnerability, and a fundamental agreement to change the nature of work and the experience of the worker. The coach challenges the new leader to see the expression of leadership in light of the journey that the learning leader is experiencing as though he or she were already playing the leader role (see **Figure 10-7**).

The new age requires a different contextual framework for the leader's role expression, from industrial-age direction and controlling mechanisms to the new expectations of leadership to engage relationships, communication, and skill transformation. In leading others (especially emerging leaders) to express their role in a transforming work environment, the coach challenges them to incorporate within the context of their own behavior a facility at exploration, coaching, dialogue, and experimentation in the arena of new practices and processes. The learning leader also incorporates into her or his behavior an ability to engage others in conflict, respond to the noise of change, and deal effectively with the pace of change.

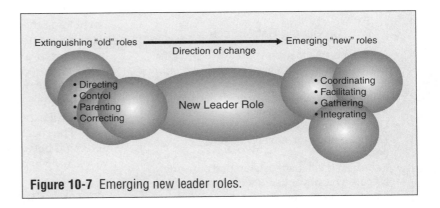

Figure 10-7 Emerging new leader roles.

The coach's role in encouraging deep change includes being able to engage others at a personal level. First, the coach must exemplify in her or his own role an understanding of the impact of change on the self. This notion of understanding one's own accommodation or challenge with regard to the impact of change is an important prototype for providing an opportunity for the coach to role model that response for others. As the coach confronts personal inadequacy and represents that challenge in the coach's own transition to change, she or he begins to represent to those learning leaders her or his role modeling for change and how adjustments and accommodation to the challenges can be well addressed. If the coach is unable to accommodate change, face the noise of transformation, or confront the challenges of conflict in his or her own role, it cannot be expected that the learning leader will be able to do so. This modeling of lived behavior is a critical coaching characteristic, especially in a time of great change. Since the language of change and transformation cannot always be clearly understood by others as they are moving through the change process, it is vital for the coach to be able to present a living example of confronting the vagaries of change and transformation. Not finding the appropriate words to describe or delineate change, feeling overwhelmed by the change events, and being uncertain of the appropriate response are all normal role characteristics that can be used to school others, through modeling, how they can be addressed and incorporated into any change journey.

It is neither important nor appropriate for the coach to have all the answers. It is far more important to be delving into the right questions than it is to have the right answers to the wrong questions. The coach plays a dominant role in raising appropriate questions that relate to the experience of change and transformation as people accommodate new rules for work. As has been identified in other sections of this book, the work environment and all the elements related to the leader's understanding of context is becoming so different that the usual responses based on historical experiences are no longer acceptable for adequate problem solving. The coach, understanding this reality, creates a safe space for emerging concerns and challenges to be better addressed. Rather than eliminate the noise, anger, and aggravation of the transformation process, the coach uses those vagaries as tools, personal instruments that help people move through their own change experience. Exemplifying her or his own experience of challenge and of noise, the coach uses these experiences as vehicles for teaching and learning modeling for others, enabling others to engage new ways of doing business and undertaking the challenge of transforming clinical work.

Leadership Vulnerability

- An openness to discuss personal pain
- Sharing insights regarding personal journey of change
- Being clear about what is not known
- Intuition regarding others' struggles
- Willing to name one's personal difficulties with change
- Gathering advice and counsel from others
- Willing to explore all options
- Good at information gathering and sharing
- Unafraid of confronting difficulties/barriers
- Recognizing the need and timing for self-renewal

Having the Right Questions

Traditionally the role of the manager/leader was tied to having the right answers to others' questions. The contemporary leader and mentor, instead of having the right answers, makes sure that the right questions are raised. Without the right question, any answer will do. The leader never takes accountability for other people's answers. In order to assure that doesn't happen, the leader makes sure that ownership of the question is established and that those being mentored are focusing on the right questions instead of simply looking for the appropriate answer. Without the right question there is no right answer.

Creating a Safe Space

- People feel free to express their own concerns.
- No retribution results from self-expression.
- A context for problem-solving is present.
- Adult-to-adult exchange is encouraged.
- There are no undiscussables.
- Conflicts are addressed quickly.
- Dialogue and problem solving are encouraged.
- Fear-based language is stamped out early.
- Negativity is never tolerated.
- Hope and encouragement are expected of everyone.
- Social interaction and humor are encouraged.

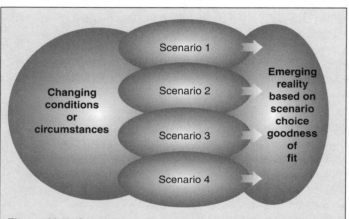

Figure 10-8 Creating and using scenarios for leader learning.

Transitioning of Leader Skills

- Coach discusses various scenarios.
- Dialogue centers on a vision of change.
- Group process is facilitated.
- Multiple insights are integrated.
- Using a flip chart, perceptions are recorded.
- Impact on leader role is outlined.
- Skill deficits are defined.
- Work plan for matching skill with demand is created.
- Learning work plans are compared with each other.
- Experiments are conducted, and the plan is implemented.
- Progress and problems are evaluated by a group.
- The plan is revised, replanned, retried, and reviewed.

In helping the learning leader accommodate his or her own struggle for change, the coach makes a safe space for that individual to address, give a voice to, and lay out the pain and struggle of adapting to change. The coach is receptive to the noise of learning as people confront the challenges of their own personal adaptations to change. The coach allows learning leaders both opportunity and time to express negative and painful experiences related to their own journey to effective leadership. The coach, by inviting this openness, creates a level of trust and interaction between coach and learner that makes a safe and productive learning experience for both.

ACTION LEARNING

The coach recognizes that learning best occurs in the process of action (**Figure 10-8**). Action learning reflects that the learning leader is an adult and will experience all that he or she needs in order to be able to undertake the appropriate role of leadership. The coach understands that the work environment creates all the opportunity necessary for learning leadership to unfold.

It is the notion that the environment continually provides an opportunity for learning that guides the coach in the role. As the change process unfolds and the environment begins to adjust, the conflict between past practices and future demand create the conditions within which new leadership is learned. Using these conditions, the coach develops scenarios and action processes that can be used in the learning dynamic to help the learning leader accommodate new rules and principles in the experience of applying new leadership processes in a changing world. It is this continuous and fluid change that creates the conditions within which contemporary leadership must unfold. The coach, using this fluid condition, challenges the learning leader to address the development of skills and talents within the context of a shifting reality. There is nothing less useful for the leader than a set of leadership skills in a context that cannot accommodate them. Furthermore, the learning leader must realize that leading others essentially involves unbundling others' attachment to their own work, providing a framework for new work, and bringing others into a new work environment able to practice their work with skill and competence. In addition, the learning leader must be able to help others in such a way that they can rise to the new work context and can do their work with higher levels of satisfaction and with personal joy. There is nothing more challenging in the work of leadership than accomplishing these goals.

People will find changing to new practices difficult. This is normal and is to be expected in all phases of any work transformation. The challenge for the leader is to help others engage the demand for a changing practice by helping them visualize the need for that change and their own personal relationship to the change. They must begin to understand the series of steps that will be necessary for them to act on the demand for change. The time available for such activity is increasingly limited. As organizations compete and struggle to be successful in a new frame of reference for work, the timeline is shorter for accommodating the demand for change. That means that a part of the demand for work is the ability to adjust and change the capacity to work in tighter periods of time. The coach recognizes that she or he is not only helping others to change their relationship to work but also guiding them as to how to alter their way of confronting the change itself. The coach, in this set of circumstances, reflects that change itself is the work and that commitment to the process of change is more important than commitment to any specific work function or activity. Since the work function or activity will change at any moment, the ability of the workers to adjust focus, attention, and effort quickly will be a critical part of their accommodation and adaptation to the change process. This expectation is appropriate for both coach and learning leader. Both must quickly adjust to their leadership practices as quickly as they expect workers to adjust their own work practices.

Leaders must be able to discern and reflect on the elements of change affecting leadership and work. The skill of reflection is a critical leadership talent often underaddressed. The wise leader recognizes the importance of being able to discern the correct fit between demand and response. As they increasingly emerge, there also is required a different response to that work. The coach with the learning leader must now take time to determine the relationship between demand and response.

The coach must be able to read the signposts of the change and to anticipate the implications of those changes on the role of leadership. The leader is always aware of the need to shift and adjust responses based on the change in expectations and performance. A part of this role in expressing leadership is found in the leader's facility with signpost reading and is grounded in the direction and pathway of change. The leader is able to understand the vectors for change and, in reading those vectors, can begin to determine the points of convergence that are indicated by the combined direction of each vector leading to an understanding of change. This signpost reading or factoring is an important leadership skill because it helps the leader anticipate the appropriateness and timing of responses. The coach requires in the learning leader an ability to read the signposts of change, to understand the compositions of movement that work in concert with each other, to be able to anticipate the appropriate responses driven by timing the events of change correctly and undertaking the appropriate action. This requires skill in reflection and discernment. The coach exemplifies this commitment through the use of dialogue and interaction. The dialogue and interaction and purposeful questioning and exploration become a subset of a directed conversation between coach and learning leader. The coach begins to work with the learning leader in a way that engages the issues as they are unfolding and invites to the table of discussion those players upon whom the change has the most impact or who have the most information related to the change. The wisdom that can be found through this collective dialogue and interaction by stakeholders begins to build an aggregate of appropriate responses. These new skills and opportunities create a database upon which the learning leader can draw as the issues demand and as the need arises. Developing skills and accessing and utilizing collective wisdom in decision making becomes a major strength and skill set of leaders as they mature and grow.

Change Itself Is the Work

Both coaches and those they mentor must realize that in the time of great transformation, the work of leadership is embedded in the change itself—recognizing change, acknowledging its impact on individuals and work, identifying and predicting the directions indicated by change, and remaining available to new insights and opportunities to literally see the change coming. Translating the elements of change into the action of work becomes the critical role of the leader, raising the level of accountability for matching performance to desired outcome in an ever-changing context for work.

Leader Discernment

- Is insightful
- Has a future investment
- Is informed
- Accesses contemporary information
- Is aware of surroundings
- Is intuitive
- Senses context change
- Integrates data
- Sees inner flow

Leader Reflection

- Can find a quiet place
- Sorts through "noise"
- Sees real from fad
- Can link concepts
- Touches internal values
- Links broad notions
- Trusts intuition
- Sees the river of change
- Finds direction
- Gives change a language

Purposeful Questioning

The coach always assumes a questioning stance, recognizing that the right question is more important than the answer. Coaching questions are deliberate and focused, as follows:

- What is the direction of change?
- What are competencies of the learning leader?
- What is the fit between learner competencies and direction of change?
- What best exercise or learning opportunity fits the needs of the learner?
- Will learning tools will be required to facilitate the learning leader?
- What time and competency demands affect the rate of learning?
- What are the performance and outcome expectations for the learning leader?
- How will change in the learning leader be evaluated and sustained?

The Coach as Teacher

Coaching involves a program of learning, calling the coach to develop a systematic approach with the learner to guiding the learning leader on the developmental pathway. Critical elements of the program are:

- Assessment of learning needs
- Organized and systematic approach to learning
- A leadership learning plan
- Identification of learning support systems
- Formation of a learning contract
- Clarification of the individual and group learning process
- Timeline and program stages
- Review and evaluation processes
- A definitive mechanism for ending the coaching relationship

---

ACCOMMODATING INDIVIDUAL LEARNING NEEDS

The leader as coach recognizes that there are many ways of learning and of accommodating learning needs. All people are individuals. They have unique approaches to their own learning and development. What is critical for the coach is the commitment to the individual in addressing learning needs and committing to an ongoing program of learning. The coach enters this program of learning as a guide, helping individuals through their learning process with tools and techniques and an awareness that sometimes cannot be visualized within the learning moment. The coach, recognizing the uniqueness of each individual learner, identifies with the learner a program of learning, reviews the processes related to the individual's best way of learning, and assesses situational and circumstantial tools and vehicles within which learning will unfold.

In the practice environment, the coach is predominantly a peer-based learner. The coach simply plays a role in helping others in their own commitment to learning and in their learning activities. The best model for this is the coach's own learning process and program. Through attending to his or her own leadership development, the coach exemplifies the elements, components, and processes associated with personal change and accommodation to transformation.

As a part of the coach's relationship with peers and learning leaders, dialogue is essential, since learning leadership and coaching involves the collective action of those members of the work team who continually relate to each other. It is appropriate that they understand their unique characteristics and practices and processes related to their own learning. This dialogue, facilitated by a good coach, helps people understand the activities and roles of others as they address their own learning processes. Furthermore, it gives all members of the team an opportunity to understand and accommodate the learning talents and unique skills of individual members.

As a part of this dynamic, the coach recognizes that each learning leader must have an action plan that relates specifically to his or her own pattern of learning and expectations for change. This coaching contract provides a framework for individual learners to identify both their goals and their processes in a way that can be realistically yet rigorously applied.

A learning contract can either be a verbal or written agreement between coach and learning leader. If it is a group contract, it is an understanding between all the members of the learning group about their relationship to their learning goals and to facilitating each other's achievement of goals. Increasingly, coaching must involve more than a one-to-one relationship in a time of increasing pace and accelerating rate of change. The coach often cannot be spread thin enough to help guide others in their developmental work. As a result, a group work team contract with the coach is becoming a more common tool for transformational work.

The agreement is more a reflection of the relationship than it is of the coach's wisdom and expertise. In times of great change and personal transformation, every member of the team, including the coach, is fully on board with regard to personal change and transformation work. The coach essentially exemplifies the role of the chief learner, acting as the facilitator who calls to discussion all new learning that is necessary for learning leaders to move individually and in concert with each other.

Coaching in the new age calls for a commitment to help others transform. New rules and new roles in the 21st century call us to reconceptualize the function and role of leadership, as well as its impact on work organization and process. The leader is critical for organizations to successfully transform and attend to a completely different framework for work. The coach–learner relationship exemplifies a mutual commitment to the growth and development of new skills and talents in expressing leadership in this new age. It is an important vehicle for advancing the work of the organization, improving the dynamics of leadership, and providing a continuous opportunity for learning leadership to occur. This relationship is a positive vehicle for both coach and learner, ensuring competence in applying leadership in a time of great change when such leadership is desperately needed.

SUGGESTED READINGS

Anderson, M.C. (2003). *Bottom-line organization development: Implementing and evaluating strategic change for lasting value.* Boston: Butterworth-Heinemann.

Bacon, T.R., & Spear, K.I. (2003). *Adaptive coaching: The art and practice of a client-centered approach to performance improvement.* Palo Alto, CA: Davies-Black.

Bench, M. (2003). *Career coaching: An insider's guide.* Palo Alto, CA: Davies-Black.

Carter, L., Giber, D.J., & Goldsmith, M. (2001). *Best practices in organization development and change: Culture, leadership, retention, performance, coaching; case studies, tools, models, research.* San Francisco: Jossey-Bass.

Cloke, K., & Goldsmith, J. (2003). *The art of waking people up: Cultivating awareness and authenticity at work.* San Francisco: Jossey-Bass.

Coens, T., & Jenkins, M. (2000). *Abolishing performance appraisals: Why they backfire and what to do instead.* San Francisco: Berrett-Koehler Publishers.

Crane, T., & Patrick, L. (2007). *The heart of coaching: Using the transformational coaching to create a high-performance coaching culture.* San Diego, CA: FTA Press.

Cullen, J., & D'Innocenzo, L. (1999). *The agile manager's guide to coaching to maximize performance.* Bristol, VT: Velocity Business Publishers.

Dotlich, D.L., & Cairo, P.C. (1999). *Action coaching: How to leverage individual performance for company success.* San Francisco: Jossey-Bass.

Flaherty, J. (1999). *Coaching: Evoking excellence in others.* Boston: Butterworth-Heinemann.

Fournies, F.F. (2000). *Coaching for improved work performance* (Rev. ed.). New York: McGraw-Hill.

Goldsmith, M., Lyons, L., & Freas, A. (2000). *Coaching for leadership: How the world's greatest coaches help leaders learn.* San Francisco: Jossey-Bass/Pfeiffer.

Kamp, D. (1999). *The 21st-century manager: Future-focused skills for the next millennium.* Dover, NH: Kogan Page.

Lenhardt, V. (2004). *Coaching for meaning: The culture and practice of coaching and team building.* New York: Palgrave Macmillan.

Markle, G.L. (2000). *Catalytic coaching: The end of the performance review.* Westport, CT: Quorum Books.

Parsloe, E., & Wray, M.J. (2000). *Coaching and mentoring: Practical methods to improve learning.* Sterling, VA: Kogan Page.

Stone, F.M. (2002). *Coaching and mentoring.* Oxford, UK: Capstone.

Thorpe, S., & Clifford, J. (2003). *The coaching handbook: An action kit for trainers & managers.* Sterling, VA: Kogan Page.

Warner, J. (2002). *Aspirations of greatness: Mapping the midlife leader's reconnection to self and soul.* New York: John Wiley.

Weiss, T.B., & Kolberg, S. (2003). *Coaching competencies and corporate leadership.* Boca Raton, FL: St. Lucie Press.

Whitmore, J. (2002). *Coaching for performance: Growing people, performance and purpose* (3rd ed.). Naperville, IL: Nicholas Brealey.

Whitworth, L., Kimsey-House, K., Kimsey-House, H., & Sandahl, P. (2007). *Co-active coaching: New skills for coaching people toward success in work and life.* Mountain View, CA: Davis-Black Publishing.

Self-Directed Learning

The learner–coach arrangement is critical to the effectiveness of the learning process. This arrangement represents a partnership between two or more individuals who are committed to each other's learning, one being facilitator (coach) and the other being actor (learner). It is essential that they meet the following basic requirements of a learning relationship in order to assure meaningful interaction and viable outcomes:

- The learner is always in control.
- The coach is present for the learner's needs.
- The learner is responsible for the outcomes of learning.
- The processes of learning are always negotiated.
- Coaching is a learning partnership.
- The coach is never a "parent" to the learning leader.
- Outcomes of learning are defined in advance.
- An agreement of learning expectations is always explicit.
- The learner determines when the coaching contract is ended.
- The coach creates a safe milieu for honest dialogue.
- Learning evaluation is performance based.
- *Change is always the work of the learner.*

Coaching–Group Learning Contract

Components

- Mutual goals defined
- Collective agreement regarding outcomes
- Regularly scheduled group process times
- Continuous peer evaluation
- Peers control group membership
- Members contract performance expectations
- Defining the timeline for performance

Relationship

- Agreement to support each other
- Developmental evaluations
- Regular group process
- Dialogue leads to change
- Trusting and interdependent

Outcomes

- Individuals feel valued
- Performance has improved
- Personal and team expectations are met
- Developmental learning is shared
- *LEARNERS THEMSELVES BECOME COACHES.*

COACHING SCENARIO 1: TEAM-BASED ISSUES

Jill was struggling to keep up with the demands of the team. The learning team had been organized as a way of building mentor support for new charge nurses who were emerging into very new leadership roles. Most of the charge nurses on the team had not been in the role for more than a year and had been in practice for less than 5 years. Each member of the team had committed to partnering with others in identifying leadership needs and skills necessary to be effective in the leadership role. The group gathered together with their coach bimonthly to deal with specific leadership development issues and to evaluate progress.

Team members had made progress, but Jill felt herself falling behind. It seemed that other team members were growing at a faster rate and catching on to the leadership role more quickly than Jill was. Whenever Jill brought up issues it seemed as though they held the team back from consideration of more important or advanced concerns. The last time the learning team had gathered together, Jill had felt a real sense of their irritation with her and the questions she raised. The coach had pulled Jill aside following the meeting and asked Jill how she felt she was progressing and if she desired additional personal time with the coach. Jill was uncertain as to whether that meant the coach felt she was lagging behind and needed special individual attention. She certainly did not want to hold the team back. Indeed, Jill was concerned whether she fit the role she was attempting to undertake and whether she should simply withdraw from the team and, ultimately, from the role.

Scenario Evaluation

In the group, discuss Jill's circumstances. Identify the issues that Jill expresses and make some assumptions about the underlying issues that your team identifies may be affecting Jill's progress. In addition, explore Jill's circumstances by answering the following questions:

1. How did Jill fall behind without other members of the team recognizing it?
2. What was the learning team's obligation as Jill fell behind?
3. Was there something the learning team could have done to be of more assistance to Jill?
4. What is the coach's role with regard to both Jill and the learning team?
5. Can Jill be rescued from these circumstances, or should she move out of the role?

Break into small teams and devise a team contract and a specific learning plan for Jill that follows up on this set of circumstances. Be creative and define what you feel is the coach's role and how that role can facilitate Jill's progress. Report back to the whole group and collectively agree upon the next step for both the coach and for Jill.

COACHING SCENARIO 2:
ESTABLISHING THE COACHING RELATIONSHIP

Ben has just been promoted to his first management position. Ben is a little concerned about how the management position and his skills will match. Never having been a manager before, Ben feels a tremendous need for growth and development in the role. Yet, he has to land on the ground running since he is already in the role, not leaving much time for learning.

Ben has a great deal of respect for his previous manager, Sandra. One day over coffee, Ben and Sandra discussed Ben's new role as manager. During the conversation Ben asked Sandra if she would mind acting as a coach and mentor for him as he began the role of manager. Ben pointed out to Sandra that, while the basics certainly were in place, he anticipated that problems and issues would arise from time to time for which he would need advice and counsel. Neither Ben nor Sandra had been in a coaching and mentoring relationship before. Sandra was a little concerned as to whether she would be competent in providing insight and guidance to Ben. She was also a little concerned as to how the relationship should be established and what the characteristics should be that defined the coaching relationship. Sandra left her lunch with Ben wondering what her first steps should be.

Scenario Exploration

As a learning team, gather together to discuss and expand on Ben's situation. Spend some time conversing about Sandra's position and the contribution that she might be able to make to Ben. Respond to the following questions:

1. What should Ben ask and/or expect from Sandra?
2. What are the basic elements of the coaching/mentoring relationship?
3. Should the coaching relationship be narrowly defined, or should it be open, available to all issues and circumstances?
4. Explain the pros and cons of a written versus verbal coaching relationship.
5. In Ben and Sandra's circumstances, what are the clear outcomes that can be defined as a result of their coaching relationship?

Break up into small groups and prepare a coaching contract for Ben and Sandra. When you have prepared it for them, compare the contract elements you have constructed, evaluate them, and together create a learning agreement for Ben and Sandra with which you can all agree.

APPENDIX 1

Elements of the Coaching Agreement

The coaching contract needs to contain specific elements in order for it to adequately address the individual performance roles and expectations of the parties to the coaching experience.

1. The coaching contract should define the role expectations of both coach and leadership learner. The role expectations and the obligations of commitments made to each other are a critical part of the faithfulness each has to the growth of leadership and the skill development both in coaching and in leader development. This contract, which identifies the expectations of each to the other, helps provide a framework within which both can perform and meet the commitments of their coaching relationship.

2. The coaching contract should specify the expectations for performance and for outcome. The agreement between coach and learning leader is one that is directed toward achieving some specific value for performance outcome. This expectation should be clearly enough explained so that it can be identified as a part of the expectation that each has for the other. Failing to accomplish the goals of coaching and learning leadership does not reflect well on the coaching/ mentoring experience. In fact, it may indicate that no real coaching relationship existed. Identifying a specific performance expectation and its relationship to mutually desired or defined outcomes helps set boundaries for the relationship and maintain its meaning and impact as it unfolds.

3. Any coaching contract should have some elements of measurement of performance and accomplishment of goals. The coach/mentor relationship cannot have much value or impact if some differences are maintained through the process of coaching and learning development. Points of demarcation, elements of evaluation, review of degrees of improvement or change over time all help the learner meet performance expectations and advances the relationship between coach and learning leader. Such evaluation keeps the process focused and directed toward specific goals and performance expectations and assures that the relationship remains one that is developmental, productive, and growth oriented.

4. A time frame should be created for the expectations of performance so that accomplishment or changes in practices or behaviors can be defined within a specific time frame. This helps define the expectations for performance and begins to set parameters around actual change behavior. Often in the coaching and learning relationship there is an open time frame with regard to performance expectations and specific changes. The problem with this is that specific changes

may not ever occur as a product of the relationship. What results instead is a high level of personal relationship interaction and a low level of substantive change and role impact. Developing friendships and an abiding relationship between coach and learning leader may be a valuable human experience, but does not necessarily advance the development of effective leadership skills or roles.

5. The coach–learner role should at some time come to an end with regard to its formal purpose and mentoring interaction. This is not to suggest that the relationship between people ever ends. However, what is important is to recognize that the coach and learner role is purposeful and directed toward achieving meaningful and viable products. It is when these ends are obtained and development has occurred and expected changes happen, as laid out in the role contract, that the relationship changes its form as well as its purpose. Reflecting this understanding of the change in form and purpose, the contract specifies a time when its formal nature ends and the expectations for the agreement have been fulfilled. This gives both coach and learner an opportunity to evaluate the effectiveness of their interaction, to determine the value of its impact on expectations, and to evaluate the outcomes and impact of the coaching relationship. In this way the real value of the coaching relationship is clearly spelled out and identified with the specific outcomes involved as a result of the contracted interaction.

Leading With Courage

CHAPTER OBJECTIVES:

Upon completion of this chapter, the reader will:

1. Discuss the significance of revolutionary behaviors as a vehicle to continuing adaptation and transition into the information age.

2. Understand the value of courageous leader behaviors and their impact on organizational performance.

3. Enumerate four strategies to develop courageous communication competence.

4. Identify specific leader behaviors that reflect courage.

INTRODUCTION

The paradox of leadership requires leaders to be creative and futuristic in their thinking while sustaining the essence of the current culture, which may be fixed and entrenched. This challenge finds leaders often stuck, sustaining the past at the expense of adapting to the changing external environment. Leading courageously requires specific skills and focus on work, in which the leader neither dwells in the past nor revels in the present. The courageous leader fully understands personal strengths and weaknesses and how best to use those skills in addressing the obstacles to the future. The leader moves forward assertively to cocreate the preferred future that reflects emerging expectations, new knowledge, and new technology.

> **Gem**
>
> The most radical revolutionary will become a conservative the day after the revolution.
>
> Hannah Arendt

In this chapter, leaders will examine the nature of courage from several perspectives. A description of the courageous leader as a revolutionary is presented from Kuhn's (1996) perspective of scientific revolutions and the phenomena surrounding the emergence of new science and new models. Several communication challenges that continually confront leaders and require much courage are presented to further examine the essence of courage and stimulate discussion. In the final section, specific challenges reflecting leader courage are offered to leaders to continue their courageous journey of healthcare leadership.

Facing Fear

I have not ceased being fearful, but I have ceased to let fear control me. I have accepted fear as a part of life—specifically the fear of change, the fear of the unknown; and I have gone ahead despite the pounding in my heart that says: turn back, turn back, you'll die if you venture too far.

Erica Jong

Courage

I do not ask to walk smooth paths, nor bear an easy load

I pray for strength and fortitude to climb the rock strewn road.

Give me such courage and I can scale the hardest peaks alone,

And transform every stumbling block into a stepping stone!

Gail Brook Burket

Courage

Few people realize that Ford Motor Company was Henry Ford's third attempt at making automobiles. He was voted out in one company and went bankrupt in another. He was ousted from the Henry Ford Company when he insisted on improving the design of the car instead of thinking of short-term profits. When he was removed by the board of directors, the name was changed to the Cadillac Automotive Company. The Cadillac was originally a Ford. Later, as we all know, Ford's quest for a better car paid off.

Dare to Revolutionize

The work expected of the leader is analogous to the scientific revolution described by Kuhn (1996) in the *Structure of Scientific Revolutions*. As the world evolves from the industrial age to the information age, the work of health care is shifting from work that requires the skill set of an employee to work that requires the skill set of the knowledge worker. Previously, the work of the employee was grounded in functional analysis, manual dexterity, fixed skill sets, an emphasis of process value and practice, and unilateral performance. This is quite different from the required skills of the knowledge worker, namely, the ability to synthesize concepts, embody multiple intelligences, demonstrate competence in providing care, skill set mobility, being driven by outcomes that create value, and the ability to function most effectively within a team model.

While the evolution to the knowledge worker paradigm may seem slow, even invisible, there is a revolution of work processes occurring. This revolution occurs through courageous leaders committed to the belief that the creation of anomalous situations, or situations that deviate from the norm, is essential to facilitate the paradigm shift from the industrial age to the information age.

Quantum leaders thrive in the work of discovery, which includes asking new questions, identifying new methods to examine processes, finding new areas of relevance, and creating new meaning for the work of health care. These processes necessarily challenge the current assumptions and industrial paradigm underpinning health care, creating the well-known anomaly or shift in scientific knowledge that changes shared assumptions and subverts existing traditions of practice. In time, the anomaly created by courageous healthcare leaders will evolve into a scientific revolution, and traditions will be shattered, thus rendering the tradition-bound activity of the current paradigm inappropriate. It is important to note that the courageous leader who assumes the role of the anomaly creator can be often lonely and sometimes scorned. However, it is only through the creation of an anomaly that new realities can be advanced and ultimately supported. New ideas tend to emerge only with difficulty in cultures strongly entrenched in current processes. Resistance is the norm to most new ideas.

Creating a sustainable revolution will result in certain outcomes. First, the current paradigm must be replaced in whole or part by an incompatible new one; second, the new approach is immune to attack by competent knowledge owners. The journey of the courageous leader is never finished. As the courageous leader moves forward and continually examines personal behaviors, values, and communication processes, new paradigms result in better ways to conceptualize and provide health care.

In summary, several challenges always remain with the leader committed to the revolution of health care. These include:

- Creation of a new reality that is better than the current reality in some way
- Appreciation for current dogma and willingness and courage to remove existing assumptions
- Commitment to changing the culture or social behaviors necessary for revolutions to succeed
- Tolerance of rejection
- Appreciation of areas of vulnerability

- Avoidance of acquiescing to the glamour of short-lived fads instead of a substantive, sustainable revolution
- Willingness to abandon the past
- Developing energy to sustain emerging revolutionary outcomes and continually move forward

An example of a paradigm shift can be found in the changing documentation of healthcare records. Computerized word processing has all but eliminated the need for the typewriter and caregiver handwriting. The paradigm shift began with upgrade from a manual typewriter to an electric typewriter, which enhanced the processes within the current paradigm of creating legible documents. The work of documentation has been transformed from a single, static entry of information to an electronic entry that is retrievable, editable, and stored as long as the author wishes and not simply modified from a handwritten entry to a typewriter entry.

The shift from invasive surgery to the use of external scope-facilitated procedures is another example of the beginning of a paradigm shift: less invasive procedures, different equipment needed, differing skills needed to complete the processes. The role of the physician and nurse has changed dramatically in this transformation, one that is incomplete, as the need for some invasive procedures still exists. The work of invasive surgery has yet to be completely replaced. As imaging technology continues to advance, the anomaly of the noninvasive procedure will become the dominant paradigm once biological and genomic therapies further complete the transformation to surgical interventions that are exclusively noninvasive.

Build a Conspiracy of Innovation

As previously noted, the journey of transformation is often paradoxical; people actively support the idea of and need for new processes and strategies, but seldom dedicate adequate time or energy to live the role of transformer. Excessively high workloads take precedence over reflective time for examination of work effectiveness and evaluation of opportunities for change. Nurses have demonstrated the ability to adapt to differing circumstances but have not demonstrated this ability as a discipline to embrace and engage in change processes. Most likely, this is due to the lack of skills in translating great clinical ideas into ways of doing business in an economically driven marketplace. The need emerges for courageous leaders to build conspiracies for innovation, to gather a critical group of people committed to seeing the good ideas through to actualization, to create passion for the work that will overcome the obstacles, and to develop relationship skills that will place the right people in the right place at the right time (Porter-O'Grady, 2003). Courageous leaders committed to innovation demonstrate the ability to manage the noise created by anomalous processes, develop a few key players, and plan or conspire to work through others to advance the innovation throughout the system. The effective leader recognizes that innovative ideas are seldom spontaneous; rather, they occur through methodical processes of creating evidence for the idea and cascading support from those in the organization. This is an often slow and lonely process. In the next section, several behaviors are presented to assist leaders dedicated to the transformation of practice through innovation.

Courage to Risk
To laugh is to risk appearing the fool.
To weep is to risk appearing sentimental.
To reach for another is to risk involvement.
To expose your feelings is to risk exposing your true self.
To place your ideas, your dreams before a crowd is to risk their loss.
To love is to risk not being loved in return.
To live is to risk dying.
To believe is to risk despair.
To try is to risk failure.
But risks must be taken, because the greatest hazard in life is to risk nothing.
The person who risks nothing, does nothing, has nothing, is nothing. They may avoid suffering and sorrow, but they cannot learn, feel change, grow, love, live.
Chained by their attitudes they are slaves; they have forfeited their freedom.
Only a person who risks is free.
Anonymous Chicago Teacher

The Daring Leader

Oftentimes, the creative and innovative leader is described as outrageous or gutsy. According to Frieberg and Frieberg (2004), gutsy leaders are not afraid of criticism or ridicule by others. They have dismantled fear-based behaviors and processes and replaced them with heart, soul, discipline, loyalty, humor, and of course, long-term

> **Gem**
>
> The art of progress is to preserve order amid change and to preserve change amid order.
>
> Alfred North Whitehead

record profits. While it might seem contradictory to have gutsy leaders in health care, where the stakes of life and health are significant and the need for consistently high-quality outcomes are expected, the reality is that current processes have yet to achieve the desired outcomes. Significant modifications of the healthcare system are still desperately needed to both create the desired outcomes and to effectively transform the system into the new age of technology and meet the greater expectations for high-quality, caring, therapeutic relationships. Consumers are demanding compassionate health care with the best of technology at a reasonable price; thus the need for much more innovation and transformation of current practices. Gusty leaders have several things in common (Frieberg & Frieberg, 2004). These include:

- An emphasis to ensure that employees are overwhelmingly enthusiastic about their organization, not just satisfied
- Promoting of a sense of ownership of the work; those closest to the point of care are recognized as the experts of the organization
- Building business literacy competency among all employees; developing skills in translating individual work through accounting processes to the bottom line of the organization and the employee paycheck
- Expecting accountability for success and failures through service guarantees
- Creating a moral imperative for doing great work for the right reason: work is more than just a job
- The ability to stand up for what is right and to admit mistakes in front of those you work with and to say I don't know when you don't!

The Vigilant Leader

In addition to being gutsy, the courageous leader must also be vigilant of the context in which care is provided and the interrelated components in the environment. Clinical vigilance is recognized as a key behavior in minimizing failures to rescue and thus improve patient outcomes. When a nurse is vigilant, he or she is likely to intervene on the patient's behalf, recognize problems early, or avert them entirely. Emrich (2004) writes, "vigilance is a collection of behaviors and activities, based on professional commitment or duty, that includes seeking or intellectually scanning within the nurse–patient relationship for situations that require nursing actions and reacting appropriately to that need." Vigilance is one of the caring acts of nursing that are deeply ingrained into the professional role and are often undetected by nonnurses. These acts often seem intangible and nonspecific, are identified as lower priority in skill development, and marginalize nursing's artful practice to the demands of efficiency and cost control.

Historically, the notions of vigilance emanate from the work of Fairman (1992) and the rationale for the creation of intensive care units. Specialized knowledge was needed, as was more frequent monitoring, identification of high-risk situations, and timely actions. Kennedy (2000) further described vigilance as a means to support normalcy, rather than a search for pathology, requiring confidence, intelligence, intellectual curiosity, and objectivity to assess the situation. Another significant attribute of vigilance is the act of doing nothing well: allowing events to progress naturally when the range of normalcy is identified. Knowing when to intervene and not to intervene is critical for the courageous leader; it involves leader actions of trusting, being competent, and recognizing past experiences of the team.

Similarly, there are opportunities for leader vigilance in ensuring that the infrastructure to support clinical vigilance is in place and is able to support current safe practice and innovation. Leader vigilance is about the commitment to leadership through the specialized knowledge of the organization's infrastructure, processes and outcomes, routine assessment of processes and outcomes, recognition of high-risk situations, and timely reaction to avoid negative outcomes. Leader vigilance, as expression of courageous leader behaviors, is more than sensitivity for conditions that will lead to error; it means being proactive rather than reactive in assuring that the conditions for innovation and quality work are always present. Leader vigilance means scanning for opportunities and taking action to advance both the work of the organization and the practice of nursing. Leader vigilance is truly an art form of nursing leadership that embodies a high level of awareness for the signals that indicate effectiveness and excellence. Those signals reflect minor variations that could lead to major issues if not investigated, and the leader must have the courage to react at the appropriate time. The characteristics and representative behaviors of leader vigilance include the following:

- Discusses minor issues regularly with employees
- Recognizes potential problems early
- Intervenes on the employees' behalf
- Builds sustainable relationship with employees
- Eliminates outdated practices early
- Adopts contemporary practices more suited to the context of health care as soon as possible

> ### Leader Vigilance Data Scanning
>
> - Status of available staff at the aggregate and daily level
> - Status of supply availability
> - Working relationships between departments
> - Presence of joy in the patient care area
> - Presence of joy in the break room
> - Patient satisfaction and perception of patient care; perception of the healthcare experience
> - Productivity measures that include variance analysis from volume and projected costs
> - Occurrence reports
> - Skill level of available staff
> - Errors/failure-to-rescue situations
> - Informal staff feedback—ask focused questions rather than general satisfaction questions

Diminished vigilance is described as incomplete vigilance relative to one of the basic components of vigilance, such as intellectually scanning the work of nursing, identifying areas for intervention or nonintervention, and reacting appropriately. An action reflecting diminished vigilance may be the result of poor judgment due to inappropriate or lack of knowledge, failure to scan the environment appropriately, or failure to react in a timely manner. Examples of diminished vigilance include:

- Inappropriate actions taken due to lack of knowledge
- Interventions that focus only on the immediate issues and do not address the situation effectively
- Undermonitoring of the critical elements of practice
- Inappropriate judgment as to the appropriate intervention to be taken or not taken
- Failure to prevent negative outcomes

Nonvigilance is the absence of professional commitment that precludes the nurse from being vigilant, namely intellectually able to scan for the critical indicators of work effectiveness and to react appropriately. Examples of the outcomes of nonvigilance include:

- Negative patient outcomes
- Negative employee outcomes
- Poor leader–employee relationships
- Potential problems become real problems
- Failure to recognize problem behaviors
- Failure to respond to significant data, leading to errors and missed signs and symptoms
- Lack of awareness of appropriate delegation practices specific to clinical and managerial tasks
- Lack of awareness of the impact of the level of secretarial support

One of the challenges for leadership is how to integrate the essence of clinical vigilance into productivity systems, or, how does one make the business case for vigilance? Historically, productivity measurement has not included calculation of preventive measures, a significant component of the nursing role. This is not because clinical vigilance has been ignored or disregarded; rather, it is because those accountable for vigilance have not been able to create objective and defensible measures that can be integrated into a productivity system. Recent published research documents the impact of registered nurse oversight and monitoring and the resultant rescuing of patients from negative consequences. According to Blakeney (2003), ANA president, the challenge is not reinventing how nursing is practiced, but how nursing is perceived and partnered within healthcare institutions. The perception of rescuing, observing the subtle changes, and continuous vigilance needs to be translated into current productivity measurement systems. While good nursing care is often seen through the absence of problems, this essence requires credible, standard metrics not currently available in most productivity monitoring systems. Measuring success on the basis of events that do not occur is possible, given the recent publications specific to pressure ulcers, nosocomial pneumonia, patient falls, and urinary tract infections. Thus the new metrics that identify the time and skill level for the definition and articulation of the minimum monitoring necessary for safe patient outcomes must be created and become an essential element in the calculations of caregiver productivity.

Dare to Revive the Nursing Uniform

Letting go of the past requires careful analysis of what we are giving up and what should be retained, which is a process of using resources more appropriately and finding better value for one's efforts. A revolution in nurse uniforms is in the making. New technology and new environmental hazards have rendered the current nurse uniform only marginally helpful to the work of nursing.

Uniforms are immediate identifiers. They represent authority and convey a sense of competency within the nursing field. The once-traditional white uniform, white stockings, and starched cap of nurses have been unceremoniously replaced with bright and colorful uniforms. Both licensed and nonlicensed caregivers have adopted similar uniforms, diminishing the use of the uniform as an identifier of the nurse.

In the spirit of creativity and utility, members of the Fabric Workshops and Museum (FWM), in association with the Center for the Study of the History of Nursing, have examined nurse uniforms and proposed a future uniform that combines the lore of science fiction with new material technologies (Houweling, 2004). Conductive fiber technologies embedded in the fabric equip it to assess a patient's vital signs at the touch of a hand. It also provides hazard protection from a biological attack or biological spill, which enables nurses to administer to patients without endangering themselves.

A computer-generated model of the intergalactic nurse uses a uniform design incorporating the acupuncture concept of chi (energy flow) (Houweling, 2004). The uniform conceptualized for nursing in the 23rd century incorporates reflective tape, magnets, and silver-plated fiber that can be wired for computers or other electronics. The antimicrobial fabric conducts heat via silver to soothe the body at the various chi points, further supporting the safe practice of nursing. The design, a collaborative effort of artists Puett, Dion, and Kerr, the Fabric Workshop and Museum in Philadelphia, and materials from 3M, Sauquoit Industries, and Noble Fiber Technologies, is an example of creativity, evidence-based decision making, and courage to change the present paradigm on the basis of the new nursing role expectations and the new hazards of the work.

Revolutionizing the uniform for the nurse may indeed be much less complicated than reworking the cultural context of the work of nursing. The courageous leader approaches rework in spite of its awesome and overwhelming nature; the courageous leader moves forward because it is the right thing to do.

Gem

Over the last 20 years, we've changed the world just enough to make it radically different, but not enough to make it work.

Anna Quindlen

Discussion

Consider the changing role of the nurse leader.

How would you design the uniform or the basic competencies of the leader to reflect the needs of the 23rd century in a technologically healing context?

What knowledge would be essential for the processes of rework?

What protective skills would be necessary for the leader?

What would you leave behind that would not compromise the future value of nursing?

COURAGEOUS COMMUNICATION

Courageous leaders continually work to communicate openly and honestly, even in the most unpleasant situations. The skills of confronting, sharing information, ending relationships, and using new technology effectively are presented in this section as guides for continuing the evolving journey to excellence.

Dare to Confront

It is trite to say that delivering unpleasant news is seldom easy, given that so many leaders continue to struggle with sharing honest, open, and caring communication. Numerous explanations for less-than-open communication have been identified and include lack of skill in confronting difficult issues, reluctance to upset the other person, unwillingness to stand out in a group, and fear of retaliation. Many strategies to confront others as caring actions have been recommended, such as skill-building workshops and increasing individual account-ability as a core performance expectation. Yet, the challenge remains. There may be no other skill that requires as much courage as giving unpleasant, but honest, feedback.

Courageous leaders have no magic strategies; rather, they practice, practice, and prac-tice some more in giving feedback to others in the most timely and caring manner.

Consider the situation in which a recently hired surgical director has been noted to be confrontational and has not been listening to others during introductory meetings. The supervisor shares the feedback and after discussion with the director advises her that this behavior is inconsistent with the culture of the organization and needs to be modified. Within 2 days, more feedback of the same negative nature is received. The supervisor does not wait for change to occur but rather once again informs the direc-tor of the poor communication style. Both expectations for change and strategies to support better communication are discussed. The first confrontation was a challenge, but the second was even more difficult. Failing to follow through on issues as they recur results in unresolved, festering issues that eventually result in a critical incident. Courageous leaders focus on addressing issues quickly and appropriately as a key strat-egy to role model expectations and to support open dialogue and effective teamwork.

Dare to Tell All

As more and more healthcare information is available and managed through the Internet, leaders are presented a new challenge of ensur-ing that the right information is shared with the right person at the right time. Legislation to limit the sharing of patient information and expectations from employees to know what is going on often seem contradictory. The principles of information-sharing specific to patient information has been defined in recent HIPAA legislation; only the patient or those designated by the patient have access to the informa-tion and are able to discuss patient information.

Knowing which information specific to organizational operations can be shared with employees continues to challenge leaders. Telling all is irresponsible, and shar-ing nothing is paralyzing. Guidelines that maximize employee involvement, protect employee confidentiality, and addresses the evolving nature of data are needed. Hesselbein (2004) has noted that rigid hierarchies, which assign people boxes and restrict information to assigned boxes, up-down, superior-subordinate relationships, are disappearing from the world of effective organizations. The new reality of fluid, flexible management systems, structures, and practices requires an inclusive, circular organizational culture in which information is shared openly with those involved in the work of the organization. The inclusionary approach reinforces that an inclusion-

> **Gem**
>
> Success is measured not so much by the position that one has reached in life as by the obstacles which he has overcome while trying to succeed.
>
> Booker T. Washington

> **Gem**
>
> There is a fine line between healthy dissent and arrogant disregard for authority.
>
> Pamela Herr

> **Gem**
>
> It is better to be a lion for a day than to be a sheep all your life.
>
> Sister Elizabeth Kenny

Discussion

Dare to Tell *All*

Much information about department or organizational operations is believed confidential. As a leader you are entrusted with information specific to clinical management, policies, pay structures, discipline criteria, costs of care, supplies, and equipment, to name a few. Carefully review the information and determine how much of the information you can share with every member of your department. When you identify information that is not currently shared but you believe should be, use your newly acquired skills in being a courageous leader and work to change the expectation to allow information sharing.

1. Who will support your recommendation?
2. What are the barriers that must be overcome?

Gem

Changes are not only possible and predictable, but to deny them is to be an accomplice to one's own unnecessary vegetation.

Gail Sheehy

ary culture is indeed about the beliefs and values practiced by all members of the organization, not just a selected few in selected boxes.

New energy and synergy emerge when organizations share operational information specific to revenues, expenses, outcomes, and strategies. In essence, leadership becomes dispersed throughout the organization, and involvement and support for the organization increases exponentially with the circle of inclusion approach. This is much different from the old departmental or boxes of control that expected communication separation and isolation. Managing from a circular model moves the organization to new levels of engagement, inquiry, performance, and results.

Dare to Move to Virtual Communication

The increasing use of electronic communication creates opportunities for increased collaboration, participation of all team members, and significant decreases of travel time to and from meetings. Online education programs have pioneered the model that results in an increased level of student participation with the required posting of ideas and feedback to reflect assimilation and comprehension of assigned materials. These processes are readily applicable to organizational group communication in which input from each participant is needed. Courageous leaders have challenged the traditional face-to-face meetings and developed new meeting processes with clear guidelines to assure the desired outcomes are achieved. Examples of guidelines to transform meeting processes to a more effective and efficient use of time and energy include:

- All meetings virtual unless there is specific, identified benefit to physical presence; first and last meetings in person to establish relationships and celebrate completion
- Identification of required participants
- Clear expectations for each member to participate and provide feedback/discussion for all issues in virtual work
- Specific time frames for project discussion and completion
- Completion of a standard evaluation for each virtual meeting

Dare to Close with Closure

Most leaders have experienced relationships that did not end well. Miscommunications, differing values, competing interests, or decision-making styles were just too different to reside together. Chinn (2004) tells us that ending relationships or asking a member to leave a group can be appropriate. As difficult as that might be, sometimes the work of the group and the individual are not harmonious. When attempts to address the differences are not successful, actions must be taken to sustain overall group effectiveness. It is unrealistic to think that everyone can live together happily ever after; this is just not consistent with reality. This is not to say the relationship was a failure; rather, one phase is ending and another is beginning. Courage is certainly required to address the issue and move on as kindly as possible. Allowing the conflict or disharmony to fester and failing to address it is less than courageous and may in fact border on cowardice!

COURAGEOUS LEADER BEHAVIORS
Dare to Rework the Work

The context for all healthcare service must change and adapt as rapidly as new technologies, pharmaceuticals, and genome innovations, which are forever changing the delivery of care. Courageous leaders are focused on advancing the practice setting to accommodate new processes and achieving the work of the day. Assumptions are challenged and rationales are validated to ensure that changes are appropriate and ahead of the curve. The courageous leader seldom waits for others to lead the way with new innovations and completion of process validation. Being a part of designing the future is an essential role for both the leader and members of the organization.

> **Gem**
>
> Life is a grindstone. Whether it grinds you down or polishes you up depends on what you are made of.
>
> Anonymous

Dare to Eliminate Your Job

As the nature of work changes, few current jobs should remain as they are. For example, using oral thermometers, sippy diets for ulcer management, and invasive chest surgeries have been replaced by ear thermometers, pharmaceuticals to control gastric acid, and endoscopic procedures that are safer and more efficient. The same evolution, while not as dramatic, is occurring for leaders. Classroom orientation has been replaced by online courses, communication has moved from phones to e-mail, and manual calculators have been replaced by complex software calculation programs. Eliminating the specific tasks but not the basic work is the challenge faced by all leaders: the work of nursing assessment, planning, intervention, and evaluation remains, while the time and tools to complete the processes evolve continually. The need for employee performance reviews is a constant, but the content, method, and frequency of the process evolves as well. No employee should have the same type of evaluation as occurred 10 years ago. Reworking the job description on a regular basis to reflect the desired outcomes of the work, not the specific approach, is an evolving process. As with the virtual meeting processes, leaders continue to ensure effective communication but move from processes that may overuse resources and decrease the number of participants and towards better processes that result in better discussion and outcomes. For example, if the bulk of new employee orientation can be online, the space requirement for classrooms decreases significantly but the need for computer terminals increases. The expectation for a quality orientation that produces competent caregivers never varies; the methods and tools used to achieve the competence often change based on advances. The leader must continually evaluate all processes and eliminate the outdated jobs while sustaining the essential values of quality, integrity, and efficiency of resource use.

Caution is noted regarding frequent changes in organizational reporting structures as the means to advance practice. Rearranging processes is much different from evolving and transforming processes. Too often, new organizational structures are created to manage unsatisfactory performance of certain individuals. Courageous leaders learn to confront the issues and avoid making complex system changes that serve only to confuse others in the organization. Only when leaders truly believe that the future is advanced should changes be made in the organizational chart.

As leaders rework the work, the significance and number of policies should be examined as well. Too often, policies that are long out of date are retained in the system for no apparent reason. All leaders should be challenged to eliminate or archive at least two policies for each new one created.

Dare to Live in the World of Information Technology

The complexities of information technology have caused much confusion for nurse leaders, who must integrate computerized systems into the work of nursing. While much has been gained in the cross-training of nursing and information technology skills, significant work remains to transform today's nurses to tech-savvy clinicians. Given that computerization is here to stay and there is no turning back to a manual world, and given the pervasiveness of computerization, the courageous leader must recognize the need to immerse him- or herself into the discipline of information technology and become tech-savvy. A toolbox of resources that guide leaders in understanding basic computer function, networking, web-based learning, Internet programs, and technical support to assure adequate functioning of computerized systems are essential skills for the quantum leader. This is not to say that leaders should develop skills in programming. They should develop expertise in the management of existing systems and the evaluation of new technology that will serve to enhance practice, rather than merely accept an additional level of computerization without specific clinical benefits.

Dare to Transform the Culture

Seldom does a leader have the opportunity to start with a new facility and create a new culture for the provision of healthcare services. However, whenever the opportunity is present for a new facility or for a new unit, it is courageous to embrace a process of *care* transformation that redesigns processes to address the problems and inefficiencies of the current system. More often than not, new construction and renovations focus on duplicating the current physical environment with only minor modifications of existing care processes. The opportunities are incredible for creating a better future that requires caregivers to examine their practice, recommit to doing the right thing for the right reason, and to improve personal satisfaction with the organization, which must translate to quality patient outcomes. The necessary changes identified by leaders creating a culture of transformation have included the following goals:

- Computerized documentation to minimize the need to interpret physician handwriting
- Streamlined documentation that can be completed by the nurse in less than 15 minutes for each shift
- Elimination of the need to ask a patient for the same information over and over
- Documentation of information only once, namely, allergies and past medical history
- An environment in which all employees provide nurturing, compassionate, respectful, creative, and excellent clinical patient care
- A patient care delivery model in which all caregivers are not only allowed but are expected to use their full scope of practice as defined by their licensure
- Equipment in the patient care area that supports patient lifting and minimizes nurse lifting
- Access to online reference sources, policies, and procedures, and a documentation system that alerts the caregiver to standards of patient care
- Adequate space for the family at the bedside
- The right computer device is available at the right time and in the right place for every patient
- Access to members of an interdisciplinary team on the patient care unit
- Ongoing research is conducted to validate processes and outcomes

It is important to note that none of these activities alone will transform the culture. Transformation will occur through the collective commitment to the majority of these behaviors.

Dare to Form New Partnerships

Leaders often wonder why we can't all just get along. Both external and internal divisions or separations of individuals, departments, organizations, and funding sources may make it difficult to work together to benefit the community at large. Facility competes with facility, for-profit organizations compete with not-for-profit organizations, and nurses compete with other nurses. In a recent, revolutionary move, two major competing universities in the same state agreed to collaborate for the benefit of the state's residents. After discussion by several courageous leaders, one very new to the state and willing to reverse and challenge existing assumptions, a new model for education was proposed that included a new medical campus to support the growing health needs of the community.

The new partnership reflects several behaviors that should indeed be emulated by others: reaching out beyond usual insular boundaries toward a world of expanded opportunities; discarding old baggage of my way and your way to pick up new baggage of our way; enhancement of the use of technology to support innovation and communication; and documentation of increased efficiencies and convenience to the citizens of the state. The reach for new levels of excellence emerges from many sources, both expected and unexpected, and always begins with the re-creation of relationships and reversal of some key assumptions.

Dare to Be Politically Competent

Elected officials make decisions that directly affect the work of healthcare leaders, often without knowledge of the pertinent issues and the impact of their decisions. In one state (Arizona) in 2004, for example, 3 of 90 legislators have previous healthcare experience; one is a registered nurse who has not practiced for 20 years, one is a licensed practical nurse working part-time in a physician's office, and the third a retired human resources executive. The hard reality is that most elected officials know little about healthcare issues and need the sage advice of knowledgeable healthcare professionals.

Energy and encouragement often are needed to develop relationships with elected officials in the district. Knowing those individuals who make decisions about allocations of revenues to health, the environment, transportation, and sanitation are certainly important, but decisions made specific to healthcare regulations directly impact the work of nurses. The courageous leader asserts him- or herself to establish communication with elected officials and gives comments on issues of interest on a regular basis. The availability of webcasts of legislative sessions and the use of e-mail communication by the legislators provide opportunities for real-time monitoring and communication of pertinent issues. Involvement in the policy-making process may seem insignificant and one might think that one call or letter will not make a difference. However, when the policy maker is unfamiliar with the topic and only one person is sending comments, one voice can indeed make a significant difference.

Dare to Reverse Assumptions

Many practices and values related to hierarchal behaviors between levels of caregivers, the location of patient care services, and the role of the patient in the provision of services have changed significantly. The physician is no longer the captain of the ship, but rather is a member of the healthcare team, with other disciplines owning their own practice as colleagues with the physician provider. Healthcare services have moved from the location of the provider much closer to the location of the patient and more recently to remote locations connected via telemedicine clinics. The patient is no longer the recipient of the values and decisions of providers but is now expected to be the director of his or her care. Each of these changes has reversed the original assumptions of care, namely that only the physician could direct care, care is delivered at the location of the provider, and the team of providers controlled and directed the care received by the patient. The shifts in assumptions require healthcare providers to learn new skills, deliver care in different locations, and communicate as facilitators of care rather than the directors of care.

Another assumption that the courageous leader reverses is the notion that being in the middle between the organization and the patient is inescapable and problematic due to the conflicting values of the patient and the system. The courageous leader thrives in the role of the in-between position, between the patient and the healthcare system; seeing it as the ideal position in which to be the translator and advocate for the patient in selecting and evaluating patient care services consistent with his or her own needs. The courageous nurse recognizes those situations in

---

Discussion

New Partnerships for Nursing

Given the need to improve resource use, share expertise, and provide services to greater numbers of individuals, how can nursing contribute to the community?

Consider the following dyads in your group and identify ways that new and different relationships between the two could address the above needs.

- Schools of medicine and nursing
- Community colleges and universities
- Nurses and social workers
- Retired nurses and working nurses
- Professional sports teams and nursing homes
- Banks and hospice facilities

Gem

Institutions falter when they invest too much in what is and too little in what could be.

Hamel & Valikangas, 2003

which the position between the system or other providers and the patient creates a moral dilemma and poses ethical challenges for the nurse and works to resolve the issues. Further, the nurse works to create better conditions in the future to ensure that the different options are addressed prior to reaching the crisis point. The courageous nurse leader does not defer to the hierarchal position of the organization; the nurse assumes the role of communication facilitator and creator of the context for safe, patient-driven care.

Dare to Retire Retirement

Have you ever wondered what is significant about the age of 65? It is optional to retire at 65 years of age and begin to claim Social Security benefits. As people live longer, as more work shifts to knowledge work and replaces physical work, and as the economy requires some to continue to work, new structures for work are needed. While it might be difficult to change the Social Security system quickly, there are some solutions worth considering so all those workers who wish to work beyond the age of 65 can do so without penalty or feelings of inadequacy. The courageous leader is challenged to adjust physically demanding jobs and create new roles that value the knowledge and experience of the older worker. The rationale is not only about addressing worker shortages; it is also about valuing the skills of individuals regardless of their age and allowing them to contribute when able.

According to Dychtwald, Erickson, & Morison (2004), the long-standing human resource policies that favor youth and push out older workers is out of date and indeed is leaving a severe shortage of talented workers. To address the need for skills, knowledge, experience, and relationships, new models of employment that honor and recognize experience are needed. Efforts to decrease the bias against older workers, create new recruitment approaches that entice the older worker, and institute flexible scheduling are strategies surely to be welcomed by older workers as bona fide efforts to accommodate their changing physical capabilities.

Finally, courageous leaders must work with policy makers to modify the current retirement plans and allow for flexible retirement that prorates retirement benefits instead of the current all-or-nothing payment strategies. Much can be accomplished to assist the older generation in being more productive, useful, and less bored—and this leads to better health and less use of healthcare insurance benefits.

SUMMARY
Courageous Self-Care: Leader Time Out

Quantum leaders can neither dwell in the past nor revel in the present. The work of the leader requires courage to know the self as best as one is able to, to overcome the current obstacles to moving forward, and to take courageous action to cocreate the future that reflects emerging expectations, new knowledge, and new technology. The need for leader resilience, the phenomenon of capacity for continuous reconstruction rather than spells of success followed by failure, and so on require a strong emphasis on one's personal energy and ability to focus at the moment. No leader can be perfectly focused and energized to do the work that needs to be done every day. Leader time out is a practice that serves the effective leader well. It is always important to remember that making no decisions is often better than making partially thought-out, emotionally charged decisions.

> **Courageous Leader Affirmation**
>
> I am able to take courageous, consistent, and appropriate management actions to overcome barriers to achieving my organization's mission.

Leader time out also allows the leader to reflect on his or her fit with the current organization, culture, and colleagues. It is a time to consider reinvesting in the work or deciding to change employment. The time to move on from one position to another is seldom planned or perfectly timed. When all efforts to reconcile the gap between the personal you and the outside organization are expended without sufficient success, the courageous leader recognizes what has been accomplished and begins another pathway in healthcare leadership, not as a failure but as a lifelong learner of the work of health care. But what is most important is that the courageous leader must leave an organization when there is a disconnection between the leader's internal values and the values of the external world.

Exercise 1 Changing Paradigms

Much evidence has been developed specific to the high cost of turnover, both financially and qualitatively. The employee-focused paradigm supports long-term employment as a vehicle to increased quality and lower costs through established relationships and organizational commitments. In the age of the knowledge worker, the value of retention is necessarily changed. Mobility of knowledge and competence is the norm rather than the exception. Workers thrive on mobility and thrive on learning new skills and team performance. Given this evolution, design a new employee management philosophy to support the new values and minimize or eliminate the previously valued paradigm.

Exercise 2 Courageous Behaviors

In this chapter, seven behaviors to assist leaders in developing courage have been identified. These include:

- Rework the work
- Eliminate your job
- Live in the world of information technology
- Transform the culture
- Form new partnerships
- Be politically competent
- Reverse assumptions

Select two behaviors from the list, one in which you are most competent and one in which you are the least competent. With a colleague, address the following:

- Share the situations specific to the courageous behaviors.
- What behaviors made you feel competent?
- What behaviors/situations made you feel less than competent?
- Given the same situations, what can you do differently?

REFERENCES

Blakeney, B. (2003). Nursing's message to the world. *Creative Nursing, 9* (3), 4–8.

Chinn, P. L. (2004). *Peace and power: Creative leadership for building community* (6th ed.). Sudbury, MA: Jones and Bartlett.

Dychtwald, K., Erickson, T., & Morison, B. (2004). It's time to retire retirement. *Harvard Business Review, 82* (3), 48–57.

Emrich, L. (2004). *Nurse vigilance and practice breakdown: A study of relationships.* Unpublished master's thesis, University of Ohio, Columbus.

Fairman, J. (1992). Watchful vigilance: Nursing care, technology, and the development of intensive care units. *Nursing Research, 41* (1), 56–60.

Frieberg, K., & Frieberg, J. (2004). How gutsy leaders blow the doors off business-as-usual. *Leader to Leader, 33,* 32–37.

Hamel, G., & Valikangas, L. (2003). The quest for resilience. *Harvard Business Review, 81* (9), 52–63.

Hesselbein, F. (2004). Circles of inclusion. *Leader to Leader, 32,* 4–6.

Houweling, L. (2004). Image, function and style: A history of the nursing uniform. *American Journal of Nursing, 104* (4), 40–48.

Kennedy, H. (2000). A model of exemplary midwifery practice: Results of a delphi study. *Journal of Midwifery and Women's Health, 45* (1), 4–19.

Kuhn, T. (1996). *The structure of scientific revolutions* (3rd ed.). Chicago: University of Chicago.

Porter-O'Grady, T. (2003). Creators & dreamweavers: Building conspiracies for innovation. *Nurse Leader, 2* (1), 30–32.

SUGGESTED READINGS

Hegyvery, S. T. (2004). New partnerships, new opportunities. *Journal of Nursing Scholarship, 36* (1); 1.

Hramec, A. B. (2001). Reflections on being in the middle. *Nursing Outlook, 49,* 254–257.

CHAPTER 12

Leadership and Care of the Self

CHAPTER OBJECTIVES:

Upon completion of this chapter, the reader will:

1. Define the issues affecting the personal role of the leader and the impact of those issues on the exercise of leadership.

2. Name at least three spiritual attributes that relate to the person of the leader and that affect the exercise of good leadership.

3. Identify specific and unique elements of the personal exercise of leadership that represent the leader's ability to manage the role through chaos, change, and challenging team dynamics.

INTRODUCTION

Leadership is demanding work. There is nothing in leadership that is inherently rewarding, nor does anything generate from leadership that guarantees a continuing level of commitment and energy in the role. In fact, there are many who suggest that leadership is more challenging than rewarding.

One of the first elements of self-focus for the leader relates to an understanding that the leader must be willing to play the key role in attending to one's own needs. Leaders cannot expect in their role any real defined personal support from followers, nor should they. When leaders look for nurturance and renewal from followers, they are often disappointed. It isn't that followers won't give positive feedback, support, or encouragement to the leader, but they are not required to do so. Leaders do not ask of those being led for support, agreement, or encouragement. While it is nice when that happens, expecting it is illegitimate.

As noted previously in this book, leaders simply have no friends. The expectation of leadership does not include under its rubric the notion of friendship. It is not that the person of the leader does not have friends; it is instead that the role does not demand friendship as a part of its exercise. Therefore the leader should not expect to get the encouragement, support, and validation that friendship can offer. The leader in this set of circumstances can feel very alone.

> **Gem**
>
> Leaders must reflect in their own roles the skills of self-care. Leaders cannot take care of others if they are unable to attend to their own needs. Modeling the ability to address one's own needs positively and with a high degree of balance is the best exemplar for the staff to do the same in their own professional lives.

Some Basic Rules for the Leader

- The buck stops here.
- You're usually always alone.
- Leaders have no friends.
- Accountability begins here.
- Others are watching you, not listening to you.
- You either create or eliminate blame games.
- It's about respect, not love.
- You are partner, not parent.

Remember

Wise leaders create coalitions and partnership with other leaders. The leader knows that the only kind of understandable leadership support one can get is from other leaders experiencing the same struggles in the exercise of leadership. Leaders do not seek support from their staff. It is not that support cannot be found there, but it is inappropriate to seek it there.

Ego Management

- Develop an accurate sense of self.
- Find a good mentor or role model.
- Check personal behavior with others.
- Do a regular 360 evaluation.
- Follow up personal conflicts quickly.
- Create a personal development program.
- Assess behavior against outcomes.
- Separate the public from the private life.
- Have interests other than work.

In truth, leadership *is* a lonely exercise. The leader stands apart from all others because the role demands that this person be willing to confront, challenge, and engage others in ways that may not facilitate the development of personal relationships. Not only does the leader not have friends, the leader also often creates conditions that do not generate positive feelings toward the leader. This can make it very challenging for the leader and increases the leadership level of difficulty.

GETTING SUPPORT

While the expression of personal leadership may be a lonely experience, leaders do have support in the system. A leader is not alone in the role. Leaders share that role with others who are also experiencing the isolation, challenges, and lack of rewards in the expression of personal leadership.

It is the obligation of individual leaders to recognize the collective support that they have in the role from other leaders. Leaders must gather together to do more than simply undertake the business of the organization. The gathering of leaders should also include opportunities for support, growth and development, and encouragement in the role. It should be a time where leaders share their personal story of leadership, including what has and what has not worked. This can only occur in a collective framework in which the story of leadership is shared among the leadership community in a way that can be understood by those who share the same experience. Leaders must come to recognize that their strength lies with each other and that this horizontal leadership community provides the foundation for encouraging, supporting, and advancing the role of the leader.

What frequently occurs as people move into the role of leader is a higher level of competition emerging between and among individuals. Leadership is historically structured in its orientation and hierarchical in its expression. Often, those who ascend the leadership ladder bring with them characteristics that represent their own personal commitment to growth and development, advancing their careers, and affirming their personal impact on the organization.

Good leaders do not come without egos. The ego is a powerful human psychological tool that encourages us to develop a personal identity, a place in the world, a sense of self and person and expresses itself in individuality and in purpose. Balanced against other personality characteristics, the ego serves a sound purpose and helps the individual assertively address the vagaries and challenges of life in a complex world.

On the other hand, an out-of-control and poorly managed ego can create a great deal of difficulties in human expression and personal relationship. The undisciplined ego runs wild and creates conditions in which individuals sacrifice the values of relationship, integrity, human interaction, and friendship on the altar of personal advancement and gain. When that happens, individuals in this circumstance run through the organization as though everything was a personal fight, creating noise, continuous challenge, and, frequently, personal and relational pain. The challenge for leaders is to find balance between the personal need to grow and make a significant contribution and the ego's need to be individually recognized. Successful leaders must establish meaningful relationships to advance the interests of the organization and to build personal and professional relationships within the context of a positive workplace. This balance is often difficult to achieve. Yet it is one of the most powerful elements of the personal work of the leader and a part of the obligation the leader takes on in assuming the role.

In the 21st-century organization, much has been learned about how organizations work, the role of individuals, the characteristics of leadership, and the needs of both people and organized systems. Part of the challenge of that experience is the recognition that all individuals, regardless of what they do in a work system, have value, seek meaning, and want to fully participate in the life of the organization. Recognizing this, the leader should never operate in a way that diminishes or in any way slights the expression of these needs. All people in the workplace depend on a disciplined ego to be well managed in terms of advancing the interests of the leader but also balanced against advancing the needs of those he or she leads and of the organization of which they are all members.

A primary challenge for the leader is the recognition of the varying degrees of ego management that must exist within the leadership role in an organization. Regardless of how the role is defined or how the organization uses it or defines it in its various leadership categories, there will be a wide variety of personal expressions of the role as it unfolds in the organization. Individual leaders should recognize this diversity as essentially healthy and should also be aware that there are times when the diversity of persons can serve as an opportunity to ameliorate the impact of the ego and keep it directed to a common purpose.

Part of the challenge is for leaders to comprehend in the 21st-century organization the differences between the categories of leadership that are not simply differentiated by level of leadership (organizational chart). This comprehension does two things: (1) it helps the leader focus on the contribution of the role; and (2) it helps the leader understand the value of the essential relationship between leaders in fulfilling the goals and objectives of the organization and the needs of those who provide its work. Every leader must recognize that every leadership role must make a contribution to the organization, regardless of where the position of leadership is expressed. The purpose of leadership, essentially, is to help the organizational community attain its mutually defined goals, achieve sustainability, and advance its interests with regard to its own future. Within the context of this understanding, every category of leader must contribute at some level to the values of the organization, to its purposes, and ultimately to achieving its goals. Therefore, whenever expressing the role of leadership, individual leaders should recognize that their specific role is always significant, valid, valuable, and important to the viability and sustainability of the organizational community.

This understanding of the role of leader should help the leader move away from a traditional view in a vertical orientation of leaders to other leaders. The old notion of leader as boss is one that is no longer viable and doesn't reflect the working of the human community network. The leader recognizes that he or she is playing a role that operates in the interests of the organization, to which that role has been directed. The leader understands that advancing the goals of the organization and assuring its success comes from the collective integration of the efforts of all leaders and those who do the work of the organization. It is this notion of collective intersection and interface that drives a clearer understanding of valuing and expressing the role of the leader (**Figure 12-1**).

Leaders must understand that they are differentiated from each other simply by their obligations to the organization. Each role has a fundamentally different impact driven by different requirements, depending on the role's position and application in the

---

Watch Out for Others' Egos

- Don't be easily manipulated.
- Find a mentor who cares.
- Validate your judgment with others.
- Process whose agenda you're supporting.
- Make sure personal goals are organizational goals.
- Watch out for those who take full credit.
- Always negotiate the value of relationships.
- Fully participate in shared decision making.
- Make sure relationships are value balanced.

The Leader's Role

Leaders are defined by role, not by position. Regardless of where the role is located, it has specific contributions to make to the people and to the organization. The role is defined by that contribution, not by the position it represents. Everyone has a right to know what contribution the role makes to the organization. Defining positional status does not answer this question.

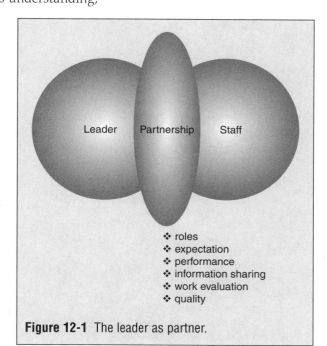

❖ roles
❖ expectation
❖ performance
❖ information sharing
❖ work evaluation
❖ quality

Figure 12-1 The leader as partner.

organization. Even with individual expectations, each role depends on the performance of other leadership roles in a way that assures the individual role contributes toward the synthesis of effort that advances both the organization and its people. No organization advances successfully upon a unilateral decision or action of the role of a single leader. Critical understanding of the mutuality and synthesis of leadership roles with regard to advancing the interests of the organization is critical to understanding organizational success. The individual leader must recognize her or his role within the context of collective leadership commitment, obligation, and purpose.

From this understanding, individual leaders come to recognize that a unilateral expression of ego at the expense of the relationship with the leadership team and others who do the work of the organization creates a deficit, not only for the organization and the achievement of its purposes but also for the exercise of individual and collective leadership. The ego-driven individual works at the expense of others and therefore fails to facilitate the relationships and interactions necessary for the collective action and wisdom of leadership.

The individual leader should bring to mind several things with regard to the balanced expression of good leadership. Each of these questions should be a part of the formation of the leader's intent in assuming the role and in expressing leadership on behalf of the organization. These questions essentially call the individual leader to discern purpose, reason, and intent for exercising the leadership role in a very personal way.

1. What personal need am I fulfilling by assuming the role of leader?
2. What satisfactions do I obtain from the expression of the role of leader?
3. What rewards am I receiving in the expression of this leadership role, and am I renewed by them?
4. How do I see my expression of this leadership role advancing the interests of the organization and the needs of those I lead?
5. How has the organization expressed what it needs from this role, and am I expressing the role as the organization sees it?
6. What difference do I think this leadership role will create for the organization?
7. What difference do I think this leadership role will make in my own life?
8. How will others' lives be better because of my exercise of this leadership role?
9. Have I written down my personal goals, needs, purposes, and expected accomplishments in my expression of this role of leader?
10. In what ways will I advance the role of other leaders in fulfilling the mission and purposes of the organization to which we are all mutually committed?

Remaining clear about one's own role and the need of that role in the expression of leadership provides a frame of reference that advances the meaning and value of the leadership role within the individual's life journey. Individuals who continually keep the above questions before them help to manage the vagaries of the ego, keep tabs on its action, and balance its force against the elements of service and purpose. Constantly attending to the need of creating an ego balance helps the individual leader keep the role in context, maintain the integrity of personal contribution, and ensure a continuing commitment to growth, development, and maturation as a good leader.

Leadership and Mutuality

Leaders are in place in organizations to achieve organizational goals. The organization is not a vehicle for the leader to achieve unilateral goals. Leaders are recognized by the extent of their capacity to advance the interests of the organization and to create a high level of success. In addition, the leader extends the same enthusiasm and commitment to the minds and the work of the staff.

Leaders Are Always Testing Their Assumptions

- About others
- About the organization
- About their role
- About individual effectiveness
- About expectations
- About understanding
- About individual responsibility
- About the direction of change
- About personal growth
- About achievement of goals

THE LEADER AS A LEARNER

Like any other pursuit, leadership is a journey. The only difference with regard to leadership is that leadership is a journey with no permanent destination. The journey that the leader represents is one of lasting commitment to personal growth, development, and improvement. What is critical for the leader is the recognition that the role requires continuous and endless personal growth and development.

No leadership role provides all that is necessary for the leader to succeed in it. The role can only be successful to the extent that there is goodness of fit between the skills of the leader and the demands of the role. This match, however, rarely occurs. Most leadership roles have demands that outstrip the ability of the leader living in the role. The vagaries and challenges of life in all of the experiences that it brings creates so much diversity and complexity that it often surpasses the skill level and the confidence of any leader, regardless of how much she or he knows and what that leader's role is in the organization.

The important issue is for the leader to acknowledge that he or she cannot know everything there is to know about the role. The more important concern is whether the leader is committed to learning and gaining insight from the expression of the role in circumstances and occasions when the demand is greater than the leader's individual skill. This is the real test of leadership.

It is not how much the leader knows. It is instead what the leader is willing to risk on the journey of development and growth in the expression of the role that is critical to effectiveness. As covered elsewhere in this book, issues of openness, vulnerability, risk taking, awareness, availability, and engagement in the role are all fundamental elements of the successful expression of the leadership role.

The leadership role reflects the journey of life. The leader is an exemplar of commitment to the full engagement of the life experience. The leader exemplifies a continuing and ongoing engagement of the vagaries and challenges of life and exemplifies in that role the willingness and ability to confront and address whatever issues life brings. They give witness for the expression of their role to those they lead, indicating thereby the appropriate mechanisms and responses to the challenges that confront all individuals in the expression of their life and their work. Leaders should exemplify the expression of the leadership role, acknowledging their openness to the unpredictability of the role and the many unfolding uncertainties and human and environmental challenges that create delight in its expression. It can be said that if leaders want to know how effective they are, they need only look at their staff: these people serve as the only valid mirror of the true effectiveness of the leader.

Leadership is not only found in the management of the rituals and routines of work. Simply engaging these routines and saying that they are successfully carried out does not signify effective leadership. In fact, managing these processes is not necessarily an expression of good leadership. This is not to suggest that good management is not necessary in undertaking the routine aspects of accomplishing work. It is. But it is important to understand that the leader's role goes beyond the basic expectations and that its expression is founded in how successfully the individual confronts those things that fall outside of the routine, challenge the normative, and raise expectations for performance. This is especially critical as the work environment continues to shift and change and increase in complexity. These many and varied situational shifts in the experience of life and work create a contextual framework for the expression of the role of leader. In fact, these variables, these challenges, and the resulting noise in the organization are the meat of the work of the leader. It is these times and these

---

Leaders Never Stop Learning

Good leaders are continually growing. Development is fundamental to the role. Good leaders are committed to personal growth and development, first in themselves and then in those they lead. Leaders should not expect competence from the staff if the leaders are not committed to personal continuing development.

Leadership Is a Journey

The good leader recognizes that leadership is a progressive and growth-driven experience. In short, it is a journey that never ends. The leader reflects this understanding within the role and acts as a beacon for those who are led so that they, too, might see the journey embedded in their own roles.

Innovation and Creativity

The work environment is continually shifting and changing, and the good leader is one who can accommodate that change. This leader:

- Adapts quickly
- Looks for subtle shifts
- Reads the landscape well
- Lives in the potential
- Is always searching for more information
- Has a diverse network of colleagues
- Continuously communicates with others

circumstances that test leadership emergence and underpin the basic constructs for leadership performance.

CHAOS AND THE DEMAND FOR LEADERSHIP

Chaos provides an opportunity to understand the operation and workings of the universe as it applies to all human life. All the vagaries of complexity, which are signs of the fundamental characteristics of the universe, have an impact on every aspect of human existence. At the personal level, chaos affects the choices that we make, the way in which we live our lives, the opportunities that are available to us, and the outcomes that result from the variety of responses we give to any demand on our energy and resources. In short, "noise" is a synonym for the operation of chaos in our lives. Noise in this case means the incongruent, sometimes inexplicable, and often unexplainable convergence of seemingly extraneous forces and factors that influence the thoughts and actions of an individual. While noise is consistent with the operation of chaos, it is not always comfortable in the context of individuals' lives. Noise represents the vagaries and inconsistencies of all processes of human experience. The wise leader, recognizing the operation of noise, functionally incorporates it into all interaction and communication.

These multidirectional and nonlinear energies associated with a quantum understanding of the universe become an important undercurrent in the expression of the role of the leader. The wise leader reflects on the reality and the permanence of noise and seeks to accommodate it through meaningful dialogue and effective processes. Early recognition that these quantum shifts and the related ebbs and flows often confound and confuse can guide the leader's thinking. The noise associated with this confusion creates a high level of incongruity and affects people's belief in their understanding and their rituals and routines. Most of the time, the leader will confront in others the pain and discomfort they feel in relationship to their own experience of chaos.

The leader must not only give evidence of accommodating the noise of chaos but also be able to exemplify a personal sense of calm in the acceptance and engagement of essential chaos. This is difficult if the leader has not concluded that incorporating chaos is a fundamental element of the role, which is necessary for incorporating both an understanding of chaos and the ability to maximize the opportunities contained therein within the context of his or her own level of tolerance and acceptance.

Personal discomfort with uncertainty and the vagaries of change require that the leader be able to reflect on his or her own personal accommodations to change. If the leader does not find adaptation to change consonant with personal expectations, it will be difficult to guide others into acceptance of their own change. This does not mean that the leader must be free from struggle or conflict associated with adjusting to major change. It does mean that the leader represents in personal behavior a willingness, openness, and engagement of the challenges, demands, and noise of change. It is this willingness that attests to and demonstrates the leader's personal engagement of the realities of change and a peaceful accommodation of their impact on the expression of the role.

This accommodation means that the leader undergoes reflection and personal dialogue, finding a place in the change experience where he or she can be at peace with the demands for change and the vagaries and inconsistencies of transformation in the chaos embedded in all

---

Gem

The leader recognizes the value of chaos in change. The leader always uses strategic opportunities embedded in chaos to create the conditions and circumstances that generate a demand for change. For the leader, chaos serves as an opportunity for personal and collective transformation and provides the vehicle for changing behaviors.

Leading In the Middle of Chaos

In the midst of the chaos the leader always:

- Remains calm
- Finds deeper meaning
- Translates meaning into action
- Engages others
- Translates signposts
- Stimulates dialogue
- Keeps people moving
- Gives form to the chaos
- Describes new behavior
- Changes expectations

The Value of Personal Reflection

Effective leaders recognize that they cannot guide others through the chaos if they find themselves unnerved by it and challenged in the way in which they fail to cope. The leader is continuously self-reflective.

- Finds time apart
- Can focus in a quiet place
- Does daily reading
- Focuses on one insight each day
- Translates insights into action
- Encourages others to reflect
- Maintains a calm demeanor

change processes. Arriving at this point is not easy. What is critical for the leader is the ability to reflect personally on those forces and factors that affect her or his ability to accommodate the chaos and noise of quantum change. There are several factors that can influence the leader's accommodation and engagement of the personal challenges in addressing the experience of chaos. They are:

1. *The willingness to look at life as a journey.* The wise leader engages the vagaries of change by recognizing the broader journey. This leader understands that life is a longer set of challenges that when looked at individually can overwhelm. However, when each challenge is looked at in the larger set of challenges and aggregated within the context of the life journey, each does not appear as daunting and overwhelming as it might without context. The leader begins to recognize that all processes in each element of the experience are dynamic, continuous, and endless. They are simply a portion of a longer journey that requires a deeper vision and more critical understanding of the link between individual action and the aggregated processes of life experience.

2. *The leader has developed highly refined reflective skills.* The ability to reflect, analyze, and evaluate individual occurrences within the context of larger occurrences is critical to the effectiveness of the expression of the leader's role and to helping others move through change. Leaders who react to change in the same fashion as their followers provide no real guidance or value to those followers. The followers have a right to expect that the leader has taken time to reflect on the issues confronting them, to have sorted through that which is viable and valuable and that which is not. Followers have a right to expect that the leader has taken all of the information and data with regard to change and has incorporated it into the larger journey in a way that is meaningful and valuable and contributes to mutual outcomes. The leader must be able to demonstrate that an accurate acknowledgment of the change process has been made, disciplined by a sound reflection of its context, its impact on the staff, and its ultimate impact on the goals and direction of the organization. This personal facility for reflection and for discernment is critical to the effectiveness of the leader's role in contemporary systems.

3. *The leader can translate the chaos of change into language followers understand.* As indicated in prior chapters, translation skills are important in the leader's toolbox. What is more important at the personal level is the leader's ability to translate the impact of change on his or her own life. Indeed, the leader sees the elements and circumstances of change within the context out of which they are unfolding rather than the window of the experience of the past. As a team leader, there are always many challenges in implementing any change. What is important to the leader as an individual is an understanding of the demand of that change and a personal adaptation to incorporating that change within the context of the individual's own personal journey of change. Leaders should never ask followers to engage in change the leader has not already engaged. Leaders reflect in their behavior what they can expect to see in their own staff. At a personal level, the leader must be able to acknowledge the personal challenges, adaptations, and experiences of a given change so as to have already translated it into personal experience and applied it to accommodating behaviors. Through this process of lived leadership, the individual leader provides a framework out of which others can witness the leader's own struggle with

---

Managing the Journey

The leader fits the particular experiences of unit, service, and department with the larger journey of the organization. This goodness of fit assures a seamless connection between person, team, and system. To do this the leader focuses on:

- Translating goals into practices
- Finding points of good fit between service and system
- Engaging individuals toward organizational goals
- Assuring internal service matches external culture
- Individual performance fulfills organizational goals
- All team members are enthused in their work

Translating Chaos

Leaders make chaos understandable to all those they lead by:

- Anticipating the changes
- Discerning the impact
- Participating in design
- Telling the story
- Sorting through the irrelevant
- Defining meaning
- Reducing "noise"
- Gathering the stakeholders
- Celebrating the moment

change, and through positive experience, be able to adapt to the acceptance skills in the lives of each follower.

4. *Leaders love the future.* Leaders give followers an opportunity to hope. It is this commitment and belief in the possibility of the future that most exemplifies the positive experiences of life. This desire to be a part of creating the future, to be a designer, is the most powerful example of truly sustainable engagement. If the leader can represent these characteristics in his or her own role, they translate into acceptance in others.

5. *Leaders embrace all of the activities that relate to creating a desirable future.* Preferable futures rarely arrive on their own. People give their future form and substance. Leaders in highly changing circumstances bear witness to the capacity to give personal form to the future so that followers may by example be able to do so in their own lives. The reflective and engaging leader stops momentarily to take stock of the impact of the change at the personal level and how that change has been translated into a way that can be reflected in the leader's behaviors. This reflected pattern of application becomes the behavior that staff see and for them exemplifies the appropriate lived application of the role to their own experience.

6. *Leaders overcome their individual fear of making bad choices.* The journey of change and moving toward the future always looks uncertain. Since the future has not been created simply because one sees it or discerns the direction toward it, its form and substance are still unclear. Whatever form the future will take depends on the individual response. There is always fear that the response will not match the demand. Leaders, however, exemplify a willingness to engage the risk of uncertainty and even failure in order to exemplify a willingness to embrace the construct, the elements that make up the journey to the future. This change process and the cycles of activities related to it call the leader to make sense of the individual components and, subsequently, the integration of each component necessary to a successful change journey. This willingness to confront the challenges and face the vagaries of an unformed future model leads the staff to more appropriate patterns of response in their own behavior and makes it safe to confront their own issues. This modeling, this openness to uncertainties and risks, is more important in making meaningful change than even the skills and successes. Time, effort, gains, and losses will all impact the effectiveness of response and will either teach or direct leaders and followers about their failures or encourage them to be successful in unfolding essential change for themselves.

It is important for the leader to understand these processes as a part of the individual adaptation to change (**Figure 12-2**). It is the leader's behavior that has an impact on followers. If leaders cannot appropriately engage

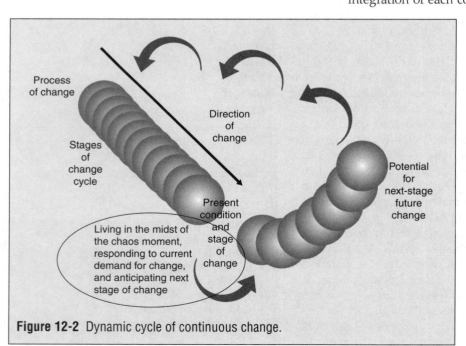

Figure 12-2 Dynamic cycle of continuous change.

the demands of change through personal reflection, adaptation, and application, it cannot be expected that followers will be able to do so. It becomes critical for leaders to note at what level of doubt and personal courage they themselves are reacting to change and then model the level of safety for the staff in experiencing the same concerns. Whether the interpretation of the change is accurate or even appropriate, it is critical that the leader give evidence of comfort and confidence with regard to the vagaries of the quantum change process. Without this level of perceived comfort there can be no translation of ease in managing change to the staff. Without an internal sense of confidence, a good compass with regard to the direction of change, and a process for discernment and reflection, the leader cannot translate to the staff the behaviors or the insights appropriate to the accommodation of meaningful change.

PRINCIPLES OF UNCERTAINTY

The leader reflects in his or her own role the accommodation and acceptance of the characteristics and elements of uncertainty as a lived experience. The leader understands the following principles, which are always conditional within the exercise of leadership and have an impact on the behavior and expression of the role:

1. *The universe is a work in progress.* It continues to unfold and become. The universe is not a finished creation and, as such, represents the dynamic associated with "becoming." The leader, therefore, understands that individuals, organizations, and systems, like the universe itself, are continually transforming and changing.

2. *Chaos and complexity are the essential constituents of the universe.* They do not go away, and they will never end. The universe can never be understood outside of its own condition of complexity, chaos, and uncertainty. This complexity and chaos as well as uncertainty relate to the endless becoming of the universe and the dynamic and inherent changes that unfold as a part of the complex interface of the array of factors acting in concert to influence whatever the universe will become.

3. *Everything in the universe is ultimately self-organizing.* All of the elements of the universe, including its patterns, mosaic, web, and intersections, create a framework requiring a high goodness of fit such that all of the elements work in concert (synthesis) to create the very next stage of change. This interconnectedness exemplifies the self-organizing and critical relationship existing at the intersection of all elements of the universe.

4. *Individuals, as a part of this universal constant, become cocreators of the future.* It is a willingness to deeply engage in the activities of transformation and change that empowers individuals in the role of cocreation. Whatever generates from their effort is the form the future will take. This understanding that every individual influences the form and substance of change is important in valuing the process of change. At this level of understanding, change activities (or lack of them), when aggregated, create the conditions and circumstances that influence the form all change will ultimately take.

5. *All individuals, teams, organizations, and systems are smaller reflections of the totality of the universe.* In each individual, the

---

The Leader's Internal Enemies

The greatest impediment to leadership success are the demons that live within. Most leaders who fail do so because of their own personal issues with regard to their role and relationship to success. Leaders need to watch out for:

1. Self-fulfilling prophecies of failure
2. Internal insecurities
3. Poor leadership vision
4. Failure to engage stakeholders
5. Inability to develop meaningful relationships
6. Internal and unspoken fear
7. Continuously hidden agendas
8. Failure to identify with the goals of the organization
9. Failing to help the boss succeed
10. A lack of personal self-belief

Unfinished Universe

The universe is unfinished work. So is the work of leadership. Leaders must never consider their work done. There is no measure of completeness; nothing is ever finished in the exercise of leadership. Leaders are in play the entire time that they are in the role. It is a role whose work is never done and whose task is never finished. Persons move through leadership, never complete it.

The Leader as Cocreator

The leader joins in the collective enterprise of creation, accessing and maximizing all resources, joining in the creative process, and working to create a sustainable future. Elements of cocreation include the following:

- A comprehension of the integrity of all things
- Empowering the collective wisdom
- Recognizing the themes of change
- Developing an aggregated vision
- Translating vision into action
- Encouraging and supporting others
- Enumerating the meaning of everyone's contribution
- Acknowledging and recognizing accomplishment
- Keeping moving

Gem

It is important for the leader to understand the rules of complexity and the quantum processes operating in the universe. Just as these principles operate at the universal level, they also act at the individual level. The more the leader understands the action of complexity in all activities of human life and applies those principles to the process of leadership, the more effective the leader becomes.

---

complexity and dynamic of the entire universe are operating. The leader understands that the same dynamic of complexity, fluidity, and convergence is occurring at the local level as it unfolds in the entire universe. Therefore, every action, every person, every situation is, in one way or another, contributing to the aggregated action of the universe as it works to continuously and dynamically construct a future.

It is imperative for the leader to understand these principles as a fundamental constituent of the expression of the role of the leader. These principles and universal forces are acting continuously. It is through this ever-present movement of the universe with the confluence of human action that essential change is sustained. The success of the leader is directly determined by the competence of his or her own actions with the principles that guide the functions of change across the universal landscape.

LEADERSHIP AND CREATIVITY

It is vital for leaders to fully understand the expectations and functions of the role in light of knowledge generation and management. If the leader cannot live in the potential that is created in the tension between the present and future, it is likely the role will be compromised. Leaders must always demonstrate in their own role a personal pattern of positive response to the challenges of change invariably embedded in every aspect of leadership expression. Leaders must demonstrate in their own behavior that they have committed to fully engaging all of their resources in addressing change and the effort to create congruence between change and people's response to it. As the universe inevitably unfolds in undifferentiated and chaotic ways, yet represents a self-organizing facility, so must the leader demonstrate a capacity for making sense out of pieces. Since the universe evidences in every aspect of its unfolding the creative and innovative characteristics of uncertainty and of movement, so must the leader demonstrate her or his ability to positively embrace the challenges and vagaries of change. A level of joyfulness, even enthusiasm, must be exemplified within the context of the leader's role so that that enthusiasm can be contagious and evidenced in the roles of followers.

The Leadership Skill of Enthusiasm

- Recognizing the positive forces of change
- Telling the story of the larger journey of change
- A willingness to embrace the stages of life
- A personal aura of joy
- An infectious level of energy
- An ability to translate idea into action

Creating New Mental Models

Mental models reflect the way of thinking and of subsequently acting. They provide a context within which structure and behavior can unfold. The leader creates this frame for thinking and acting in order to encourage followers to give form and substance, resulting in an effective applied model. This work includes:

- The description of the change context for work
- Articulation of the influences affecting work processes
- Generating new rules affecting thinking and acting
- Elucidating the impact of new concepts, technology, and applications
- Stimulating others to identify creative response to changing circumstance

---

Enthusiasm

The leader must exemplify a level of energy and joy with regard to work and relationships. If the leader does not exemplify personal joy and happiness in the role of leader, there should be no expectation that joy and enthusiasm will be present in the role of the follower. Remember, leaders create context. The context created by the leader exemplifies the patterns of behavior that will be positively generated in the organization. A part of the challenge of creating good context is a personal joy and satisfaction leaders brings to their role and relationship with others. Somber and morose leaders can expect the same in their staff. If there is a clear engagement of the challenge and excitement of change present in the responses of the leader, it is likely that those behaviors will be present in the roles of the followers.

If the mental model for the role of the leader is that life is unfair, work is overbearing, and opportunities are nonexistent, it can be expected that will be reflected in the context that is created for the staff. The staff live the context that is provided for them in the role of the leader. The staff take their cue from the behavioral pattern of the leader and represent in their own behavior the mental model that the leader creates. It is therefore essential that the leader reflect in her or her his own role a level of joy and enthusiasm in confronting the opportunities and challenges of life. If the leader sees the journey of life as an opportunity for growth and advancement, it is likely staff will feel the same.

FOLLOWERS AS COCREATORS

Just as the leader represents a clear reflection of persons as cocreators in unfolding the future, the staff are cocreators with the leader in creating and providing substance for change. This notion of cocreator empowers followers to fully invest in the options and opportunities that derive out of their own role in creating a direction and response to the future. Cocreators are originators of the future, designers if you will, and in that role, begin to give the future whatever form it will take.

This is a powerful image. The leader creates this image in order to fully enable the followers to embrace the challenges of their own experience of change, both as individuals and as a team. This gives them full control over the circumstances and influences that result from their own choice and full participation. The leader communicates to the followers that full participation is an expectation of membership on the team and of their own personhood. Through that empowerment, the leader creates a level of intensity of response that ensures generativity, originality, and innovation in the team's movement toward creating their own future.

> ### Originality and Innovation
>
> The leader values—indeed, treasures—the creative impulse present in all people. The leader creates a context in which it is safe to experiment and to risk, allowing the staff to:
>
> 1. Attempt new approaches to old work
> 2. Identify new ways of working
> 3. Challenge existing policies and practices
> 4. Evaluate work processes for effectiveness
> 5. Bring in new reading, thinking, people to raise questions about existing practices

Chaos and the Need for Order

While chaos is an essential constituent of all change, it brings with it its own embedded sense of order. The order that we usually see in organizations really acts as a synonym for stability. While stability is desirable, it is also an inadequate notion. A certain level of personal stability needs to be present if the organization is to move confidently forward. However, stability should not be offered as a replacement for the challenges of transformation. Chaos brings with it a need for order. The kind of order that the leader provides is an order of confidence, support, presence, and continuity. The leader acts in the role of stabilizer by keeping the promise of presence, of faithfulness, of continuance with the workers in meeting the challenges of change. Stability comes from the constant confidence represented by the leader's encouragement, support, enthusiasm, information, and mobilization. This constant and consistent leadership support for the activities of the followers in the processes of creativity and innovation is the only stability and consistency necessary for effective change.

The Leader as Opportunity Creator

The leader as innovator and creator always sees the future through the eyes of opportunity. The leader becomes for the follower a living example of hope in the engagement of the future. Leadership becomes for those it influences a model of living in the potential, recognizing that the future is always open to the creative act. The person of the leader sees the future as a blank slate, an opportunity to give form and direction to human effort. The leader represents in her or his own behavior a full engagement of the range of resources and the creative processes necessary to ensure that the form change takes is meaningful and viable and makes a substantive difference to individuals and organizations.

Furthermore, leadership experience is not enough for the creative process. While experience is valuable, it does not in and of itself provide the full range of skills necessary to embrace and create a new future. Education and openness to learning is as necessary to effective and

> ### Creating New Opportunity
>
> - Identify ways of changing work
> - Allow the creation of new prototypes
> - Stimulate lateral thinking
> - Reward staff for innovation
> - Share credit with creators
> - Celebrate innovation often
> - Bring in new ideas, new reading
> - Set aside time for innovative conversation
> - Include other disciplines in creative dialogue
> - Create storyboards of new work processes
> - Present creative and innovative work to others

Putting Experience in Its Place

Experience is valuable. But it can also be a limitation. The wise leader is not held hostage to claims of experience. The leader knows that experience represents a validation of the past, of what has gone on before. In a time of critical and dramatic change, experience can become a serious impediment, crippling vision and taxing the creative impulse. We build on experience; we do not limit response because we have experience. Many organizations have died on the altar of experience as it precluded their availability to the transformative action of the new and innovative and impeded their ability to adapt.

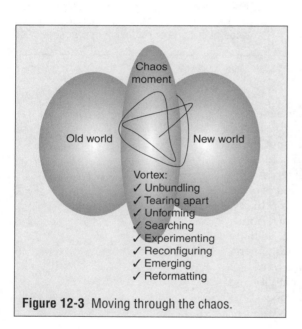

Figure 12-3 Moving through the chaos.

Projecting a Sense of Self

1. Clarity with regard to your own values
2. Understanding what the leader role means to you
3. Ability to put the role in the right context
4. Existence of a life outside of work
5. Evidence that you take time for yourself
6. Ability to hold firm to what you know is right
7. Willingness to advocate for what is true
8. Confidence in the exercise of one's role
9. Access to spiritual source of strength
10. Frequent self-renewal and time away

desirable future planning as is knowledge and experience. Experience is mostly about the past, reflective of those things already accomplished. It is insufficient as a tool for leaders to draw upon to give insights and information with regard to the direction of change. While experience can give the leader many sets of tools that he or she can use in anticipating changes, those tools are often not adequate in addressing the changes observed or the potential impact of those changes on individuals and organizations. Quite often new tools need to be created. Therefore, the leader embraces opportunities for new learning and new ways of thinking and seeing, creating, and doing. Envisioning a new context tied to past experience helps the leader translate that vision into a plan of action and implementation.

Living with Uncertainty and Mess

Change is messy. The leader, as indicated earlier, is comfortable with the mess and the noise of change and creates a place where others can be comfortable as well. However, just as important is the ability to confront the logical, systematic, organized, structured, and formal processes in the organization that themselves can act as an impediment to creativity and innovation. Also, the leader can personally impede creativity and change to the extent that he or she desires the stability and the safety of structure. In the old organization, formal structure is predicated against disarray and disorganization. Order was itself a desirable condition. In the midst of great change, order disappeared, as the ability to engender positive response out of the noise and messiness of change became critical to effective adaptation. In the midst of all change old structures and processes fall apart. Indeed, old structures are forced apart by those who are attempting to create an organized response to a demand for change in the organization. In the midst of such change, it is critical for the leader to be able to unbundle an attachment to order and to find embedded in the midst of a demand for change a creative response to the destructive process.

Positive destruction means purposely breaking apart or tearing down the organizational structures and systems in order to create the vacuum out of which new forms, structures, and systems can unfold. Without creating this opportunity for deconstruction, there is limited availability and openness for the new, the different, the innovative. The leader, understanding this dynamic, regularly examines current structures and organizational stability in an effort to challenge them when they impede new forms, structures, and innovations (**Figure 12-3**).

Leaders Always Preserve Their Sense of Self

In the midst of all of change and challenges of transformation, it is easy for the individual to lose a sense of identity and of personhood. The leader must always be aware of the struggle for identity in a changing organizational system. Understanding one's own role and meaning in undertaking change is critical to surviving it. Often individuals will identify that they have burned out because their work has changed. Work always changes. It can never remain constant. If one finds meaning in work, it is clear that one's meaning is located in the wrong place. Meaning drives work. Work is a reflection of value of purpose. If meaning becomes lost in the purpose of doing the work, the value of it gets lost, too.

It is often easy to embed one's identity within the context of work. When that happens and work changes, meaning and identity can become lost. The leader must periodically reflect in the course of his or her own activities on the meaning and purpose for those activities. As the activities themselves change, reflecting on the meaning of work and its purpose calls the leader to remain grounded in those values and principles that guide personal action and validate individual identity. Leaders who get swept up in the work of change and transformation frequently get lost in that work. As the work unfolds or as it gets completed, emotional dissatisfaction, depression, and even a lack of direction can sometimes emerge. The completion of work should not result in a loss of direction. Completing a particular job, task, or assignment does not mean that the work is ended. It means instead that the tasks associated with the continuum of transformation in change have moved on to demand a different response and unique set of emergent activities. Remaining in touch with one's meaning allows the vagaries and inconsistencies associated with changing and transforming work to continue to stimulate change without threatening value and meaning over the course of that change. Keeping in touch with this purpose and meaning ensures for the leader a grounding in values and the representation of the sustainability of personal principle. Good leaders always act in concert with the team.

> ### Sustaining a Sense of Direction
>
> The leader recognizes that any particular work falls within the context of a greater concert. Occasionally "going to the balcony" provides the leader an opportunity to develop a broader and deeper insight with regard to the context of change affecting the activities and practices of daily work. The leader regularly visits the balcony to see work at a longer distance, translate the journey in broader terms, instill meaning in the activities of the worker, and deepen the sense of meaning for all members of the team.

Individual Action Cannot Stand Alone

In moving toward meaningful change, the collective energies and efforts of all are necessary to create sustainability in the change. The leader guides all members of the team in a common direction committed to achieving aggregated value for the team and for the purposes the team is directed to fulfill. All change operates within the context of team values. The leader recognizes that if the organization changes, its people have also changed. The rules, processes, conditions, and elements of growing and changing act both individually and collectively. Whatever its work, the team moves ahead, acting in concert and working together to create the conditions of living in a new way and acting in a new place.

The Leader Constantly Assesses His or Her Relationship with the Team

The intensity of the leader's relationship and the quality of the interaction is a determinant of the success of the work of the organization. Since most of that work is accomplished through effective team action, the leader is critically aware that his or her efforts guide the organization to sustainable success. Discernment is a greater gift than definition. The leader constantly reflects on the relational needs of the team, the needs of individuals, even the need of the leader in relationship to his or her team. Leaders must recognize that they need from their team a sense of support, affiliation, and renewal, just as the team needs that from the leader. The leader must make this known to the team. This is a collaborative relationship. The ebbs and flows of personal interaction and collective action have as much impact on the leader as they do on the team. The person of the leader needs an opportunity for expression, communication affiliation, and collective action with a full understanding that those integrated activities can lead to both individual and group success. Therefore, the leader must make clear to team members the leader's needs in terms of communication, interaction, support, and performance from followers. Fulfilling the individual leader's needs as well as attending to the followers' needs creates a dynamic of interaction and intersection between leader and team that is essential to maintaining the energy and the commitment to continuous and dynamic change.

> ### Effective Leaders Always Work Through Teams
>
> Leaders are continually working with groups, attempting to move many people through the process of change and innovation. Therefore, team skills are an important fundamental for all leadership roles. Leaders need to understand:
>
> - Work always gets done through teams.
> - Teams require a lot of horizontal communication.
> - Teams need good information.
> - Teams are always looking for encouragement.
> - All teams experience conflict.
> - Facilitating teams requires great group skills.
> - Leaders must constantly remind teams of goals.
> - The major leader's work is maintaining team relationships.
> - Team outcomes are more sustainable than individual results.

Team Culture

All teams have their unique characteristics. The wise leader assesses the particular communication, relationship, and interactional dynamics of individual teams, and through that process begins to understand the team's identity. That identity is unique to the team and informs the leader what will work best in motivating and leading that team.

Leadership Is Never Easy Work

The leader recognizes that the demands of leadership are ever changing, depending on the circumstances and the need of the team and the goals of the organization.

Organizations are dynamic entities, constantly in motion, requiring continuous reevaluation and reconfiguration of the efforts of work around ever-changing goals. This creates emotional demand on both leader and follower, increasing the need for support, time away from work, rest, and relaxation.

Gem

Leaders simply cannot maintain the energy necessary to the role without a mechanism of renewal and regeneration. Whatever the spiritual values that lie at the heart of the individual leader's personal principles, they need to act as a source of reflection and regeneration. A leader with no spiritual center is a leader who acts with no soul.

Leadership Work Is Not Easy Work

No one should stay in the role of leader without a clear and discerning understanding of the implications of the exercise of leadership. All of the demands of leadership and the needs of the leader must be carefully considered every moment that leadership is being expressed. The person of the leader is like any other individual in the organization. This person has strengths and weaknesses, good moments and bad moments, ups and downs, all of which influence the effectiveness of the leader's expression of the role. The leader must attend to the person inside and address whatever specific individual needs give reason, value, and meaning for exercising the role. Continuous and constant reflection of the role, the dynamics influencing the expression of the role, the relationships necessary to maintaining the energy and commitment in the role, and the personal challenges and facilities the individual brings to the role must be renewed if there is to be any success in the expression of leadership.

SPIRITUAL INTELLIGENCE: FINDING THE COURAGE WITHIN

Spiritual integrity is an essential component of good leadership expression. Leadership is not simply a set of skills but is in fact a discipline. The term *discipline* means that leadership has its own set of rules and characteristics, demands, and criteria for its appropriate and sustainable expression. Leaders must express the role, not only to lead and direct the process of change but also to create the conditions by which change itself is experienced by others. Therefore, the leader is intimately aware of the impact of change on the leader's own person and confronts that impact with openness and personal availability. The leader must be able to adapt to the change and exemplify adaptability and fluidity in meeting the demands and the vagaries of shifting work obligations. Leaders, therefore, are always involved in seeking and reaching their own potential.

Leaders cannot, however, reach their potential without reflecting deeply on their own relationship to life and to their own personal spiritual journey. Leadership demands great courage and persistence. It confronts high elements of risk and of pervasive challenge. Leaders are constantly living in a potential between current reality and the unfolding future. This is a place of great demand and risk. The leader is called to translate the potential into a language that followers can understand. In order to do this, the leader must be able to understand the potential within his or her own experience and give it a personal language so that it has meaning in the self-expression of the role. Leaders are always making others aware of meaning and purpose in change and help others ultimately seek the direction necessary to achieve meaningful change. As a result, leaders must live on the cutting edge; they must constantly be pushing the boundaries of consciousness and of innovation. Leaders focus the staff's energies on confronting their own behaviors, perceptions, and actions in relationship to the change process. In order to do this successfully, leaders must be clear through their own expression of leadership about what the change means, the direction of that change, and the value of that change as a part of their own personal leadership expression.

Leaders are often on the cutting edge of change. When one is on the cutting edge of change, there is limited support, sometimes even limited understanding, with regard to the change. The leader is often looked at as an anomaly, perhaps as an organizational pain, and as a result doesn't have much support even perhaps from followers. Having confronted the vagaries and challenges of change and the independence needed to undertake meaningful change, the leader comes to more clearly accept the fact that leadership is often a lonely experience. However, being in touch with the spiritual values in the expression of that role and recognizing the essential loneliness of the role can cause the leader to draw on spiritual resources, which can be a source of strength.

The leader recognizes that he or she cannot take care of others if they cannot take care of themselves. Self-sacrifice, abandonment of individuality, or being long-suffering or passive are mindless energies that can take over if the leader is not fully aware of the values and purposes for undertaking any particular action. Good leaders have a strong sense of their own identity and values and stay completely in touch with those motives and intentions that relate or exemplify the values that lie at the core of their own leadership. Leaders recognize the essential elements and characteristics of change, are able to identify where individuals and organizations are in their transition to change, and are able to identify the most appropriate responses in any given time and place. Time for reflection, discernment, exploration, and clarification are all elements of the leader's spiritual skill set. The leader will draw on the conclusions and assessments made in moments of reflection and will make choices that reflect deeper meaning and ultimately respect the connection with the self that indicates the leader's ability to understand, willingness to risk, and expression of energy necessary to engage and undertake successful change.

The universe is full of mystery and creative uncertainty. The leader's individual personal beliefs and traditions bring the leader to understand that the universe is full of mystery, uncertainty, and many challenges to change. Most of our beliefs accommodate those things we do not know. However as we become clearer about what we can know, that knowledge can confront the very beliefs that are central to our fundamental value system. The leader is open to challenge and to exploring what knowledge does in terms of beliefs and past practices. Knowledge should reflect light into our beliefs so that we do not hold blindly onto those that knowledge can easily address, challenge, and change.

The leader should always remember that the universe is in continuous motion, constantly shifting and adapting and changing its own form and direction. Still, deeply embedded is a sense of order and systemness that reflects a set of principles and processes that are as ancient as creation and as contemporary as the latest creative act. No change happens simply for its own sake. All change is a reflection of the greater concert, such that when linked with all other efforts it creates a symphony or mosaic (a synthesis) that ultimately deepens the picture of understanding that we have of the change itself. Our beliefs should not be so rigid and so fixed that the revelation of science and the generation of new knowledge cannot inform and advance our beliefs. This is as much a part of the spiritual journey as any other element.

What is also important is to respect the value of prayer, whatever that might reflect for the leader. There are many kinds of religious and spiritual practices that an individual can draw on in terms of expressing meaning and value through prayer. Whatever that tradition is for the leader, it should encourage and strengthened the individual, help realign the individual's energies and principles, and continuously motivate the individual to seek higher levels of performance and to advance individual and collective levels of understanding and application. However prayer renews, strengthens, and encourages, it should refresh the individual and renew individual effort in the leadership role and in meeting the challenges of change.

Finally, the leader exemplifies in the context of his or her own role a clear understanding that all efforts, regardless of whether they are related to work or home, are all part of a larger journey of transformation change and growth. The leader

Gem

Leaders are always advocates. That can sometimes position the leader to act individually, swim upstream, confront organizational leadership, create team discomfort, and slow progress. The courageous leader recognizes these times will occasionally arise and will call for personal commitment, energy, and clarity in helping the organization perceive that which is most difficult yet essential to its own growth.

Leadership and Mystery

Not everything can be knowable or understandable at once. The leader recognizes that embedded in every activity, change and possibility are elements of uncertainty that reflect the unknowing and mystery embedded in all human experience. The leader comes to appreciate the value of this finding and sees it as a representation of the eternal curiosity that continues to motivate, encourage, and inspire.

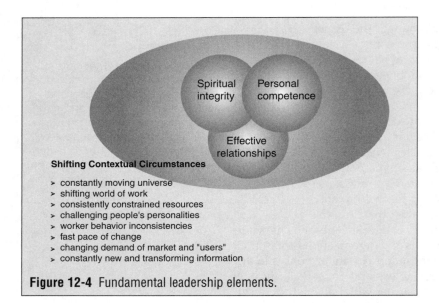

Shifting Contextual Circumstances

- constantly moving universe
- shifting world of work
- consistently constrained resources
- challenging people's personalities
- worker behavior inconsistencies
- fast pace of change
- changing demand of market and "users"
- constantly new and transforming information

Figure 12-4 Fundamental leadership elements.

Gem

The transforming leader comes to understand the leader's work as a part of a great opus. The leader recognizes in everyone's effort an individual contribution to a greater effort that when aggregated to all efforts contributes to the dance of the universe, advancing, revealing, renewing, and enhancing all of human experience. No matter how small the effort, it is an essential contributor to the mosaic of the living universe.

The Creative Leader

Leaders are the purveyors, stimulators, and energizers of organized creativity. Therefore, the leader must exemplify the creative spirit by the following methods:

- Has a love of play
- Exhibits a little craziness
- Displays an affection for experimentation
- Enjoys game playing
- Translates idea into action
- Encourages different thinking
- Creates a safe space
- Allows others to innovate
- Sees life as an opportunity

Time Is Not the Enemy

Good leaders recognize that time is a gift, not a weapon. One major gift of human life is the ability for people to control their use of time. Time is a gift, a tool, a talent, nothing more. Leaders recognize that how time is used is a universal issue and the proper use of time is the greatest vehicle for creativity, innovation, and the full experience of life.

reflects the challenges of expressing the role of the leader, substantiating that all change is normal and should be expected as a fundamental part of the exercise of work. Translating this within the context of one's own efforts creates for the leader the primary drive for the role in relationship to those she or he leads. People can change by design or by default. It is a requisite of the leader to help during change by designing so that others are not affected in a negative way, having failed to see the implications and actions of change soon enough for it to make a difference in their own lives. Therefore the discernment of potential change is a critical element in the role of the leader. By applying the skill of understanding and translation, the leader is able to give a voice to change, its meaning, and its application in the lives of all those he or she meets. To do this, the leader must be in touch with this dynamic within her or his own person (**Figure 12-4**).

The leader is a creator. As a creator she or he joins the other creators, regardless of their location in the organization, to build a frame for the creative journey in the movement toward innovation and adaptation in organizations and in people. No one can provide the meaning and value for other individuals with strength and courage if the meaning and value is unable to emerge within the context of that individual's life. Imagine the number of leaders working in the world who use the role as the exercise of their own inadequacies. How many leaders attempt to obtain the role for power, ego renewal, personal support, and adulation? Leaders who need the role for these purposes end up using it as a personal vehicle rather than an opportunity for organizational and team creativity and advancement. Often these people need the role more than the role needs them.

The journey of leadership, like the journey of life, should be an experience that is without boundaries. Leadership is life lived in the white spaces, between the lines. In this place, the leader recognizes that the work is to create an opportunity, a frame of reference, a contextual framework where others are free to create, relate, grow, and advance, both as persons and as the organization. The leader accurately reads the signposts of the journey, translates them in a language that others can understand, and then joins with those willing to engage the journey in a meaningful experience that helps create the future. To do this, the leader must be able to engage personally, have a spiritual depth and a sense of purpose and continuous renewal. The leader must set aside time for the self, the spirit, and the energy renewal necessary to continue the process of leadership. This spiritual and personal transformation is a continuous dynamic that calls the leader to an ever-unfolding dance between present and future, personal and collective, and real and potential.

In the final analysis, the leader cannot create change in others if she or he cannot engage that same change within. This ability to identify with both change and followers is an important criteria for the measurement of great leadership. Leaders must attend to their own needs, but only in the context of how those needs ultimately serve the greater good of those they lead. Self-care, self-assessment, translation of leadership skills into the language of others, and joining of all human energy in the creative act of building a preferable future is the best testament to success in the role.

SUGGESTED READINGS

Allcorn, S. (2002). *Death of the spirit in the American workplace.* Westport, CT: Quorum Books.

Bar-On, R., & Parker, J. D. A. (2000). *The handbook of emotional intelligence: Theory, development, assessment, and application at home, school, and in the workplace.* San Francisco: Jossey-Bass.

Conger, J. A. (1994). *Spirit at work: Discovering the spirituality in leadership.* San Francisco: Jossey-Bass.

Giacalone, R. A., & Jurkiewicz, C. L. (2003). *Handbook of workplace spirituality and organizational performance.* Armonk, NY.

M. E. Sharpe, Harrison, O. (2007). *The spirit of leadership: Liberating the leader in each of us.* San Fransisco: Berrett-Khoehler.

Kalakota, R., & Robinson, M. (2001). *E-business 2.0: Roadmap for success.* Addison-Wesley information technology series. Boston: Addison-Wesley.

Kennedy, S. (1975). *Nurturing corporate images: Total communication or ego trip?* Cranfield, England: Cranfield Institute Press for the School of Management, pp. 39–83.

Kilmann, R. H., & Kilmann, I. (1994). *Managing ego energy: The transformation of personal meaning into organizational success.* Jossey-Bass management series. San Francisco: Jossey-Bass.

Kincaid, J. W. (2003). *Customer relationship management: Getting it right.* Upper Saddle River, NJ: Prentice Hall PTR.

Mitroff, I. I. (2004). *Crisis leadership: Planning for the unthinkable.* Hoboken, NJ: Wiley.

Monroe, M. (2004). *The spirit of leadership.* Kensington, PA: Anchors Press.

Owen, H. (1999). *The spirit of leadership: Liberating the leader in each of us.* San Francisco: Berrett-Koehler.

Rubin, H. (2002). *Collaborative leadership: Developing effective partnerships in communities and schools.* Thousand Oaks, CA: Corwin Press.

Spitzer, R. J. (2000). *The spirit of leadership: Optimizing creativity and change in organizations.* Provo, UT: Executive Excellence, Publication 344.

SCENARIO 1: COMFORT WITH CHAOS

Jane sat in the strategy meeting and began to feel the rising pressure of tension within. The hospital was outlining a whole new direction for clinical services. This meeting involved establishing a different framework for the delivery of clinical services and was reemphasizing mobility-based and outpatient clinical services in place of the past focus of inpatient clinical care. For Jane, this meant a complete shift in the service structure and orientation of her clinical unit. Her concern was heightened as she reflected on a recent shift in the focus of her clinical service and the reorientation of the medical staff to different models of medical care. On top of this change, a new electronic medical record had been introduced and the clinical staff was struggling with adapting to documenting and recording of care in that new model. New challenges with regard to quality priorities had also been initiated in the past year, calling all clinical providers to refocus their activities using a new quality format that would better document clinical process and the achievement of outcomes. In addition, a new staffing and workload management system was being introduced in order to better undertake patient care assignments, distribute staff across the shifts, and initiate better control mechanisms with regard to the use of overtime.

Jane was beginning to have feelings of panic and a sense of being overwhelmed by the pace and the complexity of change. She didn't know if she could continue to cope. If she couldn't continue to cope, Jane wondered, how in the world will the staff be able to handle this level of intensity of change? And how would Jane lead them through it?

Scenario Exploration

As a learning team discuss together in detail the following questions:

1. Is this the pace of change in today's healthcare environment?
2. Are leaders today becoming overwhelmed with the rate and pace of change?
3. Are the number of changes that are occurring in today's world too much for leaders and workers to handle in the workplace?

Following the exploration of these questions, break up into small groups and explore the following questions in relationship to Jane's experience of change:

1. What has caused Jane to feel particularly overwhelmed as a leader?
2. What should be Jane's best first response to the feelings she is currently experiencing?
3. Is Jane capable of dealing with the level of complexity that leadership now requires, or should she change roles?
4. How we do break down and establish priorities for how Jane might approach her issues of complexity?
5. What advice would you give Jane in dealing with workplace issues and leading staff through the complexity of change?

Following the small-group process and response to the aforementioned questions, regather in a larger group and compare and contrast your responses. At the completion of your dialogue, construct a leadership charter that would guide the leader in establishing a set of principles and priorities in living in a time of complexity and chaos and leading others through it. Reflect on the group charter, and as individuals, construct a personal leadership charter that will guide your own leadership development and application as you unfold your own leadership role.

SCENARIO 2: BECOMING OVERWHELMED

Nora has been the department manager for 10 years. She is a good manager. A lot had been accomplished over the past 10 years as the technology of the service advanced and as clinical practice improved. Patient care had advanced, length of stay had declined, therapeutic intervention had been highly successful, and patient satisfaction scores had remained consistently high.

Yet Nora feels depressed with a decreasing level of energy. She had worked hard over the past 10 years, taking little time for herself in order to build the department to the level of success it had achieved. She found the work exciting and energizing and found every opportunity to be creative and innovative in building this new service. Her work had been her source of energy and satisfaction. Nora felt she did not need to take weeks of vacation like so many other people. She had seen her work as fun, constantly energizing her, and acting as a source of creativity and of joy. Lately, however, joy has been missing. Her energy doesn't seem to reach as high a level. She still finds the work satisfying and somewhat energizing, but something seems to be missing. The pace of change seems to overwhelm more than it used to. Staff complaints seem to irritate her more than they did in the past. She can't quite understand what is happening with her and what to do about it.

Scenario Exploration

In reviewing the scenario, break up into teams of four to five members. In your team, process and respond to the following questions:

1. What are your feelings about Nora's work practices?
2. Was Nora's satisfaction with the challenges of her work sufficient to encourage, renew, and motivate her?
3. How did Nora renew herself, and was it sufficient to sustain her?
4. What three things, in your judgment, did Nora ignore or fail to recognize in her approach to leadership?
5. At this stage in Nora's circumstances, what would you recommend that she do?

After completion of your individual team sessions, rejoin with a larger group and compare your responses to the previous questions. After completion of the discussion together, break into smaller groups again and undertake a role play with one member playing Nora's role and another acting as mentor to Nora, guiding and advising her with regard to what she might do with her circumstances. Pay special emphasis on helping Nora to develop personal insights and skills in relationship to her own leadership self-care and support.

Index